AF893765

Daily Communication

Strategies for Adolescents with Language Disorders

(Second Edition)

LINDA R. SCHREIBER, M.S., CCC-SP
NANCY L. MCKINLEY, M.S., CCC-SP

THINKING PUBLICATIONS
EAU CLAIRE, WISCONSIN

© 1984, 1995 by Thinking Publications®
A Division of McKinley Companies, Inc.

Thinking Publications grants limited rights to individual professionals to reproduce and distribute pages that indicate duplication is permissible. Pages can be used for student instruction only and must include Thinking Publications' copyright notice. All rights are reserved for the pages without the permission-to-reprint notice. No part of these pages may be reproduced in any form, electronic or mechanical, including photocopy, recording, or any information storage and retrieval system without permission in writing from the publisher.

Published 1984. Second Edition 1995

02 01 99 98 97 96 95 12 11 10 9 8 7 6

Library of Congress Cataloging-in-Publication Data

Schreiber, Linda R. (Linda Rose)
Daily communication : strategies for adolescents with language disorders / Linda R. Schreiber, Nancy L. McKinley. — 2nd ed.
p. cm.
Includes bibliographical references.
ISBN 0-930599-35-7 (alk. paper)
1. Speech therapy for children—United States. 2. Language disorders in adolescence—United States. 3. Oral communication—Study and teaching (Secondary)—United States. I. McKinley, Nancy L. II. Title.
LB3454. S37 1995
371.91'4'0973—dc20 95-24325
CIP

Printed in the United States of America
Cover Design: Kris Madsen

THINKING PUBLICATIONS®
A Division of McKinley Companies, Inc.

424 Galloway Street
P.O. Box 163
Eau Claire, WI 54703
(715) 832-2488
FAX (715) 832-8092

DEDICATION

To my parents, Jerry and Shirley Kortendick,
who have taught me to love
and taught me to give
and
To my sister Christine,
who in her short life, brought smiles and laughter
to me and to all who knew her

LRS

To my best friend and husband, Michael,
who understands firsthand
the importance of teaching strategies
to adolescents who are struggling

NLM

TABLE OF CONTENTS

Page

PREFACE

In the early 1980s, a professional colleague of ours commented that there was no resource for speech-language pathologists working with adolescents that addressed the delivery of intervention without materials. She had clients who blatantly refused to use 99 percent of the materials she attempted to present. In her years of work with adolescents at a residential juvenile detention center, she found she had spent much of her time talking with her clients about communication. Her comment was typical of those who have worked with the adolescent population: 50 percent of her time was spent in language intervention activities, and 50 percent was spent in counseling. We had noticed the same phenomenon in our work with adolescents in public junior/senior high schools. And the same phenomenon persists in the mid-1990s, as adolescents struggle with even more complicated personal and social issues.

What is meant by *counseling* in the sense we are using the term? We mean talking about the nature of communication disorders and how it affects a person's personal, social-emotional, academic, or vocational well-being. We have experienced few sessions that do not include discussing why a particular strategy will improve the adolescent's well-being and how it can be applied in daily communication. *Daily Communication: Strategies for Adolescents with Language Disorders* is an attempt to fuse language intervention and counseling for adolescents who have language disorders. Although counseling appears as a separate chapter, users of this book will notice questions included throughout our strategies that reinforce discussing the adolescent's communication.

Although we attempted to meet our colleague's request for a resource requiring no materials, some of the suggested activities do need them. In some cases they are optional; in others they are necessary to complete the task. In most cases, the materials needed can be prepared by duplicating the appropriate pages in the appendix section.

It is only fair to inform users of *Daily Communication* that our basic philosophy of education is that students should learn how to learn. We have been influenced by the work of Jean Piaget, Reuven Feuerstein, Gordon Alley, and Donald Deshler, and we draw heavily on their theoretical premises. Their questioning-and-strategies approach to intervention appears throughout this book. In the first edition of *Daily Communication,* we had drawn from *Adolescents' Communication: Development and Disorders* (Boyce and Larson, 1983) in our selection of problem solving, listening, conversational skills, and survival language as major intervention areas. *Language Disorders in Older Students: Preadolescents and Adolescents* (Larson and McKinley, 1995) continues to support the selection of these intervention areas. Within individual chapters, readers will note many other sources. When we have drawn from the ideas of others, we have provided the references for users who wish to retrieve original books or articles.

Daily Communication is the culmination of many years of combined experiences in mapping out an intervention approach that is successful with adolescents. As the first edition is revised, we reflect on the appropriateness and relevance of this intervention approach. Many of our students have since graduated from high school and have gone on to lead successful and productive lives.

The second edition of *Daily Communication* has been revised to reflect the needs of adolescents in the mid-1990s. Recent literature concerning adolescents has been reviewed and cited, and activities have been revised when necessary to reflect the new information. Strategies contained within this book will continue to be refined, revised, or deleted as new research data become available and as we respond to the changing nature of adolescence in our culture.

ACKNOWLEDGMENTS

So many people have contributed to the completion of this project, counseled us in its development, and coped with our frustrations when we failed. First and foremost, we want to thank the adolescents with language disorders who allowed us to field test new ideas, agreed to participate in revised activities, and offered unbiased criticism. We thank Sue Gallager, Vicki Jensen, Paula Flater, and Carol Nelson, who eagerly tried our ideas and shared results with us. We are indebted to the administrators of the Whitehall (Wisconsin) public schools for supporting the concept of secondary-level speech-language intervention and for providing the necessary time and resources to make it a reality.

We gratefully acknowledge the impact that Vicki Lord Larson has had on the content of this publication and the pioneering work she has done in the area of adolescents with language disorders. We appreciate the initial spark that Sylvia Robertson supplied this project.

Shelley Sweeny, who spent hours and hours struggling with our dictaphone tapes and scrawled inserts for the first edition, deserves a medal for going "above and beyond the call" for us many times. Karen Welsh, Bob Baker, and Mary Lou Albrecht made the first edition possible.

Robin Powell, Jenny Severt, and Kellie Hiess diligently rekeyed the original manuscript to an electronic form for this second edition; we appreciate their energy and efficiency. We thank Julie Poquette for "fine tuning" our writing and Kris Madsen for adding her creative touch to the book format and cover.

Our families deserve special accolades for putting up with our schedules the many months of the first writing and enduring the revisions of the second edition. Thank you to Kevin, Mary, and Christopher McKinley and to Tyler and Ian Schwartz for all they have taught us about adolescence. Finally, we thank our mates for the many pats on our backs, for their words of encouragement, and for not changing addresses without telling us while we were away writing.

1 HOW TO USE THIS BOOK

OVERVIEW

Daily Communication: Strategies for Adolescents with Language Disorders is a resource for professionals working with students with language disorders who are between approximately 10–20 years of age. Its goal is to teach learning strategies in seven critical communication areas for older youth: problem solving, listening, conversational speech, question asking, nonverbal communication, study skills, and survival language. In addition, the topics of motivation and counseling are addressed since they can play such a key role in promoting a cooperative attitude during intervention.

THE ADULT MEDIATOR

Throughout *Daily Communication,* the term *adult mediator* is used interchangeably with the terms *professional* and *educator.* These are generic titles referring to any professional working with adolescents on daily communication strategies. In most cases, the adult will be a speech-language pathologist or a learning disabilities specialist, although other special or content educators at the secondary level may find specific chapters to be appropriate for their use.

Mediator is a captive term in that it means someone who provides mediation, focusing on an experience and anchoring it in time, space, and/or affect. A simple example of a mediated experience versus a nonmediated one is saying, "Please run to the store and buy some milk. We're almost out and the store is not open tomorrow," versus saying, "Go buy some milk." Although the concept of mediation may appear "simple," Feuerstein (1980) maintains we have many adolescents who grew up with a minimum amount of mediation from parents and, in some cases, even from elementary teachers who said, "Do this worksheet" but gave no reason or never talked about the content of the page.

It is not too late to mediate experiences for adolescents and to have them learn skills that were previously unattained due to a lack of experiences or mediation (Feuerstein, 1980). The Stanford Research Report (Larson and Dittman, 1975) concurs that early adolescence is a prime time for students to acquire knowledge, skills, and strategies that they failed to learn in their younger years. To do this, adolescents need a concerned adult mediator.

TARGET AUDIENCE

The adolescent who has an oral language disorder is the target audience for strategies presented in this resource. The activities have been used with students in grades 7–12. Modifications occasionally do need to be made as one moves from early adolescence (approximately 12–14 years) to later adolescence (approximately 16–20 years). In general, younger students may need more concrete, "hands-on" experiences than will older students. Although the word *student* frequently appears, readers should be aware that the strategies presented are appropriate for adolescents who are in settings other than school.

STRATEGIES—NOT CONTENT

Daily Communication is based on the belief that intervention for adolescents who have language disorders should emphasize functional communication skills and teach strategies rather than tutor students in specific course content. *Strategies* are defined as "techniques, principles, or rules that will facilitate the acquisition, manipulation, integration, storage, and retrieval of information across situations and settings" (Alley and Deshler, 1979, p. 13).

Early adolescence is a prime time for instruction of learning strategies (Rowher, 1971). While general strategies are presented throughout *Daily Communication,* they may require modifications to meet individual learning needs. Some students will discover new strategies that work better for them. The professional is urged to assist this development of strategies in every possible way to facilitate the adolescent's "learning how to learn."

GROUP VERSUS INDIVIDUAL SETTING

The majority of activities in *Daily Communication* assume a group setting; however, most of them can be adapted for use in a one-to-one setting. Discussion tends to be more limited in the latter situation, but it could be supplemented by the adolescent gathering experiences others have had and sharing them with the adult mediator. This could be done as an outside assignment.

Since discussion is a major factor in a number of the activities, the educator who is not accustomed to guiding discussions may wish to develop skills in this area. Open-ended questions appropriate for a discussion format have been provided throughout *Daily Communication.* The discussion-for-insight approach is strongly influenced by the authors' training in mediated learning experience, basic in Feuerstein's (1980) theory of cognitive modifiability.

PROCESS—NOT PRODUCT

The user of *Daily Communication* will notice quickly that no right or wrong answers are provided. In some activities, example answers are given, but after those, professionals are "on their own." In other activities, adolescents are asked to create and solve their own problems, thus making an "answer key" impossible. At first, this may feel uncomfortable, but in reality, there are no right or wrong answers for many of the questions posed in this resource book. There are better answers and more relevant answers in many cases, but a variety of possible "right" answers.

The value of this for adolescents comes from realizing the diversity of options. Concrete thinkers see only a few options, all of them anchored to the present time frame. Formal thinkers see many options. They are not anchored to the here and now but are free to consider past and future events, real or hypothetical. One of the major tasks of the educator is to "push" the adolescent into formal levels of thought if he or she is not already there. Emphasizing awareness (i.e., metacognition), problem solving, and communication processes will assist adolescents in achieving higher levels of cognitive functioning.

INTEGRATION—NOT SEGREGATION

To treat the strategies in this book as if they existed in isolation from each other would be a great disservice to adolescents. Although the topics are artificially divided into chapters, they should be integrated during intervention. For example, appropriate conversational skills require listening and nonverbal communication skills. It could be argued that question-asking and problem-solving skills are also necessary. Although the professional may initially emphasize only problem-solving strategies or only listening strategies, eventually adolescents must be guided toward the combination of what they are learning. To assist in this process, activities from several different chapters may be selected for the same session or combined with other resources (see Appendix A).

BRIDGING

Engaging students in the tasks in *Daily Communication* without having them realize the pragmatic value will reduce the effectiveness of intervention. A basic premise underlying each of the strategies is that adolescents will take what they learn during intervention sessions and bridge it to their daily communication. *Bridging* is synonymous with the idea of transfer or generalization. To facilitate bridging, adolescents are frequently asked to suggest where they could apply specific strategies, discuss what happens when someone does not have a particular communication skill, and generate additional examples that illustrate application of a strategy. Bridging should be a part of every session and is the backbone of discussions for insight, mentioned in the "Group Versus Individual Setting" section on page 3.

COUNSELING CONSIDERATIONS

Intervention with adolescents is different from that with younger children in a variety of ways. Primary among the differences is the lack of a "hidden agenda" with older students (Larson and McKinley, 1995). Adolescents need explanations about the nature of their problems, the objectives of intervention, and the reasons why objectives were chosen. As much as possible, adolescents are involved in helping to pinpoint their individual difficulties and to determine the course of intervention. Adult mediators not only guide adolescents through appropriate activities to learn specific strategies, but they spend considerable time talking about communication disorders and their effect on daily functioning. As much as 50 percent of intervention time might be spent counseling adolescents (Simon, 1981). The nature of this counseling is talking about the adolescents' communication disorders, and it is an ongoing part of intervention. Although counseling appears as a separate chapter in *Daily Communication*, its principles should be used throughout the intervention process.

LEARNING STYLE

Each human being uses a different way to achieve optimal learning (Dunn, 1983). Some prefer background noise; some prefer silence. Some prefer hard chairs; some prefer soft pillows. Learning styles are specifically addressed in Chapter 9, "Study-Skill Strategies," but should be kept in mind as much as possible throughout all intervention sessions. Whenever possible, adapt the environment to facilitate learning for specific individuals.

ECLECTIC APPROACH

The strategies in *Daily Communication* are derived from a variety of sources. Activities are sometimes adapted from other authors and are sometimes the authors' own creations. Not only does this resource combine the ideas of many people, but combining this resource with other current communication programs for adolescents is recommended. Appendix A includes a listing of additional resources that are appropriate for adolescents. Users should refer to it to supplement and combine with activities in this resource book. No one resource will provide total direction for an effective intervention program for adolescents with language disorders.

PRE/POST ASSESSMENT CONSIDERATIONS

Daily Communication is most appropriate for older youth (10+ years of age) who have been diagnosed as having deficits in oral communication skills as measured by standardized assessment instruments and/or by informal observation of performance in real-life situations. As students participate in the activities in this resource, they are prompted through questioning to realize when and why they need to use certain communication skills and strategies. To document the change in their awareness of the strategies needed and their success in acquiring them, adolescents could be asked to respond orally or in writing to questions like these:

- What is a strategy you now know and when would you use it?
- Why is it important to develop appropriate communication skills?
- Explain (or describe) the importance of what you're learning in this class.
- How do you think you've changed (or improved) in the last month?

Responses should be kept in a portfolio (either as a written paper or an audiotape) and used to document progress along with actual day-to-day performance notes by the educator.

Day-to-day performance notes should include class meeting summaries. The concept of holding a class meeting whenever older students convene has been discussed by Larson and McKinley (1995) and consists of three main components: a self-report on generalization of goals, a chance to give and receive compliments (which helps to establish a positive atmosphere), and an opportunity to air communication concerns and frustrations.

APPENDICES

The appendices are included as a convenient time saver for those who use *Daily Communication*. They contain materials needed or suggested for activities used to teach various strategies. Permission is granted to duplicate the appendix section for educational use with students. The appendix pages are perforated for ease in removal and duplication.

2 MOTIVATIONAL STRATEGIES

MOTIVATION'S BEGINNING POINT: COMMON SENSE

People communicate when there is a need or desire to do so. Although this statement is common sense, it is too often forgotten when planning intervention strategies for adolescents. One must establish a reason for the adolescent to communicate, both as a listener and as a speaker. Motivation is not established by the "how to communicate" or the "when," but centers totally on the issue of "why communicate?" If the purpose of an intervention task is not firmly rooted within the mind of the adolescent, little motivation to change is generated. The bottom line of any intervention is change. Adolescents need to either add certain behaviors to or remove certain behaviors from their repertoires.

Change will not occur unless there is a perceived need to do so; providing appropriate learning experiences and framing them for the adolescent will allow such changes to take place.

Professionals seeking to help the adolescent improve communication skills, before establishing the need or desire for those skills, are spelling the demise of the intervention program and perpetuating the adolescent's ineffective and/or inefficient communication.

EXTRINSIC/INTRINSIC MOTIVATION

Motivation for learning can be either intrinsic or extrinsic. Cromwell (1963, 1967) developed a success-approach (SA) and failure-avoidance (FA) motivational system. Children are initially motivated to attain immediate gratification and to avoid unpleasant situations, both of which are extrinsic motivators. Following this, they reach the SA-FA stage, characterized by an increased ability to delay gratification and a lower vulnerability to frustration and failure. Western-culture adolescents acquire an increased tendency to see themselves as instrumental to outcomes of events rather than to assume that outcomes are beyond their control and result from fate, luck, or an external agent (i.e., they exhibit an internal locus of control).

Nothing has a more crippling effect on motivation to learn than repeated failures (Wong, 1980). It is critical for adults working with adolescents to carefully structure sessions that allow feelings of success most of the time. Simultaneously, no professional should ever put another person down, especially since "most of the trouble and friction among people, in and out of school, is caused by putting others down" (Glasser, 1993, p. 36).

CREDIT AND GRADES

A growing number of adult mediators have succeeded in offering intervention as a course for credit at the secondary level (Larson and McKinley, 1987, 1995). The authors strongly endorse this concept. The result of offering intervention for credit frequently has increased motivation within the adolescent student. Along with credit goes the privilege of grading. Options can include satisfactory-fail or use of the traditional system employed by the school. Some educators assign daily grades based on the number and appropriateness of students' responses. These grades are then averaged at the end of the term. Some establish contracts that specify what must be done to earn a particular grade. An activity appearing later in this chapter provides guidance in establishing contracts.

FACTORS THAT AFFECT MOTIVATION

In addition to establishing firmly the reason to communicate, these actions can positively influence an adolescent's motivation:

- Organize tasks in a way that will help the adolescent succeed.
- Give feedback that not only addresses what the adolescent does, but that interprets the meaning of tasks and how they affect competence (e.g., "You did a great job asking me to clarify those directions.

That skill will really help you on a job someday. If you ask your supervisor to explain in more detail what to do, he or she will know you really want to do your job well").

- Model sharing of feelings, perceptions3

, and points of view, and encourage the adolescent to reciprocate.

- Demonstrate that all people experience frustration and that it is not unique to adolescents.

- Keep records of student progress and emphasize the adolescent's role in his or her own progress.

- Train adolescents to evaluate their own work and trust their ability to defend correct answers.

- Be sensitive to your expectations as the adult mediator; do not inadvertently communicate that you expect failure by either your affective manner or trivial goal setting.

Glasser's (1993) concept of control theory is extremely germane to this discussion of factors that affect student motivation:

> Control theory explains that we will work hard for those we care for (**belonging**), for those we respect and who respect us (**power**), for those with whom we laugh (**fun**), for those who allow us to think and act for ourselves (**freedom**), and for those who help us to make our lives secure (**survival**). (p. 30)

When adult mediators address the basic needs (listed in parentheses above) of their students, the harder they will work for those adults.

ACTIVITIES TO ENHANCE MOTIVATIONAL STRATEGIES

MOTIVATIONAL SKILLS

● Participation when an extrinsic motivational system is used

●● Development of intrinsic motivation that positively influences communication behavior

TOKEN ECONOMY: BEYOND STICKERS

PURPOSE

To establish an appropriate and effective token-economy system for adolescents, if needed

If at all possible, avoid establishing a token-economy system for adolescents or establish one for a limited time period. If a token economy is needed before the student develops intrinsic loci of control, consider these points:

- Determine with the student, or group of students, what is extrinsically motivating. What prizes or privileges would they like to buy with their tokens? Do not make this decision in isolation from the adolescent(s). Consider extrinsic motivators that do not cost money, such as earning time to play a computer game or inviting the student to select the intervention activity.
- Determine for what specific behaviors tokens or points will be awarded. How many?
- Decide if the system will include response cost.

All behaviors for which points may be earned should be clearly posted in the intervention room. At the adolescent level, it is particularly appropriate to include points for using conversational rules. (See Chapter 6.)

To make a token-economy system more appropriate for adolescents, obtain savings and checking account record books from a bank. Rather than simply adding up tokens or points after each session and logging them into a notebook, have students make deposits into their savings or checking accounts. When sufficient "money" (tokens/points) has been accumulated, require students to write out checks to obtain any earned prizes. In this way, not only is an extrinsic reinforcement system implemented, but also adolescents are gaining practice in a very essential survival skill.

To make the system even more reinforcing for adolescents, give large numbers of tokens or points. Give 1000 points instead of the 10 that might go to a younger student. (It costs nothing more!) At the end of a session, a student may have earned 50,000 points. Of course, prizes and privileges are similarly structured. Getting excused for a drink of water might cost 40,000 points. Many students think twice before "spending" such a large number of points. Maintaining the savings and checking records also becomes more challenging as additional zeros are added to traditional point values.

●
LEARNING STRATEGY
The adolescent willingly participates in intervention activities when an extrinsic motivational system is used.

NEGOTIATING CONTRACTS

PURPOSE

To establish expectations for performance by jointly agreeing on objectives

Contracts can be useful extrinsic reinforcement tools. When used, a contract should be jointly negotiated by the student and professional. Components of the contract need to include answers to these questions:

1. What is the task/objective?
2. When must it be done?
3. To what extent will it be done (i.e., level of performance)? (This should be tied to grades, if appropriate.)
4. How will evaluation be completed?
5. What are the consequences of completing or not completing the contract?

Contracts should be signed by all participants, and a time line should be established for completion. Make the contract look as adult-like as possible. A sample contract format follows and a blank contract can be found in Appendix B.

CONTRACT

I, ______________________________
Name

will do the following by ____________________
Date

1.

2.

3.

Level of Performance:

Evaluation Plan:

Consequences:

Signed: ______________________________

____

Date: ______________________________

LEARNING STRATEGY

The adolescent willingly participates in intervention activities when an extrinsic motivational system is used.

ESTABLISHING REASONS

PURPOSE

To verbalize the pragmatic value of particular communication skills

This activity transcends all others. Before an adult mediator facilitates the acquisition of any communication skill, this question needs to be asked:

WHY IS IT IMPORTANT THAT THE ADOLESCENT KNOWS THIS COMMUNICATION SKILL?

If sound reasons do not readily emerge, the pragmatic value of teaching the skill becomes suspect.

When introducing a communication skill believed to have pragmatic value, ask adolescents one or more of the following questions:

- When would you use this communication skill in your life?
- Why is it important to learn this communication skill?
- Who have you seen using this communication skill? What was the situation?
- What would happen if you didn't use this communication skill?
- How would your life be made easier if you had this communication skill?
- Would it cost you any time or money if you did not have this communication skill?
- What would be a fair reward/reinforcement for developing this communication skill?

Initially, adolescents may have a difficult time responding to these questions. If they do, try these approaches:

- Describe a situation in which you were required to use the skill. Invite them to share similar experiences.
- Describe a situation in which the skill was not used and resulted in a problem and/or communication breakdown. Invite them to share their experiences.
- Immerse adolescents in a situation that requires the communication skill. (Referential communication activities described in Chapter 5 are particularly helpful in this regard.)

●● LEARNING STRATEGY

The adolescent develops intrinsic motivation that positively influences communication behavior.

- Role-play a situation that illustrates the presence and/or absence of the communication skill. Create dialogue for students who initially do not create their own.
- Interview other adults who use a particular communication skill in their day-to-day living. Tape-record responses. Have students engage in the interviewing once you have modeled it for them a few times.

SELF-EVALUATION

PURPOSE

To verbalize what is correct and incorrect about one's speech-language performance

Adolescents who have experienced continual school failure frequently believe they cannot succeed at anything. Furthermore, when they do have the right answer and are asked to defend it (i.e., "How did you get that answer?"), they scramble to change it. Why? Because for years teachers have asked them only about their wrong answers.

Adolescents will learn more communication skills when they believe they can learn. If they think they cannot learn, or do not want to learn, indeed, learning will not take place. It then becomes the role of the professional to guide the adolescent toward

- success in communication skill acquisition;
- belief in his or her ability to learn;
- recognition of correct and incorrect performance; and
- verbalization of what made the response correct or incorrect.

How is this guidance provided?

PROVIDE FEEDBACK

Give specific feedback to the adolescent. A steady diet of "very nice" and "good job" is ineffective. With excitement, tell adolescents what you noticed them doing correctly. Say, for example, "I like the way you were nodding your head to let me know you understand." Include "good listening" comments.

DISCUSS SUCCESSES

Although it is important to make certain the adolescent feels success during initial activities, the task should not be at such a low level that boredom sets in. When the student provides a correct response, discuss how he or she figured it out. This may be difficult initially for the student, so be prepared to model. Describe how you went about solving the problem. This will require you to be very aware of your own communication and problem-solving strategies.

●●
LEARNING STRATEGY
The adolescent develops intrinsic motivation that positively influences communication behavior.

DISCUSS MISTAKES

After some success has been established, explore why mistakes were made. Again, be prepared to model a mistake and explain why it happened to you.

After adolescents have had experience explaining their successes and failures, phase out any modeling. Continue asking these types of questions:

- How did you figure out that response?
- How do you know it's correct?
- How can you tell whether you made an error or not?
- How could you check your work?

Encourage students to positively reinforce themselves. Practice complimenting your own good performance so that you serve as a model for the adolescents with whom you work.

3 COUNSELING STRATEGIES

COUNSELING: A WORKING DEFINITION

Definitions of counseling range from self-exploration to therapeutic conversation to the teaching of problem solving and decision making (Arbuckle, 1970; Benjamin, 1969; Glasser, 1965; Parker, 1968). The authors share Thompson and Poppen's (1972) perspective that the counseling relationship involves one person helping another resolve a conflict or problem that he or she has not been able to handle alone.

Group counseling is an interpersonal process focusing on thoughts, feelings, and behaviors (Hunt and Smith, 1980). The important ingredients include acceptance, support, trust, caring, understanding, and permissiveness. At the same time, some amount of tension must be maintained for change to occur. Change takes place when there is conflict, disequilibrium, and meeting of opposing views (MacLennan and Felsenfeld,

1968) and when youth can see advantages to altering behaviors that are resulting in pain (Selekman, 1993). Selekman (1993) reminds professionals, "If you expect that change will occur with your clients, your expectancy of change will influence their behavior" (page 30). Change talk is composed of suppositional language such as "when" and "will," rather than "if" and "would" (Selekman, 1993).

COUNSELING AS IT APPLIES TO ADOLESCENTS WITH COMMUNICATION DISORDERS

The professional providing intervention for adolescents does not counsel in the traditional sense of handling any problem that arises. Rather, the counseling is focused upon problems within the communication process itself, exploring how this communication problem impacts upon personal, academic, and vocational performance and potential. In this sense, counseling involves giving information to the adolescent, obtaining information, and providing release and support for feelings. Simon (1981) observed that a significant amount of time may be spent in counseling the adolescent with a communication disorder, perhaps as much as 50 percent some days (i.e., 50 percent of the professional's time is spent counseling about the communication disorder, and 50 percent is spent in direct speech-language intervention activities). When the counseling begins to move beyond communication problems, the educator must be keenly sensitive to the need for referral of the adolescent to professional counseling services.

MAJOR COUNSELING BEHAVIORS

Reciprocal trust and respect are cited as the most necessary factors for effective counseling (Thompson and Poppen, 1972). Other key behaviors include encouragement at all times and active, empathic listening. The professional most likely to succeed in counseling has mastered the art of paying attention (Smith, 1969).

Baggett (1969) found that adolescents reported these behaviors to be most supportive:

1. suggesting ways to solve the problem;
2. taking time to sit down and talk;
3. spending time to discuss the problem;
4. listening to what the student has to say;
5. asking the student questions about the problem; and
6. sticking to the problem about which the student wants to talk.

These behaviors were found to be least supportive (Baggett, 1969):

1. jumping to conclusions before the student finishes giving the facts;

2. changing the topic immediately after the student introduces concern;
3. hurrying the student through the telling of an experience;
4. avoiding talking with the student about the problem;
5. sitting there "like a bump on a log"; and
6. looking at something else while the student is talking.

When working with adolescents, it is also critical for the professional to monitor his or her language for the occurrence of "we" and "our" (e.g., "Have *we* finished *our* homework?"). This is considered very degrading to adolescents (Thompson and Poppen, 1972). Use first- and second-person pronouns as appropriate (e.g., *I* gave *you* a homework assignment to do last night. Did *you* finish it?). As a general rule, avoid third-person pronouns when discussing work for which the adolescent is responsible. (E.g., "Each student is responsible for *his* or *her* own work." Instead say, "You are responsible for your own work.")

The activities presented on the following pages are not meant to be presented as a "counseling unit" during intervention. Rather, some of the activities are to be interspersed as appropriate and necessary within intervention, while others can be used in all interactions with adolescents.

ACTIVITIES TO ENHANCE COUNSELING STRATEGIES

COUNSELING SKILLS

● Recognition that different types of information are shared with different people

●● Engagement in self-counseling behaviors

INNER-CIRCLE TECHNIQUE
(adapted from Lazarus, 1969)

PURPOSE

To identify what information adolescents will share with which individuals

LEARNING STRATEGY

The adolescent will recognize what types of information can be shared in the speech-language intervention setting and in other interpersonal settings.

The inner-circle technique can be used to let the adolescent know that the adult mediator will not be overpowering nor expect to exchange private thoughts unrelated to the immediate concern. Using the inner-circle strategy generally helps overcome resistance and increases the adolescent's willingness to discuss real concerns. Illustrate the inner-circle technique for the adolescent by using concentric circles.

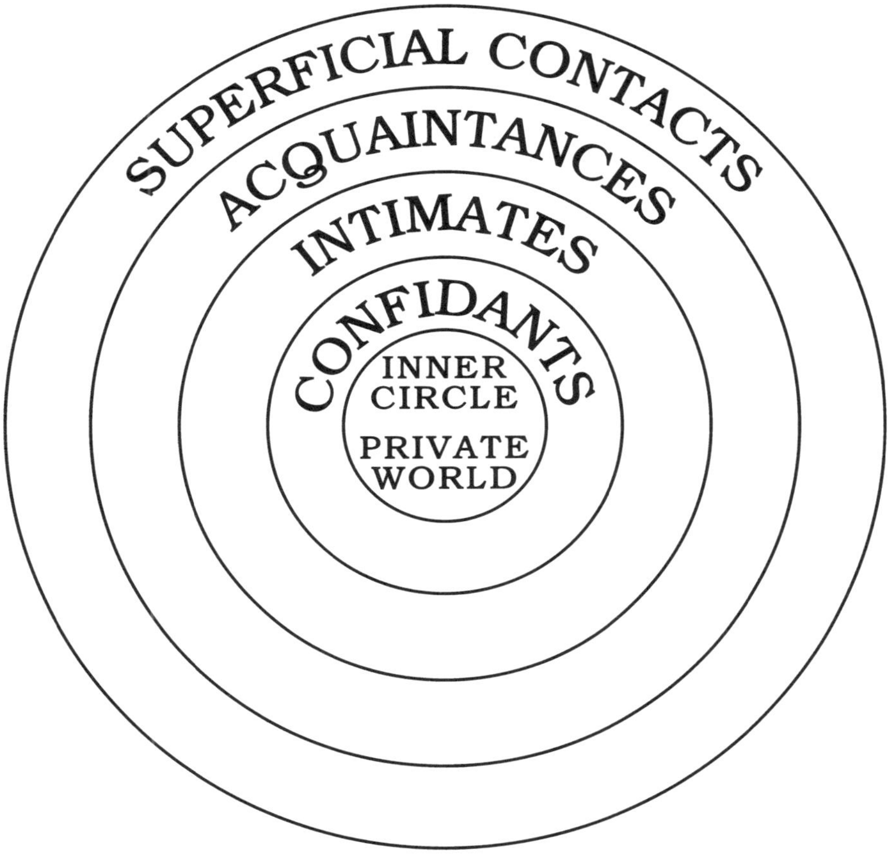

The adolescent's private world is represented by an inner circle into which no one enters. Next to that circle is a ring open to confidants with whom personal information and feelings can be shared. This circle represents those inseparable friends who "stick with you no matter what." The next level is called "intimate." At this level are friends or relatives who are allowed access to most information, but who would probably not be informed about confidential material. Next to the circle of intimates is a circle of acquaintances. These people are occasional companions, but the adolescent has no real friendship with them. The outermost circle represents those persons with whom the adolescent has only superficial contact. These are the people whose faces are recognized, but with whom the adolescent seldom speaks.

The inner-circle strategy assists adolescents in identifying when they lack a private world. These individuals "tell all" to anyone who will listen. By including nearly everyone in their inner circle, they become unable to discriminate between the levels of relationship with others. Often those with a very large private world really have nobody with whom to share personal thoughts. They lack a real confidant.

The relationship of the adult mediator and the adolescent typically starts at the outer circle and moves inward as trust and shared experiences increase. Pushing too fast toward the center generally does not work. As the adolescent begins to share feelings about his or her communication disorders, the relationship changes to an "intimate" level and sometimes even to a "confidant" level. The relationship also changes as the professional relates personal information to students. Glasser (1993) encourages educators to look for natural occasions to tell students who you are and what you stand for. As students get to know you better, and like what they know, they will develop more trust and put out greater effort.

The inner-circle technique will assist adolescents in seeing what their social relationships are and how other people deal with matters of disclosure and confidence. Feelings, which are the substance of most "inner circles," should be shared only with someone who is trusted. The inner-circle technique can help some who complete it to disclose more to those they trust; others may decide to restrict their private world to fewer people.

Guide adolescents to attach names to each of the concentric circles. Observe especially the quantity of confidants and intimates listed. If no confidants can be listed, for example, this should be noted in the student's file. If a "gang" of confidants is listed, this should also be noted. The exercise will help adolescents determine if they like how they are relating to those around them and if they think they need to change. Repeat the exercise at six-month intervals if deemed appropriate.

THE "WHAT DOES IT TAKE" DISCUSSION
(adapted from Thompson and Poppen, 1972)

PURPOSE

To explore information that might be shared in speech-language intervention sessions by participating in a role-reversal activity

LEARNING STRATEGY

The adolescent will recognize what types of information can be shared in the speech-language intervention setting and in other interpersonal settings.

Assist adolescents to answer the following question as specifically as possible:

What does it take for a student, teacher, or principal to be a successful communicator at your school?

Any of the three roles may be discussed first. Ideally, both the principal (or an administrative representative) and a teacher would be present for this discussion. The discussion follows five phases:

1. Determine a discussion leader for this activity, or the adult mediator can assume that responsibility. Select the role to be discussed first (e.g., student). Have each student offer an opinion about what it takes for a student to be a successful communicator in school. Ask the principal and the teacher their perceptions too. Direct the leader to keep notes of the responses or appoint someone to do so. A second role is then discussed (e.g., teacher). Now everyone offers opinions and observations on what it takes for a teacher to be a successful communicator in school. Next, the third role is discussed.

2. Each student in the discussion then takes one of the other roles. For example, half the students take the perspective of teachers, and half take the perspective of principals. Meanwhile, the teacher and principal both assume student roles. The discussion begins again, this time with each person offering suggestions on what it takes for a student to be a successful communicator. Thus, students, taking the perspective of teachers, respond now as if they were teachers talking about students. The teacher responds as if he or she were a student talking about students. Again, all three roles are ultimately discussed, but this time participants are taking a perspective other than their own. The discussion leader or designee takes notes throughout the discussion.

3. As the adult mediator, guide the group in discussing what each member learned from assuming a different perspective.

4. Based on the discussion notes, create a summary of the qualities needed to be a successful communicator as a student, teacher, or principal. Where everyone can see it, write three headings: student, teacher, principal. Under each heading, list the specific qualities needed to be a successful communicator. Review the lists for acceptance by the group.

5. Encourage each group member to select a new communication behavior he or she would like to try in the next week. Written commitments or contracts can be used if desirable.

Note: If a teacher and /or principal are not able to be physically present during the discussion steps of this activity, arrange to have tape-recorded responses that you can play to the students.

THE SIX-STEP PROCESS
(adapted from Thompson and Poppen, 1972)

PURPOSE

To outline and implement a six-step self-counseling process as a guide to problem solving

●●
LEARNING STRATEGY
The adolescent will engage in self-counseling behaviors.

The six-step process can be used within the intervention session or as a homework assignment. (Please note that it is a shortened version of the problem-solving process described in detail in Chapter 4.) The activity lends itself to finding solutions for intermediate-level problems that are blocking progress (e.g., communicating ineffectively with a teacher, crying when getting teased). The six-step self-counseling process is conducted as follows:

1. **Write out the problem on paper.**
If the adolescent has difficulty isolating the problem and/or writing it on paper, provide assistance for either or both of these tasks.

2. **List all the blocks to solving your problem.**
These blocks may be both internal (student difficulties) or external (environmental difficulties).

3. **List any means you have for solving the problem.**
Include the adolescent's own resources as well as resources of others who could help.

4. **List all possible alternatives for solving the problem.**
With the adolescent, list as many solutions as possible without pausing to evaluate them. Extend this brainstorming activity over several days to allow time for the mental processes to focus on the situation.

5. **Predict possible consequences of each alternative plan.**
Guide the adolescent in applying what has been learned from past mistakes or from those others have made. Some solutions might be so far off target that they can be omitted immediately. However, some of the most creative approaches may seem, at first, to be the most ridiculous.

6. **Make a commitment to a plan of action that seems to have the most potential for helping you.**
The plan is developed after possible outcomes of each alternative are evaluated. Whatever plan is chosen should be pursued and given a chance to work. Consider assigning a commitment partner who will check on the progress of the plan. If the plan is not producing the desired results, a student must assess if he or she is following the plan correctly or if the plan itself is faulty. If it is determined that the plan was given a fair try and that it still does not work, the six steps can be repeated, using the knowledge gained from the failure.

SOLUTION FOCUSING

PURPOSE

To capitalize on strengths and engage in "change talk"

Review the problem that was focused on during the last activity ("The Six-Step Process"). Explain to students that they have the strengths and resources to change, and the problem typically doesn't happen all of the time—there are exceptions to the rule (Selekman, 1993). Rapid changes in beliefs and behaviors can occur when the "miracle question" (de Shazer, 1988) is asked:

> Suppose you were to go home tonight, and while you were asleep, a miracle happened and this problem was solved. How will you know the miracle happened? What will be different? (p. 5)

Many times, the students' "miracles" may be behaviors they can perform or already are performing some of the time. Answering the miracle question often generates useful exceptions to when the problem happens and helps the student formulate goals, which in turn results in change. Asking the miracle question in relationship to the communication problems manifested by adolescents who have language-learning disorders may give adult mediators insight as to how to proceed during intervention.

If the student does not respond to the miracle question, other tasks might be posed:

1. **Formula first-session task** (de Shazer, 1985)
   Say, "Between now and next time, notice what is happening that you would like to continue happening" (i.e., in relationship to the problem at hand). (This task usually results in the identification of some exceptions to when the problem occurs.)

2. **Prediction task** (de Shazer, 1988)
   Say, "Predict whether you'll have an 'up' day without the problem tomorrow. Then during the 'up' day, try to account for what is making it that way." ("Prediction tasks are based on the idea that what you expect to happen is more likely to happen once the process leading up to it is in motion" [p. 184, de Shazer, 1988].)

3. **Pretend the miracle happened task** (de Shazer, 1991)
   Say, "Pretend to engage in some miracle behaviors that someone else is asking you to do. Don't tell anyone about the pretending, but notice the difference in responses that occurs." (In the process of pretending to engage in behaviors that someone else wants the student to do, he or she

LEARNING STRATEGY

The adolescent will engage in self-counseling behaviors.

experiences positive responses that serve to reinforce the "pretended" behaviors.)

All of these tasks allow students to view their problem situations differently. In the process, they can often set realistic goals for change.

VALUE JUDGMENTS

PURPOSE

To assist adolescents in evaluating their own behavior

●●

LEARNING STRATEGY

The adolescent will engage in self-counseling behaviors.

8 STEPS FOR ENHANCING STUDENT SELF-EVALUATION

Glasser (1969) has offered excellent ideas for enhancing student self-evaluation and modification of behaviors. Steps 1, 2, and 8 are directed primarily at the adult mediator.

1. **Involve the student.**
   Develop positive relationships with adolescents that communicate "I care" and "I believe in you."

2. **Focus on present behavior.**
   When dealing with the present incident, do not bring up past mistakes.

3. **Encourage value judgments.**
   Have students evaluate their own behaviors. Is the behavior helping you get what you want? Is it helping others? Is it against the rules? Why do we need rules?

4. **Make a plan.**
   Help students develop strategies to deal with similar situations in the future. Put these plans on paper.

5. **Get a commitment.**
   If appropriate, use a written contract. Follow up, check back, reinforce.

6. **Don't accept excuses.**
   If things go wrong, replan strategies rather than accept excuses.

7. **Seek responsibility, not punishment.**
   Students need help in developing a sense of ownership of, and responsibility for, their behaviors. Punishment relieves students from responsibility.

8. **Never give up.**
   Persist with adolescents so they know you care. Giving up can reinforce negative self-concepts.

These eight steps are reprinted in Appendix C so they can be easily reproduced and taped to the wall or desktop for ready reference during discussions with adolescents.

Most of the actual verbal interaction with the students takes place in steps 3, 4, and 5. The "Encourage value judgments" step and the "Make a plan" step interface closely with the problem-solving strategy described in Chapter 4, as well as with the six-step process described earlier in this chapter. Major check-points for developing strategies to discuss with students include the following:

- Will it harm anyone?
- Is it too risky?
- Is it OK for now, but not in the long run?
- Will it work?

These questions are captured visually in Figure 3.1. This figure is also available in poster form. (See the last page of this book for details.)

FIGURE 3.1

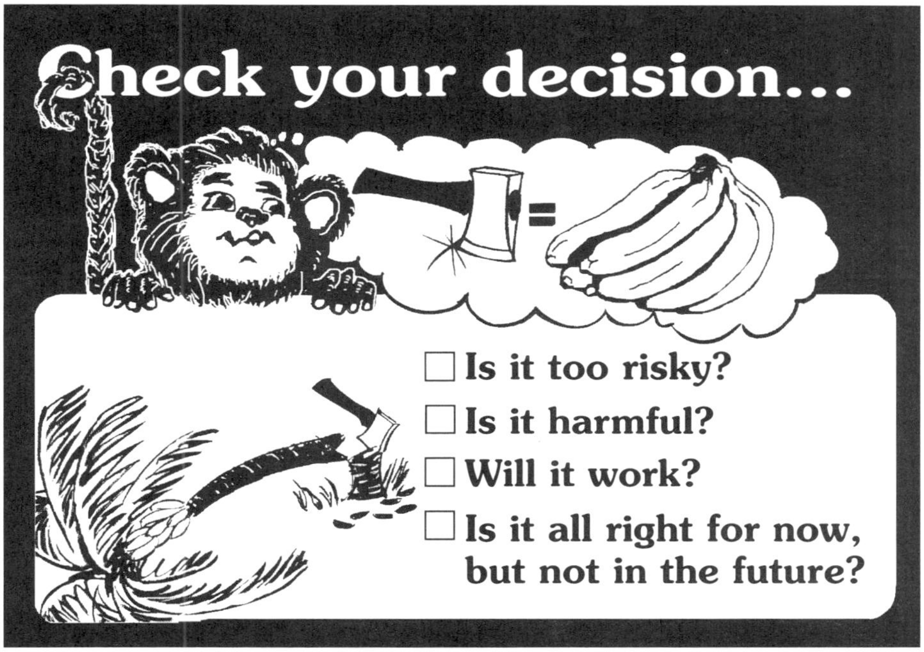

© 1984, 1988 Thinking Publications

Adolescents need to be guided in, first, identifying their problems, and second, evaluating them. Adult mediators who tell adolescents about the problems that youths have and how they should be feeling leave them unaffected and unchanged.

COMPLAINTS AND CONFRONTATIONS

PURPOSE

To illustrate how complaints and confrontations can maintain emotional health rather than destroy it

While there are occasions when the adult mediator might complain to and confront the adolescent, there are also times when the adult may need to assist the adolescent in determining how to complain to and confront others. Modeling should facilitate the latter task of teaching adolescents to appropriately complain and confront.

CONFRONTATIONS

A general principle for developing positive confronting behavior is to identify clearly what message is intended by the confrontation. There are different types of confrontations (Berensen, Mitchell, and Laney, 1968):

1. **Experiential Confrontation**
   This type of confrontation points out a discrepancy in the way two people feel about their relationship and interaction. The purpose is to share one's view with another person. For example, "You act as though I hurt you by coming home late; however, I feel I had no choice but to do what I did."

2. **Didactic Confrontation**
   This type of confrontation deals with misinformation on the part of one person in a relationship. The disagreement is over a matter of fact. For example, a teacher might confront a poorly performing student who claims he cannot do better even though his grades have been average until the present school year.

3. **Weakness Confrontation**
   A paraphrase of this type of confrontation is, "If your best friend can't tell you, who can?" Many commercials advertising mouthwash, toothpaste, and dandruff shampoo contain examples of this kind of confrontation. The simple message is, "I want you to do something about a particular characteristic."

4. **Strengths Confrontation**
   In this type of confrontation, the simple message is, "I see you as having abilities you are not using." It focuses upon a person's unused potential rather than upon a weakness. This type of confrontation identifies an obstacle to overcome.

LEARNING STRATEGY

The adolescent will engage in self-counseling behaviors.

5 Encouragement Confrontation

This type of confrontation is aimed at encouraging the individual to act. The simple message is "You can do it" or "You will improve things if you do something." Some strongly suspect that motivation to act is triggered because of encouragement from another person (Thompson and Poppen, 1972).

During confrontation tasks between the educator and the student, the type of confrontation should be clearly identified, and steps should be taken to guarantee that the appropriate message is communicated. Likewise, the adult may help adolescents sort out the types of messages they wish to deliver to someone else when confrontation is determined to be the best solution.

Ineffective confrontations include sending "solution messages" and "put-down" messages. A *solution message* "solves" the problem for the other person and does not allow that person to decide how to stop infringing on the rights of the other in the relationship. For example, if a guest in your house put his feet on one of your best chairs, you would likely communicate your concern for your chair rather than order him to put his feet down. Ordering him to put his feet down is sending a solution message. It may be helpful for us to grant the adolescent the same degree of respect we have for a house guest in order to help us avoid sending solution messages.

In a *put-down message*, one person in the confrontation wants the face-to-face meeting to be a duel in which one is clearly victorious and the other becomes embarrassed or hurt. Some adults engaged in confrontations with adolescents feel they have a responsibility to win in a fair and benevolent way. If the adult does not win—does not "put the adolescent in his place"—the adult is afraid of losing the respect of the youth (Thompson and Poppen, 1972). The adult may also think that adolescents need to learn they cannot have power over adults. Adults who think that only embarrassment and low self-regard will make the adolescent thoroughly learn the lesson and stop misbehavior often feed into the problem rather than help resolve it. The adolescent is likely to become resistant and use subtle ways to avoid developing the desired behavior. While the adult may win the first round, subsequent rounds will result in a long series of clashes designed to put the adult down. The adult providing intervention should avoid this approach to confrontations and should also help adolescents realize the same cycle will affect their lives when they give put-down messages to adults and peers around them.

COMPLAINTS

A complaint is usually less emotional than a confrontation. It may also be premeditated, but not necessarily so. The first step in complaining is learning to identify the feelings associated with someone infringing upon one's rights. This feeling does not have to be logically defended. While we all may be tempted to spend time venting our feelings, the time may be better spent examining the source of those bad feelings. We know that much of our emotional behavior results from the "bad" things we tell ourselves about an experience. A bump on the elbow to one person is dismissed as inconsequential, while to another person it may be quite a problem and probably would result in a complaint. Adults providing intervention need to help adolescents determine when they could help themselves and their situations by making effective complaints and when complaints are unnecessary.

The second step in making an effective complaint is elaboration. Elaborating the complaint helps the person who feels injured to be very specific about a complaint and to clarify all the details about the situation. Kelly (1955) listed seven basic questions that might be addressed during elaboration of a complaint:

1. With what problem do you want help?
2. When was this problem first noticed?
3. Under what conditions did this problem first appear?
4. What action has been attempted?
5. What changes have come with your action or the passing of time?
6. Under what conditions was the problem most noticeable?
7. Under what conditions was the problem least noticeable?

Most adolescents are probably familiar with being told to stop complaining. The suggestion offered here is that they can start complaining in ways that will get results. Have students discuss examples of things accomplished as a result of people complaining (e.g., women's right to vote, laws against drunk driving, compulsory education for all children). Also discuss the similarities and differences between complaints and confrontations. Is it possible to have both complaint and confrontation at the same time? How can you tell whether you are complaining or confronting?

The third step in effective complaining is making the actual complaint. Weinberg (1969) gives guidelines for making effective complaints:

1. **Complain to whomever is infringing on your rights and to no one else.**
It is a common mistake to complain to the wrong person or persons. Adopting the general rule of talking to the person who is upsetting you assures you of talking to someone who can do something about the particular concern.

2. **Avoid comparisons.**
Treating people as inferior can make them very defensive and can preoccupy their minds with self-preservation. Compliments, although desirable, are generally avoided while the complaint is in progress. While complimenting along with complaining seems right to the complainer, it frequently gives unclear messages to the receiver. Thus comparisons, whether positive or negative, are best avoided during a complaint.

3. **Put a statute of limitations on complaints.**
It is sometimes tempting when making a complaint to rehash the past. Outdated complaints need to be disallowed to help ensure clear messages.

4. **Make only one complaint at a time.**
Discuss only the major issue at hand. Watch for statements starting, "and furthermore..." or "and another thing...."

5. **Object only to things that can be changed.**
This is probably the most difficult suggestion to implement. Often complaints are focused on past behavior or situations that cannot be changed. Instead, focus upon future behaviors.

6. **Do not ask a person why he or she is doing something.**
The only request the complainer should make is that a person stop what he or she is doing or rectify the mistake, if possible. While disclosure

of motives may help the person who is harmed accept the other person's mistake, "demanded disclosures" are probably less helpful than disclosures initiated by the person who did the offending.

7. **Rehearse the complaint.**
A trial run of the complaint will help ensure that the previous suggestions are being followed. During rehearsal, the complainer may wish to determine the worst possible thing that could be said or done during the complaint. This may prevent making the actual mistake while the complaint is being registered.

Some people lack the courage to enter a complaint. Courage might be bolstered by asking these questions:

- What could be the worst possible result of my complaining?
- What will happen if I don't complain?

Often the worst possible outcome is not that great a catastrophe. The answer to the second question may point out that complaining may be quite acceptable. At the other extreme, there are people who complain too much of the time; in their cases, the answer to the second question might reveal that their complaints are really unjustifiable and detrimental to their relationships.

Have students think of complaints they have made recently. How did they feel before making the complaint? After making the complaint? Did they follow any of the suggestions outlined in this activity? Is there anything they could do differently to better make that same complaint in the future?

Have students think of recent times when other people have complained to them. Were they the source of the complaint, or was the complaint really intended for another person? How did it feel to be the receiver of a complaint? Did the person complaining to them follow any of the outlined suggestions?

As a summary activity, have students identify a complaint they want to make (either as a group or individually) and develop a plan to deliver it.

4 PROBLEM-SOLVING STRATEGIES

PROBLEM SOLVING: DEFINITION

The ability to solve problems emerges early in childhood. As young as 12 months of age, infants attempt to solve problems such as pulling a string attached to a toy to bring it closer to them (Ratner and Harris, 1994). Solutions to problems at this level are discovered through trial and error; however, as children mature, having a systematic method for solving problems is imperative for survival, growth, and success in their personal and academic lives.

Problems are confronted daily and can be as routine and familiar as deciding when to get up, what to wear, or what to or eat, or as complex as deciding how to pay for a traffic ticket when you haven't the money to pay the fine. Any disruption in an ongoing state of affairs presents a problem (Drake, 1976). Whenever there is a gap between where you are and where you want to be, and you're not sure how to close that gap, you have a problem (Hayes, 1981, 1989).

COMPETENCE IN PROBLEM SOLVING

Kurfiss (1988) observed that competent problem solvers "monitor their work using executive control strategies; they make plans, set goals and subgoals, ask questions, take notes, observe the effectiveness of their efforts, and take corrective action when necessary" (p. 27). He further observed that expert problem solvers tend to spend more time planning and analyzing while the novices impulsively implement solutions.

Expert problem solvers also tend to monitor their own problem solving and thinking better than less-experienced persons (Bransford and Vye, 1989). They are better able to judge the difficulty of the problem, manage time needed to solve the problem, assess their progress in solving the problem, and predict the outcomes of their decisions.

Chi, Bassok, Lewis, Reimann, and Glaser (1988) explored the learning strategies employed by academically successful college students and less-successful college students in solving problems. They found that successful students engaged in more self-explanation (i.e., examining why the solution worked and when the solution related to other problem situations) than did the less-successful students.

Dweck (1986), when examining what students do when they encounter difficult situations and continue to meet roadblocks in solving problems, observed that some individuals accepted the challenge while others attempted to remove themselves from the situations, thus depriving themselves of an opportunity to learn. The difference between accepting the challenge and giving up, Dweck concluded, was in how students thought of their intelligence. The students who believed that intelligence, as a trait, can change with practice were more likely to accept the challenges of the problems and solve them with persistence than students who felt that intelligence was static. The latter students gave up after failure of their first attempts to solve the problems.

Research examining the strategies and attitudes characteristic of successful and less-successful problem solvers provides some guidelines for instruction. Problem-solving success can be improved by focusing on these strategies and attitudes directly (Bransford and Vye, 1989).

TEACHING PROBLEM SOLVING AS A PROCESS

As in other activities and strategies presented in *Daily Communication,* teaching problem-solving strategies requires the professional to help students reflect on the thinking processes used while solving problems and to compare and contrast one approach with another. This includes having students think aloud as they attempt to solve a problem and having students share strategies used to solve problems with each other (Bransford and Vye, 1989).

An important element in encouraging use of systematic problem solving is modeling. Modeling helps adolescents to see how others approach problems and how they hypothesize consequences of alternatives. Modeling can be provided by the professional or by other adolescents in a group. Bransford and Vye (1989) think it is especially relevant for educators to model, aloud, while working on a novel problem. Most often, even for adults, dead ends occur when one thinks about a novel problem. The process used to deal with the roadblock is an effective model for the adolescent. These models are more relevant to adolescents than models of problem solving with perfect reasoning.

Professionals are encouraged to create problem situations that allow students to experience roadblocks and problems that seem impossible to solve, to invite problem finding as well as problem solving, and to encourage problem solving in groups where students can share alternatives and model strategies for each other.

COGNITIVE PREREQUISITES FOR PROBLEM SOLVING

The process of solving problems requires numerous cognitive functions, including the following:

- clear, precise accumulation and retention of information relating to the problem;
- accurate identification of the problem;
- expression of alternative solutions in clear and precise ways;
- comparison of alternatives;
- recognition of relationships; and
- execution of the solution in planned, systematic, and thoughtful ways.

PROBLEM-SOLVING MODEL

To become competent problem solvers, adolescents will need a systematic plan for approaching problems. Professionals couldn't possibly "rehearse" solutions for the many problems students will face in the future. Encouraging adolescents to develop systematic strategies for solving problems is essential if the adolescent is to adapt to the world as it changes. Figure 4.1 on the following page presents a problem-solving model with strategies for each step in the model. Professionals are encouraged to display this model where adolescents can see it and refer to it frequently throughout this unit and then whenever necessary to help students focus on a particular problem. This figure is also available in poster form (see the last page of this book for details).

PROBLEM SITUATIONS

While individuals face many types of problems, adolescents seem most often to face problems that are academic, personal/social (e.g., relating to family and friends), personal health/financial

FIGURE 4.1

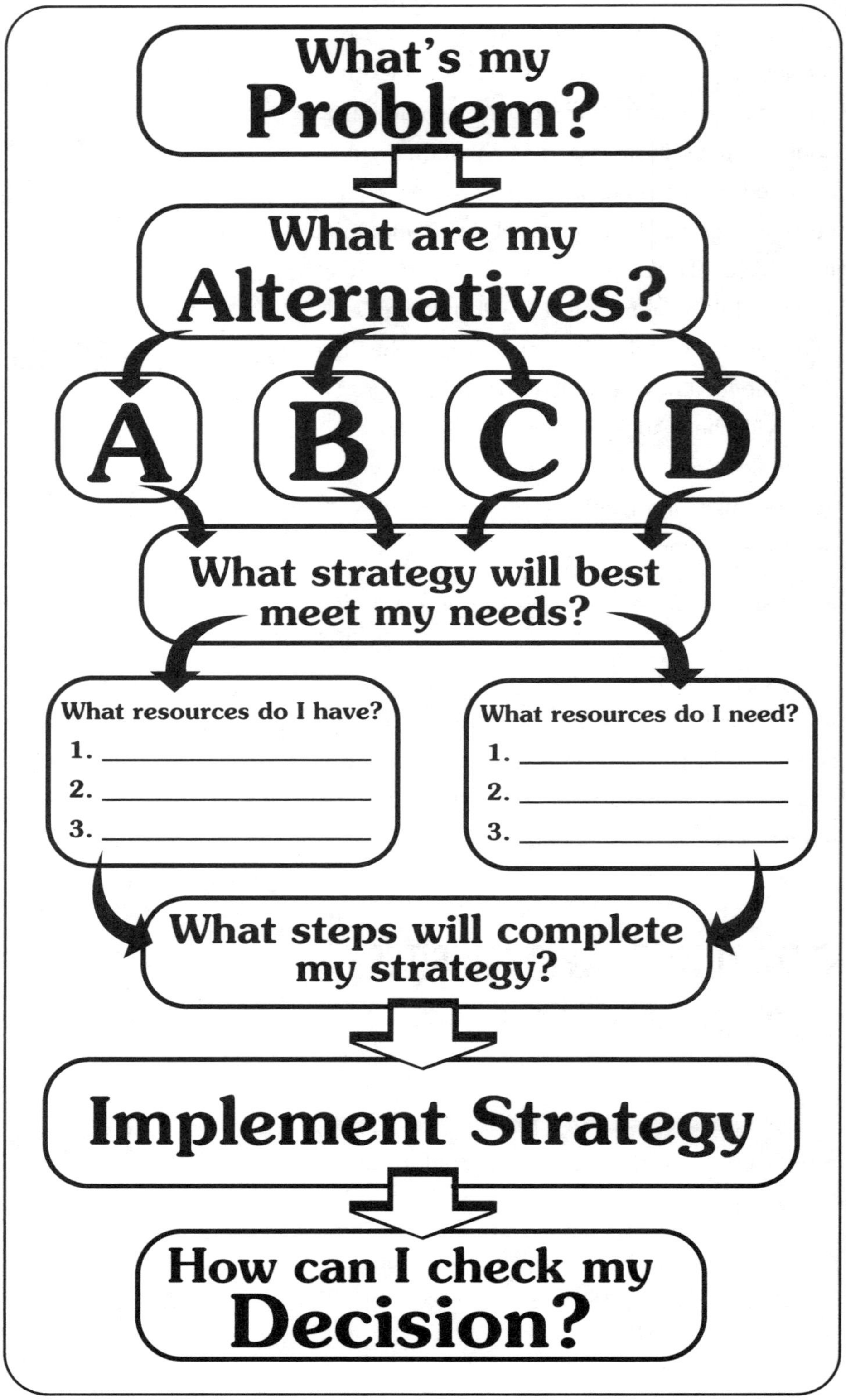

© 1983 Thinking Publications

related, and/or advanced level (e.g., problems relating to career choices or jobs) in nature. The problematic situations listed in the next three sections are typical of those encountered by adolescents. They are presented here for problem-solving application activities. Keep in mind that given a problem, event, or phenomenon, people will represent the problem in terms of what they already know (Kurfiss, 1988). The following problem situations are presented as examples. However, creating problem situations that are relevant to the adolescents receiving intervention is recommended.

ACADEMIC

1. Your father promised to take you on his annual fishing trip if your next report card shows improvement. Your report card arrives in the mail, and you open it before your father gets home from work. You are failing two subjects.

2. You were in trouble in school today, and the principal called your home. You know that you'll be in big trouble when you get home from school.

3. On your way home from school, you stop to talk to a friend sitting at the bus stop. You end up forgetting your books there. When you return later to get them, they're gone.

4. Your science project is due tomorrow. Your brother was going to help you with it but he has to work late and won't be home in time to help you.

5. You have a terrible problem remembering to bring what you need to class. You are also forgetting to do things at home.

PERSONAL/SOCIAL

6. Your class cannot attend the field trip unless the principal finds out who wrote the graffiti on the restroom wall. You know your brother did it, but your parents will punish him severely if they find out.

7. You see a good friend of yours buying drugs. You feel upset about it.

8. A friend wants to borrow your new CD. Her friendship is important to you, but whenever you loan things to her, she returns them damaged or just keeps them.

9. A boy from your algebra class keeps calling you on the telephone and talks for a long time. You don't really care to talk to him anymore and your sister wants you to quit tying up the telephone.

10. The junior high dance is coming up. Every time you go to a dance, you end up standing around with no one to talk to.

PERSONAL HEALTH/FINANCIAL

11. You think you are overweight but you find it too hard to stick to a diet.

12. After saving for three months, you have $50 to spend on a pair of new sneakers that cost $47.95. While shopping, you notice a more expensive pair of shoes on sale. "Today only! $89.95." They're the kind of shoes you really want.

13. Your mother wants you to purchase some medication she needs at the drug store on your way home from school. She gives you

the money. On the way, you meet a friend to whom you owe money. He spots the money in your hand, takes it, and runs.

14. Someone broke into your locker and took your library books. You'll have to pay $21 to replace them.

15. Your friend is planning a sleepover Friday night, but it is also your mother's birthday. Your aunt has planned a family celebration. You'd like to attend both activities.

ADVANCED-LEVEL PROBLEMS

16. You'll be graduating in four months and you still haven't decided what you'll do next.

17. There's a job opening at the local grocery store. If you were to work there, you would need transportation. You're not sure if you could afford to buy a car.

18. Your boyfriend is getting into drugs and is pressuring you to try them too. You really like him but you don't want to take drugs.

19. You've made the decision to move out of the house when you turn 18. You realize there's going to be a confrontation when you talk to your parents about it.

20. You're the only person in your group of friends who owns a car. Everyone borrows it, but you pay for the gas, the insurance, and the repairs.

ACTIVITIES TO ENHANCE PROBLEM-SOLVING STRATEGIES

PROBLEM-SOLVING SKILLS

● Identification of problems as a strategy to solving them

●● Generation and consideration of alternative solutions to problems

●●● Comparison of alternative solutions to choose the strategy that best meets needs

●●●● Development of a plan to reach a solution

●●●●● Evaluation of problems solved and decisions made

"WHAT'S MY PROBLEM?" DISCUSSION

PURPOSE

To discuss a rationale for identifying problems

Before the process of solving a problem begins, adolescents must decide that a problem exists. It is not always easy, however, to decide "what the problem is." Success as a problem solver depends on accuracy in identifying the problem, and problems are sometimes hidden in commonplace events or situations. If the existence of a problem is not realized, individuals cannot be expected to look for solutions (Bransford, Sherwood, Rieser, and Vye, 1986). Reflecting on our own educational histories, the authors recall many problems that needed solving, but recall fewer opportunities for identifying the problems.

To identify a problem means to determine its full scope and to clarify the obstacle to something desired or planned (Drake, 1976). According to Hayes (1981, 1989), to understand a problem, the problem solver creates a representation in the mind of the objects, restrictions, and relations presented in the problem. This internal representation is particularly important when the problem solver hasn't personally had experience with the actual situation. Occasionally, the internal representation is not sufficient, so the problem solver also creates an external representation in the form of a diagram, drawing, sketch, or written description of the problem.

Adolescents might need to represent some problems externally, at a concrete level, through an activity such as role-playing. The goal, however, would be an eventual decrease in the use of external representation and an increase in internal representation.

Share this information with adolescents, allowing time to discuss it.

LEARNING STRATEGY

The adolescent will identify problems as a strategy to solving them.

APPLICATION TO PROBLEM SITUATIONS

PURPOSE

To identify problems in given situations

Using the problem situations listed on pages 39–40 or other problem situations created, carefully analyze what needs to be solved using the model question, "What's my problem?" If the problem is accurately defined, the student should be able to formulate a question. Theoretically, when that question is answered, the problem is solved. For example, refer to the first problem in the Personal/Social area:

> Your class cannot attend the field trip unless the principal finds out who wrote the graffiti on the restroom wall. You know your brother did it, but your parents will punish him severely if they find out.
>
> The problem might be identified as, "How can we attend the field trip?"

Engage the adolescents in a discussion of what might happen if the problem is left unsolved.

Require students to bring to class current assignments, projects, or worksheets. Have them identify the problem or problems to be solved on the page. Cover the written instructions and require the students to predict the possible problem.

Encourage students to begin *every project or assignment* by identifying the problem to be solved. Discuss the cost of solving the wrong problem (e.g., wasted time, money spent unnecessarily, feelings that are hurt).

To further reinforce the strategy of problem identification, pair students. Provide each pair with sets of directions, recipes, meeting announcements, party invitations, etc. that have a missing component. For example, the recipe could be missing a key ingredient or the meeting announcement could be lacking the meeting's location. Direct the student pairs to identify whether a problem exists, and if so, what the problem is.

● LEARNING STRATEGY

The adolescent will identify problems as a strategy to solving them.

"WHAT ARE MY ALTERNATIVES?" DISCUSSION

PURPOSE

To discuss the rationale for generating alternatives

When the problem is discovered and the question is asked (i.e., "What's my problem?"), direct the students to consider various options for solving the problem. Some problems may seem to have no alternatives, while in other situations, the solution may seem obvious. In either case, considering all alternatives prevents later saying, "I wish I had thought of that," "I wish I had known that," "If only I hadn't said that," etc.

By 10 or 12 years of age, developing the skill of generating and considering many alternatives becomes crucial (Agency for Instructional Television, 1979). Problem solvers who respond to problems in habitual ways, with first-reaction/one-alternative solutions, will continually find themselves in predicaments they may feel to be beyond their control.

Encourage adolescents to think about generating at least three to six alternatives when solving their problems. Discuss the rationale for generating more than one alternative to solving a problem.

To encourage flexibility in the adolescents' thinking, have them generate alternative solutions for problems they have already solved. This activity helps students realize that at times more than one solution is appropriate for solving a problem.

●●

LEARNING STRATEGY

The adolescent will generate and consider many alternative solutions to problems as a strategy for solving them.

APPLICATION TO PROBLEM SITUATIONS

PURPOSE

To generate alternative solutions given problem situations

Brainstorming is one method of generating alternatives. Brainstorming requires a group discussion in which all members contribute ideas freely and search for every possible solution to a problem. Ideas generated by group members are paraphrased and listed on paper. Group members withhold comments regarding the appropriateness of the alternatives at this stage. Although students may feel tempted to automatically eliminate alternatives that seem impossible, all "solutions" to the problem should be generated, since additional ideas may flow from them. Encourage the listing of at least five alternative solutions to each problem during the activity. Using the problem situations listed on pages 39–40 (or other problem situations created), and the questions formulated during the "Application to Problem Situations" activity on page 43, generate alternative solutions.

> *Example:*
>
> Identified problem—
>
> "How can we attend the field trip?"

Generated alternatives:

1. Talk your teacher into letting the class attend even though the graffiti artist has not been identified.
2. Tell your teacher your brother did it, and let your brother worry about the consequences.
3. Tell your teacher your brother did it, but talk him into not calling your parents.
4. Organize the class to walk out.
5. Wait and see what happens. (After all, the teacher might not really mean it when he says the class can't attend the field trip.)

During regularly held class meetings (daily or weekly), allow students to express issues or problems of concern to them. Class members can contribute alternatives to aid their classmates, acting as excellent models, or they can act as sounding boards for possible alternatives.

●●

LEARNING STRATEGY

The adolescent will generate and consider many alternative solutions to problems as a strategy for solving them.

For instance, during a class meeting held by one of the authors, a student expressed the problem of having to face an instructor who was upset about his missing a scheduled meeting. After presenting the problem to the class, the student discussed his alternatives and decided that he would not become involved in an argumentative power struggle. Instead, he would try to talk to his instructor, accepting the blame for being irresponsible. Class members agreed that his choice was a "mature choice," and the student seemed more confident in his decision.

Keep in mind that thinking aloud to solve your own problems acts as an excellent model for adolescents who have trouble seeing alternative solutions to their problems.

"WHAT STRATEGY WILL BEST MEET MY NEEDS?" DISCUSSION

PURPOSE

To discuss the rationale for developing skill in making comparisons

Feuerstein (1980) views the cognitive function of comparison as a prerequisite to successful decision making; comparison is the basis of all decisions and judgments. Comparing involves considering what two or more alternatives have in common and what differentiates them (i.e., a recognition of the relationship between the items or ideas being compared).

A comparison can involve all characteristics, attributes, or qualities of items or ideas, or it can deal with just one characteristic, attribute, or quality. When considering one particular characteristic, attribute, or quality, the comparison is based on a *criterion*. In making decisions, the critical criterion or criteria (i.e., attributes, characteristics, qualities) that are relevant to one's needs are considered (Feuerstein, 1980). Consideration of these criteria, or of what's important to an individual, leads to a better decision.

COMPARING ON A CONCRETE LEVEL

Developing comparative skill initially involves focusing on two or more concrete objects. Comparing objects that can be seen or with which an individual is familiar is easier than comparing abstract ideas (Feuerstein, 1980). The objects or items considered should be compared on the same criteria. For example, when comparing an airplane and a train, the group might agree that in using the criterion "forms of transportation," the train and the airplane are similar. When considering the criterion "requirement for operation," the group might agree they are differentiated by points of arrival and departure, the plane requiring an airport/runway and the train requiring a depot/track. However, if the group were to say, "The train requires a track, and the plane weighs ten tons," they would not be comparing the same criterion, and the comparison would be inadequate.

COMPARING ALTERNATIVES TO MAKE DECISIONS

Comparing alternative solutions becomes a more abstract task. Sometimes the similarities and differences of alternatives are obvious; at other times, investment of time and effort to discover the similarities and differences is required (e.g., in deciding which CD player to buy, one might spend some time shopping, comparing prices, researching consumers' guides, asking friends' opinions, etc.). Sometimes minor differences in alternatives may become obvious only through comparison.

●●●

LEARNING STRATEGY

The adolescent will compare and contrast alternative solutions and choose the solution or strategy that best meets his or her needs.

Many everyday decisions are made without "extensive" comparison and considerations, such as what shoes to wear, what to eat for breakfast, or what radio station to listen to. One relies on feelings, emotions, or intuition, but there also exists a degree of reasoning and comparison, even for these decisions (Gelatt, Varenhorst, Carey, and Miller, 1973). For instance, when deciding what to eat for breakfast, one might consider criteria such as what is available to eat in the cupboard, how much time there is for preparation, how long it will be before the next meal, what the next meal might be, or what is healthy to eat.

Other decisions require investment of time and energy to do the following:

- gather information about the alternatives;
- identify needs, priorities, and criteria for comparison;
- compare alternatives and predict outcomes; and
- weigh risks.

DECISION MAKING

Fulcher (1965) describes four types of decision making:

1. impulsive decisions—impulsive, emotional reactions to situations that occur without much thought
2. routine decisions—decisions made in accordance with familial habits, customs, or rules
3. casuistic decisions—decisions determined by ethical, moral, or religious principles; and
4. thoughtful decisions—decisions made after careful consideration of the problem, alternatives, and consequences.

Daily Communication presents information to encourage thoughtful decision making, but professionals should be aware that adolescents may make choices governed by other factors. Share the above information with adolescents, allowing time to discuss it.

APPLICATION TO CONCRETE COMPARISONS: OBJECT COMPARISON

PURPOSE

To compare and contrast concrete objects

●●●

LEARNING STRATEGY

The adolescent will compare and contrast alternative solutions and choose the solution or strategy that best meets his or her needs.

To encourage student discrimination of similarities and differences among alternatives, a first step of comparing and contrasting concrete objects might be required. Using objects at a concrete level allows students to become familiar with vocabulary terms that will be helpful in later discussions regarding decision making (e.g., *attributes, characteristics, qualities, criteria, equivalent, identical).*

Present any two objects to the group. Allow group members to decide on which characteristics the comparison will be based. For instance, the following characteristics could be used to compare a pen and a pencil: size, color, permanence, diameter, and appropriate use.

Challenge students to name any two objects (e.g., an elephant and a lamp). Then compare and contrast them, being certain that students name at least one similarity and one difference for each combination of objects. Discuss the following concepts:

- Do objects that are similar also have differences?
- Do objects that are different also have similarities?
- Is it ever possible for two objects to be completely identical?
- What does it mean to be similar? Identical? Equivalent? The same? Equal?
- Why do we have so many words for the same basic phenomena?

If desired, complete this activity by comparing more abstract concepts or ideas (e.g., a fact and an opinion, a wish and a dream, a high school and a middle school, a teacher and a student).

GROUP SIMILARITIES

PURPOSE

To compare and contrast group members

People are alike and different in many ways. To reinforce the concept of comparison in a concrete activity, continue with the following activity. Focus a group discussion on the possible characteristics for comparing members of the group. Encourage the group to also list ideas that are more abstract than what can physically be observed.

Examples:

height	exciting things in their lives
sports interests	birthdays
eye color	rank in family
hair color	family size
favorite clothing	favorite foods
interests	nicknames
hobbies	grade in school
weight	feelings about school

Pair group members. Direct partners to address the characteristics generated by the large group and then to list commonalities and differences between each other. Require each pair to report their findings to the group. Discuss the following concepts with the group:

- What things do most of the members have in common?
- What are some of the differences?
- Do persons who have differences also have similarities?
- What conclusions can be drawn about persons who are similar but who also have differences?

●●●

LEARNING STRATEGY

The adolescent will compare and contrast alternative solutions and choose the solution or strategy that best meets his or her needs.

APPLICATION TO COMPARING ALTERNATIVES

PURPOSE

To demonstrate and use systematic approaches to making decisions

●●●

LEARNING STRATEGY

The adolescent will compare and contrast alternative solutions and choose the solution or strategy that best meets his or her needs.

Again referring to the problem situations on pages 39–40, which by now have an identified problem and alternatives generated, answer these questions.

HAS ENOUGH INFORMATION BEEN GATHERED?

If an individual has limited experience in the area of consideration (such as that in buying a bike or deciding on a medical treatment), having more information is advantageous when judging the risks and predicting the outcome of the alternatives.

Determine sources for gathering more information. There are limitless sources for solving many problems. Some traditional examples are professional services such as those of a lawyer, doctor, or counselor and references such as encyclopedias or dictionaries; some nontraditional sources include best friends, consumer guides, U.S. government pamphlets, do-it-yourself books, local experts, electronic bulletin boards, or advice columns.

Returning to the example problem—"How can we attend the field trip?"—consult traditional and nontraditional sources of information that might help answer the question. Possibilities include

- talking to the principal about the situation;
- talking to another teacher who knows your teacher well;
- talking to the guidance counselor;
- reading a book on psychology;
- talking the situation over with a friend; or
- talking the situation over with your brother.

Is the source of information objective? Are the facts clear? Is the information distorted?

ON WHAT CRITERIA WILL THE ALTERNATIVES BE COMPARED?

People will make different decisions because they have different priorities, values, and information. Allow students to identify the criteria they would use to compare the alternatives and then rank order the criteria from the highest priority to the lowest priority. Have students share their criteria and identify the differences among class members.

FIGURE 4.2

	ALTERNATIVES					
	CRITERIA	1	2	3	4	5
Highest Priority	1.					
↑	2.					
↓	3.					
Lowest Priority	4.					

The grid presented in Figure 4.2 is a model for displaying advantages and disadvantages of various alternatives. Using several problem situations, direct students to apply this process. An illustration of the process applied to the example problem (i.e., "How can we attend the field trip?") is displayed in Figure 4.3 on page 54.

WHAT OUTCOME CAN BE PREDICTED FOR GIVEN ALTERNATIVES?

Engage students in a discussion of the risks involved and the possible consequences of each alternative. Since individuals do not have complete control over their environments, favorable outcomes to decisions cannot be guaranteed (Gelatt, Varenhorst, Carey, and Miller, 1973). Every decision made involves risk; however, the more accurate the comparison of the alternatives, the more likely the hypothesis will approximate the actual outcome (Gelatt et al., 1973) and the more likely the decision will be pleasing.

Allow adolescents to eliminate some alternatives at this point if their outcomes may be undesirable. Discuss risks involved for the remaining alternatives by considering some of the following: Will the decision harm anyone? Will it work? Will it work in the long run? Have students continue to eliminate any alternatives with risks not worth taking, those that will harm someone, or those that won't work in the long run.

Before instructing students to make a decision regarding the problem situation, discuss the following common approaches to making decisions (Gelatt et al., 1973):

- Ignore risks and choose the alternative with the most desirable outcome.
- Avoid risking the worst and then choose the alternative that might eliminate the worst possible outcome.
- Choose the alternative that is most likely to bring success.
- Get the best combination of low risk and desirable outcome; choose the action that has high probability and desirability.

If an alternative is chosen that is not thought "best" or "safest" (the so-called "risky decision"), at least the consequences will not be a surprise. The reaction might be, "I wanted to take the risk even though I knew this might happen." Sometimes individuals have to take a risk! Returning to our example problem, direct students to choose an alternative solution or strategy to solve the problem (i.e., make a decision).

Recall the example alternatives that have been generated:

1. Talk your teacher into letting the class attend even though the graffiti artist has not been identified.
2. Tell your teacher your brother did it, and let your brother worry about the consequences.
3. Tell your teacher your brother did it, but talk him into not calling your parents.
4. Organize the class to walk out.
5. Wait and see what happens. (After all, the teacher might not really mean it when he says the class can't attend the field trip.)

While there's no one right answer, students might choose alternative 2. It solves the problem of going on the field trip with little risk or harm to anyone, except to the brother who might be punished (and who perhaps deserves it).

Conclude this process by having students list other situations when there is no one right answer. Draw conclusions about making decisions by discussing conditions that make decision making easy or difficult (e.g., two alternatives are equally desirable, such as choosing between pieces of your favorite desserts; or two alternatives are equally undesirable, such as choosing between cleaning your room and doing homework).

FIGURE 4.3

Identified Problem: *How can we attend the field trip?*					
	ALTERNATIVES				
CRITERIA (in order of priority)	1	2	3	4	5
Attendance on the field trip	yes	yes	yes	unsure	unsure
Risks involved?	yes	No risk to class.	Unsure of teacher's reaction to this.	Unsure of consequences of such an action.	Yes, not sure what might happen.
Anyone harmed?	Teacher may not back down.	Brother may be punished and may be angry but the class still attends.	Possibly your brother.	unsure	unsure
Solve the problem in the long run?	yes	yes	yes	no	unknown
Save brother from punishment?	yes	no	yes	yes	yes
Hypothesized outcome…	Class attends but possibly receives different punishment. Brother not punished; might continue doing this action.	Class attends. Brother pays conse-quences. Brother will know you told that he did it and he will be angry at you.	Brother not punished; may continue action. Teacher may call parents anyway. You may be in trouble for discussing home problems with school teachers. Class goes on field trip.	May be more consequences to pay in addition to not going on the field trip. May ruin all chances for going.	Teacher won't back down. Your class doesn't attend the field trip. Brother may continue this action.

"WHAT RESOURCES DO I HAVE OR NEED? WHAT STEPS WILL COMPLETE MY STRATEGY?" DISCUSSION

PURPOSE

To discuss various approaches to implementing strategies

Planning is an important metacognitive strategy that requires thinking about the consequences of choices and alternative solutions. The planning step helps to increase the effectiveness of problem solving.

Once a solution or strategy is chosen, the planning process begins. Conduct a discussion that leads to comparing various implementation approaches, including the following:

1. **Trial-and-error approach**—a "hit or miss" system of implementing a solution, permitting trials and errors until the problem is solved.

2. **Systematic approach**—a system of ordering the steps to a plan by identifying the starting point and continuing in an orderly pattern, being always aware of what's been completed and what needs to be done.

Have students generate specific examples of both approaches. Sometimes either approach works; consequently, involving students in a discussion of which system is most efficient in terms of time and energy is imperative. (Example: In an effort to find lost keys in the morning, you frantically go from one room to another, searching in a trial-and-error fashion. A systematic approach would have been to retrace your steps of the night before from the time you left the car.)

As a daily routine, encourage students to describe what they thought about as they solved various problems. Can they describe how they reached the solution? This may be the most overlooked step in the problem-solving process, particularly by educators who are often "product" oriented. The authors have observed students who, when encouraged to defend their answers or to describe how they solved a problem, quickly change their solution as though it were incorrect.

●●●●

LEARNING STRATEGY

The adolescent will make a plan that includes steps and resources necessary to reach a solution.

APPLICATION TO PROBLEM SITUATIONS

PURPOSE

To list steps in a plan and identify available or necessary resources

Using the problem situations from pages 39–40 (or other problem situations created), instruct students to list the steps for implementing each solution. Have the group consider the following questions:

- Will the solution require a systematic approach or will a trial-and-error approach be adequate?
- Will the solution require one strategy or will the problem require flexibility (switching from one strategy to another)?
- What will the reaction be if the original plan doesn't work? (E.g., in planning a picnic for a holiday, a friend and you mutually decide to meet at the park at noon. At noon, however, it begins to rain and storm. Can you flexibly adjust to a change of plans?)

Referring to the problem situation, instruct students to identify the resources or materials that have been given or are available and then decide which resources need to be gathered before implementing the solution/strategy. Encourage students to continue planning the steps necessary for implementing the strategy.

Returning to the example problem, ("How can we attend the field trip?"), assume the decision was made to "tell your teacher your brother did it, and let your brother worry about the consequences."

Implementation of this solution might include these steps:

- Plan to meet your teacher after class.
- Request a private place to talk.
- Plan what you will say.
- Explain to your teacher "how" you know your brother did it; prepare to give proof of your accusation.
- Explain to your brother that you told the teacher.

Figure 4.4 on page 57 displays the resources available and resources needed for solving the problem.

●●●●

LEARNING STRATEGY

The adolescent will make a plan that includes steps and resources necessary to reach a solution.

FIGURE 4.4

RESOURCES AVAILABLE	RESOURCES NEEDED
• time to meet with your teacher (after class) • proof of your brother's guilt	• a quiet, private place to talk

Another option for enhancing the planning process is to have adolescents identify missing steps in a planned solution. Read the following situations and have students identify the missing steps, resources needed, and available resources.

1. You are looking forward to Saturday's fishing trip and have arranged to borrow your dad's car. You bought the fishing license, packed a lunch, and placed your rod, reel, and tackle box in the car. Identify the missing steps in this plan. (E.g., this plan has omitted the place, the means for fishing [boat, shore, etc.], the departure time, etc.)

2. In planning your holiday shopping, you decide to take the shuttle bus to the mall. Identify the missing steps in this plan. (E.g., this plan has omitted the bus schedule, amount of money needed, number of gifts to buy, stores to visit, etc.) What strategy could be implemented before leaving home (e.g., list making)?

3. You decide to talk to your mother about a new jacket you would like her to buy for you. You tell her it's at Jergen's Department Store.

4. You're a bus driver and your bus has a flat tire; you decide to stay with the bus until the wrecker comes.

5. You've decided to purchase that new 18-speed all-terrain bike you've wanted for so long. You withdraw money from your savings account.

6. To get ready for bed, you brush your teeth, wash your face, and then crawl into bed.

7 Upon receiving your math worksheet, you begin with the third problem because it looks easiest.

8 You've lost your wallet; since you've looked everywhere, you give up.

9 Your dog needs a rabies shot. You show up at the veterinarian's office at two o'clock.

10 You're planning a trip with friends. You pack your suitcase, pick up your friends, and head toward the highway.

11 In registering for fall classes, you sign up for all the classes you like.

12 A conflict in your schedule puts a physical education class at the same time as your English class. You decide to attend physical education instead of English.

13 You've made the decision to take a shortcut to your friend's home; you're trusting you will remember the way since you've gone this way before.

14 The English exam you've dreaded is on the desk in front of you. You answer questions that are easy and turn in your paper.

15 While sitting in your social studies class, you recall leaving your jacket in the lunchroom. You walk out of class to get it.

16 You show up to vote on election day, but you are not familiar with the candidates.

17 You accidentally run into a vehicle with your bike. The scratch you made looks minor, so you walk home.

18 You need to talk to your teacher about a problem in class. It upsets you that he's never in his office when you need him.

19 On the day of your biology exam, you begin to read the four chapters included in the test.

20 You are planning a special spaghetti dinner. You heat the water, set the table, and sit down to eat.

"HOW CAN I CHECK MY DECISION?" DISCUSSION

PURPOSE

To discuss the rationale for evaluating decisions

The final step in any problem/solution is to evaluate the decision made. Evaluation requires determining if the solution answers the question formulated in the identification stage. Does the solution meet the limitations or priorities set by the problem? Identifying past decisions that may be considered "inappropriate" or wrong is appropriate at this step of the problem-solving process. Results of wrong decisions are called *errors.* According to Gelatt et al. (1973), errors can occur in decision making for some of the following reasons:

1. not choosing an alternative because you do not see it as a possibility;
2. choosing an alternative even though you don't know the possible outcome;
3. underestimating or overestimating the importance of certain information; and/or
4. collecting unnecessary information.

Fulcher (1965) describes a *best decision* as one with the most desirable outcome based on the decision maker's highest standards. He describes a *sound decision* as one in which the decision maker made a reasonable effort to determine the facts and to accurately determine the consequences of alternatives, and to use logic and sound beliefs. Discuss this information with students.

There may be considerable costs involved in not evaluating decisions—costs in terms of time and energy, finances, reputation, health, or even life. Students often rely on teachers, parents, or friends to check their work or decisions. While that certainly is a strategy available, encourage the students to be responsible for checking their own decisions, the most "independent" strategy. Professionals can demonstrate their own metacognitive processes in reflecting upon a problem solved by "thinking and reflecting aloud" in the presence of the adolescents.

Adolescents need to know the roles that analysis and evaluation play in problem solving; that is, these skills can be used to solve problems and also to prevent them in the future. If students evaluate their solutions, it will help them to anticipate problems in the future; if they learn to recognize trends or cause and effect, solving new problems will be easier (Atwood, 1974).

Discuss with students the rationale for evaluating decisions made and allow time for students to identify the cause and effect of past problems.

●●●●●

LEARNING STRATEGY

The adolescent will evaluate decisions and solutions as a strategy for problem solving.

APPLICATION TO PROBLEM SITUATIONS

PURPOSE

To evaluate decisions made

Continue using the problem situations from pages 39–40 (or other problem situations created) to decide which of the following evaluation techniques can be used in the various situations:

1. reversing the process of the problem-solving strategy (e.g., subtracting as a way to check addition, retracing steps when searching for a lost article);
2. using a counting strategy (e.g., counting books before returning them to the library); or
3. asking yourself questions or referring to a checklist (e.g., Did I remember to turn off the lights and lock the door? Do I have a map to help me find my way?).

Encourage students to share additional techniques for checking decisions made. Using decisions made in the previous activities, discuss some of the following concepts:

- Which decisions can be reversed? (E.g., the decision to paint a room blue can be reversed by repainting the room another color.)
- Which decisions cannot be reversed? (E.g., a decision causing harm to someone cannot be reversed.)
- With which type of decision—reversible or irreversible—would you be less inclined to take a risk?

Return to the example problem situation. Assume the decision was to "tell your teacher your brother did it and let your brother worry about the consequences." In evaluating this decision, the third technique listed above might apply. Require students to think about these questions:

- What were the consequences of this solution?
- Was the class allowed to attend the field trip?
- Was anyone harmed?
- Was this the best decision in the long run?
- Is this decision reversible or irreversible?

●●●●●●

LEARNING STRATEGY

The adolescent will evaluate decisions and solutions as a strategy for problem solving.

Asking students to consider the cause of problems is also a form of evaluating decisions. Determining the relationships between causes and effects may help students to prevent certain problems from occurring in the future. Posing questions such as, "Can you think of reasons that...?" and "What do you suppose would explain why...?" is asking students to evaluate decisions.

5

LISTENING STRATEGIES

LISTENING: EDUCATION'S ORPHAN

Of the four language arts skills—reading, writing, speaking, and listening—listening is learned first in children's development, used most in the course of our lives, and taught least during our years of formal education (Steil, 1991). Markgraf (1966) found that 46 percent of classroom time for high school students was spent in listening. Goodlad (1983) found the average junior/senior high school day has 150 minutes of talking, 7 of them initiated by students (i.e., 143 minutes of listening). At least 75 percent of our daily communication is oral (Wolff, Marsnik, Tacey, and Nichols, 1983). If there ever was a basic survival skill, listening is it. As Nichols (1995) reminds us, "Listening is so basic that we take it for granted. Unfortunately, most of us think of ourselves as better listeners than we really are" (p. 11).

DEFINITION OF LISTENING

Experts remind us that a definition of listening is still being developed (Wolvin and Coakley, 1982; Ridge, 1993). *Listening* is a complex act whereby a listener derives some type of meaning from the speaker's intent. Nichols (1991) observed: "Effective listening is conceived to be an active and dynamic process, with clearly identifiable rewards for energy expanded" (p. vi). Furthermore, listening is a collection of identifiable skills that can be improved through training and practice, just as our reading, writing, and speaking can (Nichols, 1957; Wolvin and Coakley, 1993). Good listening requires empathy, achieved by entering into another person's experience and suspending preoccupation with our own (Nichols, 1995).

LISTENING TRAINING: HISTORICAL PERSPECTIVE

Below is an illustration of how most of us were taught to listen by our teachers. The sorry fact is,

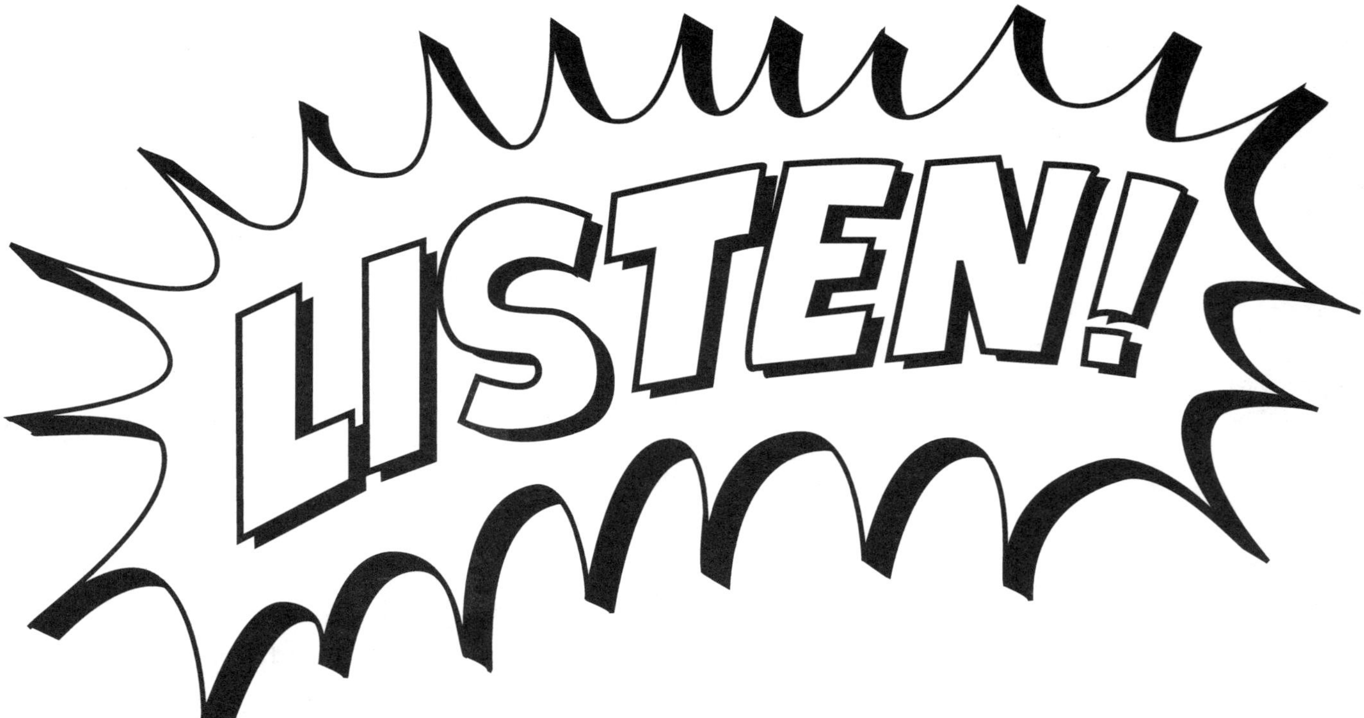

no one learns to listen by being commanded to do so. Interestingly enough, the momentum behind many of today's listening programs came first from businesses such as Xerox Corporation and Sperry Rand, not from educational sources. In 1978, the federal government mandated that listening instruction be included in the school curriculum by passing an amendment to the Primary and Secondary Education Act. Listening and speaking were included in the definition of basic skills for K–12 students and were added to reading, writing, and arithmetic as determinants of literacy.

TYPES OF LISTENING

Listening is primarily an activity of the mind, not of the ear or eye. If the mind is not engaged in the process, then one is hearing, not listening (Adler, 1983). The term *listening,* as used in *Daily Communication,* presumes the skills of auditory acuity, auditory perception (e.g., discrimination, figure-ground relationship), and comprehension of linguistic processes (e.g., syntax—understanding how word endings affect the meaning of words). Such skills are prerequisite to these types of listening:

- discriminative (also called "informational");
- evaluative (also called "critical");
- appreciative; and
- empathic.

These four listening types—discriminative, evaluative, appreciative, and empathic—focus on listening to learn, to evaluate, to relieve our tensions, and to relieve the tensions of others (Wolff et al., 1983). This resource focuses on the first two types—discriminative and evaluative—since they are needed daily in the educational system.

TEACHING ORDER

Discriminative listening skills should be intact before establishing evaluative listening objectives. Some sources also refer to evaluative listening skills as critical thinking skills, requiring that basic cognitive processes such as classification, conservation, spatial and temporal relationships, and analytical perception be intact. The educator needs to be aware of prerequisite skills for initiation of critical listening activities.

MISCONCEPTIONS ABOUT LISTENING

Ten misconceptions about listening have been identified by Wolff et al. (1983):

1. **Listening is a matter of intelligence.**
   No. Our ability to listen will be limited no matter what our intelligence if we have not learned specific skills through experience or training. Certainly, some correlation exists between intelligence and listening skill, but it is not the only determining factor.
2. **Good hearing and good listening are closely related.**
   No. It is important to find hearing difficulty within students, but "curing" them will not cure listening difficulties. Two people with the same hearing acuity may be vastly different listeners.

3. **Listening is an automatic reflex.**
   No. Listening is not innate; it is not a hereditary trait. It is not automatic like breathing. We need to learn to listen as we learn to speak, read, and write.

4. **Daily practice eliminates the need for training in listening.**
   No. Because we are in a position of listening much of the time, it is easy to think we do not need specific time to train ourselves to become better listeners. Some of us may need to take into account how much nonlistening training we had in the form of statements such as "Don't pay any attention to her," and "We don't listen to that kind of talk in this family."

5. **Learning to read will automatically improve listening.**
   No. Reading and listening are two distinct skills. Readers have many advantages that listeners do not. They can go back and reread a section for clarification, they can control the rate at which they read, and many times they can choose the place where they will read.

6. **Learning to read is more important than learning to listen.**
   No. There is no denying that reading is an important communication skill. But the fact remains that we listen three times more than we read, which places listening in a very crucial position.

7. **The speaker is totally responsible for success in oral communication.**
   No. Efficient listeners know that they must expend energy for communication to be successful. Both speakers and listeners are equal participants during an exchange.

8. **Listening is essentially a passive activity.**
   No. Nobody would consider spectators at a sporting event to be passive. Likewise, listeners actively need to attempt to grasp the facts and feelings the speaker is trying to portray. Adler (1983) emphasizes that listening involves much more than keeping quiet while the other person speaks.

9. **Listening means agreement.**
   No. Both speakers and listeners must differentiate between "He won't listen to me" and "He won't agree with my point of view." Active listening does not imply active agreement. First we listen, then we agree or disagree.

10. **Consequences of careless listening are minimal.**
    No. In fact, we pay a high price for not listening. Poor listening skills are often the basis for failure in homes, schools, and businesses.

It would be worthwhile to share and discuss these misconceptions with students.

In addition to these misconceptions, Jalongo (1991) points out these myths:

1. Listening is a passive activity.
2. Good listeners pay attention to everything they hear.
3. Children's listening is improved by admonishments to listen.

4. Good listeners keep their eyes fixed on the speaker at all times.
5. Compliance and listening are synonymous.
6. The difficulty in teaching children to listen is that they have such short attention spans.
7. Children are listening if they can repeat the message or recall a sequence of events or directions.
8. Expectations for listening behavior are the same in all societies.

In all cases, these myths can be dispelled based on evidence that exists.

1 ACTIVITIES TO ENHANCE LISTENING STRATEGIES

GENERAL LISTENING SKILLS

● Awareness of the importance of listening

●● Generation of interest in the speaker's topic

●●● Adjustment to listening distractions

●●●● Abstinence from faking attention, along with preparation to listen (especially in the school environment)

●●●●● Use of the differential between listening and thinking speeds

WHICH SKILL WOULD YOU CHOOSE?

PURPOSE

To discuss the relative importance of speaking, listening, reading, and writing

Many students need to become more aware of the impact that listening has upon them. Adolescents can be asked to discuss which of the four language arts—reading, writing, speaking, or listening—they would give up first. Phrased another way, the questions could be, "Which skill do you think is most important in your day-to-day functioning? Why?"

The questions will result in thought and discussion among students and create a greater awareness of the importance of listening. Information about the overwhelming amount of time spent listening may provide motivation for students who are skeptical of the importance of learning to listen. (Note: Do not impose the choice of listening as the most essential of the four language arts. The purpose of this task is awareness, not coercion.)

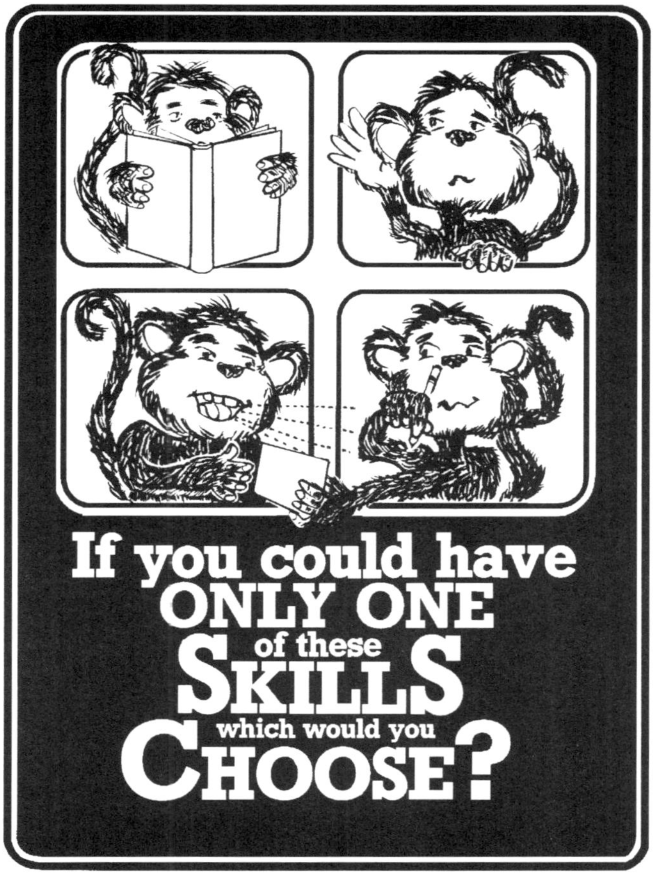

© 1983, 1988 Thinking Publications

●
LEARNING STRATEGY
The adolescent demonstrates awareness of the importance of listening and listening training.

LISTENING QUESTIONNAIRE FOR ADOLESCENTS

PURPOSE

To recognize individual beliefs and attitudes toward listening

The Personal Analysis Questionnaire proposed by Wolff et al. (1983) and Wolff and Marsnik (1992) inspired the questionnaire that follows, which can assist adolescents in recognizing their individual misconceptions about listening. The questionnaire is reprinted in Appendix D and can also be administered orally, requiring the student to listen rather than read.

LISTENING QUESTIONNAIRE

Mark each statement as true or false.

1. ____ Teachers or friends who don't listen to me aren't smart enough to appreciate my ideas.
2. ____ Teaching students to listen is like teaching them to breathe.
3. ____ I've already developed good listening skills because I have to listen all the time in school.
4. ____ It is more important to be good speakers than good listeners because we learn by talking.
5. ____ It is more important to be good readers than good listeners.
6. ____ I think I have been adequately trained to listen at school and home.
7. ____ Students should not have to work at listening to class lectures.
8. ____ I can't stand to listen to people who talk about ideas that sound crazy.
9. ____ It doesn't matter if I stop listening because I don't miss much.
10. ____ I'm a good listener when I want to be.

Each true answer reveals a misconception about listening. Have students count their number of true responses and compare it to the scale below:

0, 1	=	You are free of false information about listening.
2, 3, 4	=	You have a positive attitude toward listening training.
5, 6, 7	=	You are aware of listening training but misconceptions are warping your thinking.
8, 9, 10	=	BRICK WALL. Misconceptions have kept listening information from being useful to you.

Compare and discuss results within the group.

LEARNING STRATEGY

The adolescent demonstrates awareness of the importance of listening and listening training.

BOREDOM: WHOSE FAULT?

PURPOSE

To increase awareness that listeners are in charge of their interest level

Students need to become more aware of their responsibilities as listeners. While speakers (teachers) may attempt to select interesting topics, there will most certainly be times when listeners feel bored. Assuming the information is necessary for listeners to obtain, the logical option is to change their attitudes toward the topic. Students may need to be reminded that most topics seem uninteresting to people who are disinterested. Students need to be counseled to have an interest, to attempt to broaden their horizons, and to control personal prejudices that influence them to turn off the speaker.

Discuss one or more of the following questions within the group:

- What topics are most boring to you?
- What could be done to make this topic more interesting?
- What do teachers do, or not do, that makes a topic boring? (Attempt to have students isolate specific characteristics, such as monotone voice, lack of eye contact, or reading to the class rather than using spontaneous, natural language.)
- Have you ever been bored when one of your friends is talking with you? What was the topic?
- Do you think you have ever bored anyone else while you were talking? How could you tell if someone else was not interested in what you were saying?
- How do you feel when other people are bored with your talking?

●●

LEARNING STRATEGY

The adolescent generates interest in the speaker's topic.

LISTENER JUDGMENTS

PURPOSE

To illustrate how it might feel to be prejudged by a listener before one even has a chance to speak

Sometimes adolescents will judge adults and determine whether or not to listen to them based upon their dress, their hairstyle, or their age. To help students develop a perspective on what they are doing, it may be helpful to turn the tables on them.

When students enter the room, chat with them about how you just heard a rumor that the school day was going to be lengthened by 45 minutes each day, and there was talk about requiring summer school for all students whose grade-point averages were below B-minus. Ask the students how they would feel about these changes. When they attempt to argue for or against the changes, tell select students you are not going to listen because, for example, one student's hair is greasy and another student has gotten Ds on his report card. After some students have felt frustration, interrupt the activity and discuss what happened. These questions might be asked:

- How did you feel when someone refused to listen to your point of view?
- What did the adult's objection to your appearance (e.g., your greasy hair) have to do with your point of view and what you had to offer to the discussion?
- Has anyone else ever refused to listen to your side of the story? Why do you suppose that happened?
- Have you refused to listen to someone else because of how that person dressed or acted? Describe the situation.

Sometimes, it is not until students experience bias in reverse that they become aware of how they might have been discriminating against speakers.

●●

LEARNING STRATEGY

The adolescent generates interest in the speaker's topic.

INTERNAL DISTRACTIONS

PURPOSE

To isolate specific internal factors that influence the student's listening

Internal distractors that might interfere with listening include hunger, fatigue, and anxiety.

- Have students list and discuss those internal factors that most affect their listening ability in a negative way.
- Have them cite specific examples of times during which internal factors contributing to poor listening resulted in loss of time or money.
- Were there ways in which the internal distractors could be controlled so they did not interfere with listening?
- What might have been said to the speaker to alert him or her to the internal distractors? When is it appropriate to do this? When is it inappropriate?

●●●

LEARNING STRATEGY

The adolescent overcomes and adjusts to listening distractions.

EXTERNAL DISTRACTIONS

PURPOSE

To isolate external factors that influence the student's listening

External factors that might interfere with listening include noise, pollution, room conditions, and relative position to the speaker. Other people around may be whispering, coughing, sneezing, or laughing. The room may be too hot, too cold, too smoky, too big, or too small.

- Have students discuss which external conditions most disrupt their ability to listen.
- Have them cite specific examples of times in which external conditions contributing to poor listening resulted in loss of time or money.
- Discuss what, if anything, they could have done to improve their listening.
- Practice polite ways to request changes to one's listening environment (e.g., asking someone to turn down the sound on speakers, to turn down the heat, or to open a window).

●●●

LEARNING STRATEGY

The adolescent overcomes and adjusts to listening distractions.

FAKING IT: HEARING WITHOUT LISTENING

PURPOSE

To develop beginning awareness of characteristics of good and poor listeners

Adolescents need to become more aware of times when they are hearing but not listening. All of us drop out mentally and pretend to listen for milliseconds. We do not physically walk out on the speaker, but we do so in our minds. It is normal listening behavior. However, listeners who leave their speakers mentally for longer than a few milliseconds lose track of what is being said and forget that they can be detected by their lack of feedback. Persons who are actively listening give the speaker continuous feedback such as head nods, eye contact, and frowns or other indications that messages are or are not being understood. Students frequently underestimate the power they have, as listeners, to control speakers.

Have two students who share the same class agree ahead of time that one will give an obvious amount of positive feedback (e.g., head nods, smiles) to the teacher and one will give negative feedback (e.g., frowns, no eye contact). At the next session, ask the students to share their experiences and observations of teacher reactions. What was learned about the importance of listener feedback?

Have the students describe situations when changes occurred because listeners gave feedback to speakers. If they cannot generate any examples, watch for a moment when feedback occurs among students and use the event to teach how listeners can modify speaker behavior.

In a group, let members take turns being the speaker. Other group members can draw cards to decide who will be good listeners and who will be poor listeners. (Be careful that "poor" listening is not confused with "negative feedback." For example, frowning at the speaker when confusion occurs is actually "good" listening. "Poor" [i.e., ineffective] listening would consist of avoiding eye contact, interrupting the speaker, acting disinterested, etc.) Give each group member a chance to speak to the different types of listeners. Discuss how the speaker reacted to the good and poor listeners. Could the speaker discriminate between the two groups? How?

●●●●

LEARNING STRATEGY

The adolescent abstains from faking attention and prepares to participate in listening.

LISTENING PREPARATION

PURPOSE

To identify and discuss physical, emotional, and mental preparation to listen, particularly in a school environment

Students need to become aware of their responsibility to prepare themselves for the task of listening:

1. **Physical preparation**
   Obtain adequate sleep.
   Exercise.
   Eat a balanced diet.
   Control caffeine intake.
   Keep stress levels manageable.
   Maintain general good health.
   The bottom line is to feel and look like a listener (Wolff et al., 1983).
   Physical preparation also means not forgetting classroom equipment (e.g., notebook, textbook, etc.).

2. **Emotional preparation**
   Eliminate thoughts/emotions irrelevant to the speaker's message.
   Rid the mind of immediate concerns.
   Ask, "What's my motive for being involved in this class?" "What do I stand to gain by having an open mind during the minutes ahead?" (These questions are important on days when powerful personal issues are interfering with listening concentration. On such days, personal issues need to be put into perspective and temporarily blocked for active listening to occur.)

3. **Mental preparation**
   Reinforce your determination to be attentive.
   Tell yourself you'll concentrate only on the speaker and message.
   Increase your mental capacity to listen (e.g., increase vocabulary, study to understand human nature).

Discuss why it is important to listen. Communication is a fundamental human need. No one has any reason to speak if there is no listener.

●●●●

LEARNING STRATEGY

The adolescent abstains from faking attention and prepares to participate in listening.

AWARENESS OF THE DIFFERENTIAL

PURPOSE

To illustrate how the time differential between listening and thinking can be used

The fastest speaker can produce gusts of words at around 200 words per minute, yet our brains are capable of handling information at $2\frac{1}{2}$–3 times that speed. The efficient use of this time differential determines how well the listener receives and retains the message.

Our brains naturally flip away from the speaker momentarily while we think about our friends, what we did last night, or what we're going to eat after school. If we leave the speaker for milliseconds, return is easy, but if we remove our minds for seconds or minutes, it is impossible to retrieve the spoken information without repetition.

Have students deliberately concentrate on the following topics. Pause while they think, then deliver a piece of information to them orally. Next ask a question about the data given.

	Topic (to think about)	**Information** (spoken to students)	**Question**
1	What you want to eat tonight	Brian wants to take Michelle to McDonald's.	Who does Brian want to take?
2	A new piece of clothing you'd like	It takes three teaspoons of salt to make one table-spoon.	What is being measured?
3	What you will do next Saturday	The diameter of a circle is the distance across the middle and the radius is one-half the diameter.	Which is smaller, the diameter or radius?
4	Your favorite TV show	Sean wants Heather to meet him at 6:30 in front of his house.	What time will they meet?
5	The last time you were sick	The doctor wants you to take three pills a day right after your meals.	Can you take all the pills when you get up in the morning? (When are you to take them?)

Ask "When else have you been thinking about one thing while listening to a completely different topic? Does it make listening easier or more difficult? Why?"

●●●●●

LEARNING STRATEGY

The adolescent uses the differential between listening and thinking speeds.

TAKING ADVANTAGE OF THE DIFFERENTIAL

PURPOSE

To practice concentration on a specified topic

Have students practice mentally preparing themselves to listen. State a topic and ask them to tell associated ideas that come to mind. Encourage them to visualize closely related categories. The task is to orient themselves to topics selected by others and to "let go" of topics currently occupying their thinking space.

	Topic	Associations to Bring to Mind (Examples)
1	Nutrition	Vitamins Minerals Food Pyramid
2	Civil War	Union Confederacy North vs. South
3	Percentages	Numbers % symbol Based on 100
4	Computers	Hardware Software Cyberspace
5	Government	Democracy Dictatorship Rulers

Now, go back and see how long students can concentrate on the topic before slipping into thoughts on another topic. Thoughts such as, "I need to keep thinking about nutrition. Nutrition. Don't think about anything but nutrition," qualify as "on-topic" thinking. Agree on a signaling system for "off-topic" thoughts (e.g., raising a hand, holding up an index finger). Next, when off-topic thoughts do creep in, challenge students to have them last milliseconds. Students may indicate the need to signal off-topic thoughts after they have come back on topic, since part of going off topic includes neglecting to signal.

●●●●●

LEARNING STRATEGY

The adolescent uses the differential between listening and thinking speeds.

Discuss with students the power of control they can have over their listening. Through self-talk (e.g., "Keep listening. The teacher is talking about molecules. Keep thinking about molecules"), the student can improve concentration.

Finally, students need to move from concentrating on the main idea of the lecture (e.g., molecules) to the specific details being shared. Through self-talk, students can use the differential to repeat information the teacher just said. This rehearsal will assist students in retaining the information. Later, as students become even more adept listeners, they can critique and organize information in more efficient ways.

2 ACTIVITIES TO ENHANCE LISTENING STRATEGIES

DISCRIMINATIVE (INFORMATIONAL) LISTENING SKILLS

● Identification of main ideas

●● Discrimination of relevant details

●●● Recognition of a speaker's pattern of organization

●●●● Comprehension of how examples and illustrations relate to global idea(s)

●●●●● Following a sequence of instructions

MAIN IDEAS: DEFINITION

PURPOSE

To heighten awareness of how main ideas are signaled

Discuss with students what a main idea is. What are ways to paraphrase the term *main idea* (e.g., "the point," "the key issue")?

Assign students to listen to ways that teachers cue them about main ideas. What specifically do they say or write? Is it easier to identify main ideas while listening to some teachers than to others? If so, why? Does it have more to do with the teacher's organization or the student's interest in the topic and willingness to listen actively?

Compare results of the assignment. Is there always agreement among listeners about the main ideas presented by speakers?

●
LEARNING STRATEGY
The adolescent listens to and identifies main ideas presented orally.

DEDUCTION OF MAIN IDEAS

PURPOSE

To determine the main purpose of a short spoken passage

Extemporaneously generate a 15-second to 1-minute exposition on the following main ideas. (Using free speech rather than generating passages to be read will approximate lecture situations and conversational exchanges more realistically.) Explain to students that their job is to reduce what is being said to one sentence. A beginning example is provided.

1. Main idea: People in different locations see different patterns of stars. Free-speech exposition example: "Now, the fact is, depending upon where you are standing on earth, you would see different stars at night. For example, not everyone living on the planet can see the Big Dipper at the same time. People in South America see the Southern Cross, which is a pattern not familiar to people in North America."
2. Main idea: House exteriors are usually built with the most available and least expensive materials (e.g., wood, brick, mud).
3. Main idea: Music can be relaxing.
4. Main idea: Students cannot charge lunch tickets at school.
5. Main idea: Pets require consistent care and attention.
6. Main idea: My brother hates mathematics.
7. Main idea: Computers are commonplace in homes.
8. Main idea: We can learn from past mistakes.
9. Main idea: Hard work is usually, but not always, rewarded.
10. Main idea: People can learn to listen better (than their present skill level).
11. Main idea: We have no definite proof that life exists on other planets.
12. Main idea: Citizens have a responsibility to their country.

LEARNING STRATEGY

The adolescent listens to and identifies main ideas presented orally.

13. Main idea: All colors are tolerable, but my favorite one is red.

14. Main idea: Athletes should be required to adhere to strict academic standards.

15. Main idea: Schools should be open 12 months a year.

16. Main idea: Loud music can cause hearing loss.

17. Main idea: Seat belts save lives.

18. Main idea: Football practice can be boring.

19. Main idea: Money doesn't buy as much as it used to.

20. Main idea: Helmets protect motorcyclists from injury.

An alternative activity involves writing the main ideas above, and others that have been generated, on index cards, or cutting apart the pages pertaining to this activity in Appendix E. Have each student select a card and talk for 15 seconds to 1 minute on that idea. Let others identify the main idea being transmitted. Preferably, only the student speaking has prior knowledge of the main idea card selected. Compare the main idea identified with the assigned main idea. If a discrepancy exists (e.g., the assigned main idea was "Music can be relaxing," and the identified main idea was "Music is always relaxing"), identify the discrepancy and discuss why it occurred.

IDENTIFYING DETAILS

PURPOSE

To separate relevant details from the main idea in spoken messages

When a message is conveyed from one person to another, there is usually a main idea and supporting details. One who is listening to a message needs to answer at least the following basic questions:

- Who?
- What?
- Where?
- When?

If one part of the message is missing, action is not possible. For each message below, have students identify the four pieces of information that answer the questions set out above, the main idea in each message, and relevant details. Analyze: Do the relevant details always answer one of the four questions?

1. Brett wants to see you. He said to meet him at his office at noon and he will go to the police station with you.

2. You're supposed to go the west door of the shopping mall, and Kia will see you there at 6 o'clock. She said to bring plenty of money for clothes shopping, since you need to buy so many.

3. Mrs. John says the parent meeting is at Central High School at 7:30. It's important to be there because they're talking about new graduation requirements.

4. I understand your sink is still clogged. Denny will come to your house to fix the plumbing tomorrow morning at 7.

5. I guess volleyball season has started. Lizzy says to meet her at 5 p.m. sharp at the YWCA for the meeting.

6. Go to the pizza place on Main Street at 9 o'clock tonight. He sounded really upset on the phone.

7. Tell Jon that pictures are at 5 o'clock tomorrow night at school. He's to wear his uniform with the red shirt, not the gold one.

●●

LEARNING STRATEGY

The adolescent discriminates relevant details in spoken messages.

8. He called back to see if you could meet at 9 a.m. Friday, October 3, in the Luker Office Building. You need to have your loan approved before you see him.

9. Meet your dad at the donut shop for a treat at 10 o'clock. He's leaving on a long trip and wants to see you before he goes.

10. Ask Jim if 6 a.m. is good for him. Can he meet me by the bus stop and go running from there? Tell him to bring a jacket.

Are any of the messages ambiguous? If so, which ones? What makes them less clear than the others? Discuss whether a message could be clear and complete to one person but not to another person (i.e., someone not as familiar with a situation or a routine).

Have each student generate a message that answers who, what, where, and when. Direct the others to listen and critique the completeness of the message.

MESSAGES: MISSING DETAILS

PURPOSE

To identify which information is needed for someone to answer:
Who?
What?
Where?
When?

Write the four basic questions, from the "Identifying Details" activity on page 84, where everyone can see them. Read the following messages. Tell students to assume they have been given no information preceding the message. What details are missing to answer the four questions?

1. Tanya wants to meet you at the restaurant, and then she'll go home with you.
2. You are supposed to drive to the ballpark and meet Jesse there.
3. Mr. Timms called and wants to be certain you'll be at that special meeting at Concord High School.
4. Tammy is bringing her children to your house.
5. At 3 o'clock pronto, you are to meet Jeff.
6. Sean said to meet Tracey at the game.
7. Go to 2150 Water Street at 7 o'clock.
8. Tell Barbi it's tomorrow night at school.
9. He called to see if you could meet at the bank instead.
10. Mom wants you to ask Andrea if 5 p.m. is better than 4.

Now presume that the messages above were said in context. Discuss what *in context* means.

- Could any of the above messages be complete if in context?
- Would all of them be complete if in context?
- What assumptions need to be made within each message for the listener to identify who, what, where, and when?
- How do we know when details are redundant and when they are relevant?

●●
LEARNING STRATEGY
The adolescent discriminates relevant details in spoken messages.

MESSAGES: TOO MANY DETAILS

PURPOSE

To differentiate between relevant and irrelevant details in a spoken passage

●● LEARNING STRATEGY

The adolescent discriminates relevant details in spoken messages.

Sometimes, too much information is given rather than too little. Have students identify which details are irrelevant or redundant in short passages read to them. How did they determine that the details were superfluous (i.e., extra and not needed)? (Note: These activities can continue to emphasize identification of main ideas as well as details.)

1. Mrs. Lyons, that thin older lady two blocks down, wants to come over here and pick some flowers. She says she really likes daisies. Is 10 o'clock tomorrow OK? She really needs to put on some weight.

2. Tell your mother that college students needing help in basic skill areas are becoming more and more plentiful. More than one in four entering freshmen now need help on some campuses. This 25 percent of the student body needs help with reading, writing, and study skills. I wonder what their family lives are like. Tell your mom, too, that many students successfully complete college once they have acquired basic skills.

3. In the spring of the school year, students register for their fall classes. Each student is required to take one credit of English and one credit of math. I wonder what time the cafeteria will open. Everyone needs to register for one-half credit of physical education also.

4. I think you should hire me for this job because I am dependable, I am always on time, and I like people. I think I would get along well with the customers, and I have already done waitress work in another restaurant. Besides, my brother, is a big star on the high school football team. I can work any night of the week after school.

5. I would like to baby-sit for you tomorrow night, but I can't. I already made plans to go to a movie with a friend, and it's the last night the movie is showing. The movie is *Traveling Light*, and I've really wanted to see it for a long time. We are going to the early show and then probably somewhere after that. We might go to Lee's house and have pizza. So I guess by the time I got home, it would be too late to baby-sit.

6. I would like to buy a car with four wheels and headlights. I would like it to be a Toyota with an automatic transmission. I don't really care what color it is, but I would prefer green or blue. I hate black cars, and I really don't care for red either. I want it to get good gas mileage.

7 I went out for pizza last night. I wanted to get sausage and mushroom, but my friend wanted pepperoni and green pepper. The last pizza I had was mushroom and onion, and it was awful. We ended up ordering pepperoni and sausage and skipping the vegetables.

8 I need to buy a new sweater. I want it to be navy blue with long sleeves and a turtleneck. I can't wait to throw away my green pants. The sweater can't be wool because I am allergic to it.

9 I heard Mr. Hoiman is a really good teacher. He writes everything you should know on the chalkboard and lets you take tests when you want to. He is married and has four kids. He never calls on students to embarrass them in his class.

10 I had to wash my dog in a special solution to get rid of fleas. I could tell he had fleas because he kept scratching and scratching behind his ears. He sure likes the new dog food I have been buying for him. I hope this solution works and it's the last I ever see of fleas.

11 I sure hope my room gets painted soon. My mom says she will do it, but she is too busy. I have a real big window in my room. Before the room can be painted, we have to take the wallpaper off, and that's a really big job.

12 I didn't like the math teacher I had last year. He yelled at us a lot and never smiled. He was ugly to look at. He always had bad breath and I flunked most of his tests. My brother is going to a new school next year.

13 We went on a camping trip last summer. We slept in sleeping bags in a tent and roughed it. Our sleeping bags had zippers. We did a lot of swimming and hiking and had campfires every night.

14 A boy was standing outside and there was a dog in front of him, a cat in back of him, a bird to his right, and a tree to his left. The boy was standing in his front yard. There were three animals near him.

15 History books say that Christopher Columbus discovered America in 1492. He and his crew sailed in three boats: the Nina, the Pinta, and the Santa Maria. The sails on the boat were big and they had many

ropes. Native Americans were already living along the shore when they landed.

16 If you have one-half of a bushel of red juicy apples and buy another bushel from me and one-half of a bushel from the grocery store, how many red juicy apples do you have? The grocery store is a mile away.

17 You have one-half of a bushel of red juicy apples and buy another bushel of yellow apples from me. Then you discover one-fourth of your bushel of red juicy apples is actually brown rotten apples. How many red juicy apples do you have? You like to eat apples a lot.

18 The object of football is to move the ball down the field across the goal line any way the team can. There are hundreds of rules about what the defense can and cannot do, and what the offense can and cannot do. Fans sit in the bleachers. Penalties are given to teams when they break the rules.

19 I want you to go through this passage and circle all the nouns in red and all the verbs in blue. Remember, yesterday we circled adjectives in red and adverbs in blue. The day before we circled prepositions in yellow. When you get through, put your papers on my desk.

20 The test tomorrow will have 20 true-false statements, 10 fill-in-the-blanks, and 10 multiple-choice questions. There will not be any essay questions because of the difficulty you had with them during the last test. So many of you confused *compare* and *contrast* that we need to talk about those terms before I include them on a test again. To study for tomorrow's test, look at your notes and skim the chapter again.

Discuss student performance on these tasks. How do we know whether a detail is relevant or irrelevant? What makes a detail irrelevant? Can details be relevant in one situation and irrelevant in another (e.g., compare and contrast the necessity of including the phrase *red juicy* in tasks 16 and 17).

Guide students to think of situations in which too many details have been given to them (e.g., a friend is describing a movie and goes on and on describing every little piece of action throughout the two-hour movie).

RELEVANT DETAILS: CLASSROOM SURVIVAL

PURPOSE

To facilitate the student's ability to focus on relevant details in classroom lectures and instructions

Like the messages in the previous activity, teachers may include too many details in lectures. Secondary-level teachers sometimes persist in sharing large amounts of information through a lecture format. Even if main ideas can be grasped, it is frequently the "relevant details," as defined by each content teacher, that become test questions. The adolescent with language disorders, still struggling with main ideas, is often ill-equipped to pick out the important who, what, where, and when (and perhaps the how, why, and to-what-extent) questions answered in a lecture.

Ideally, classroom teachers could provide study guides for their students highlighting details relevant to the subject matter. This is an excellent strategy for helping students discriminate details. At the same time, educators are encouraged to move from producing study guides to teaching their students to generate their own study guides from class notes, lest dependency on adult teachers becomes even greater than it currently is. After all, the major aim of education is to assist students in continuing to learn after they have left us.

Students with language disorders would certainly need assistance in first using and then establishing study guides, since their notebooks are characteristically sketchy or nonexistent. Resources are available for teaching note-taking strategies (Allen, Mason, and McKean, 1982; Bragstad and Stumpf, 1982, 1987; Devine, 1981; Gall, Gall, Jacobsen, and Bullock, 1990; Wolff and Marsnik, 1992). Tape-recording information or duplicating notes may be useful strategies for many. A "buddy system" can be implemented between students whose note-taking skills are especially problematic and those who excel in this capacity.

When listening to a lecture, students need to be aware of details that answer the basic wh-questions. If a detail is being presented and a student is having difficulty grasping it, a strategy for gaining the information needs to be applied:

- The student who is willing to talk in class can ask for clarification from the teacher as close in time to the breakdown as possible. The student's question should be *specific* by focusing on a key word. Rather than saying, "I don't get it," the student should say, "You lost me when you talked about 10x."
- For students not willing to talk in front of others, provide clarification before or after class. Emphasis is still on being specific. Have students indicate in their notes *where* they became confused. A "?" or "*" in the margin will help remind students of what they did not understand.

●●

LEARNING STRATEGY

The adolescent discriminates relevant details in spoken messages.

- Students can also be taught tactful ways in which to ask for clarification of relevant details given during lectures. Rather than saying, "What do I gotta know for the test?" they can say, "How should I study for the test? I have the details. Which ones are important?" Rather than saying, "What do you want me to know for your test?" they can say, "I want to make sure I study the right things for the test. Can you help me?" (See also Chapter 7, "Question-Asking Strategies.")

Students who show positive signs of wanting to understand the information are at a tremendous advantage with teachers who may feel few rewards working with secondary-level students. If students try their best to listen to teachers, 9 times out of 10 the favor will be returned. That is one of the best "facts" we can teach adolescents with language disorders about listening.

BASIC PATTERNS

PURPOSE

To label the most common patterns of information organization

●●●

LEARNING STRATEGY

The adolescent recognizes the speaker's pattern of organization.

Students become better listeners when they are alerted to the organizational structure of spoken messages (Wyatt, 1989). Jalongo (1991) cited five structural patterns in messages:

- Chronological—the pattern relies on time sequences (e.g., past, present, future)
- Procedural—the pattern relies on explanations or step-by-step directions (e.g., first, then, next)
- Categorical—the pattern relies on classification by types, kinds, purposes, functions, etc. (e.g., three factors; five characteristics)
- Comparative—the pattern relies on similarities and differences (e.g., the same as; compare; pros and cons)
- Causative—the pattern relies on answering how and why by presenting causes and effects (e.g., because; reasons)

Combinations of patterns may also occur (Wolff et al., 1983).

Read messages 1–20 below and have students identify the structural pattern in each message:

1. We'll talk about three time periods: 1850, 1900, and 1950.
2. Should the government cut back on health care? Yes or no?
3. I would like to talk about the major economic impact of war.
4. We'll talk about labor unions from the beginning to the present day.
5. Today we're going to talk about the causes of fungus.
6. There are many types of conifer trees.
7. What, then, were the causes of World War I?
8. First of all, this computer has an internal modem and you need to dial our on-line service before beginning your data search.
9. Let's talk about how to write a business letter.
10. Now, why do you suppose 16-year-olds can't vote?

11. Three favorite sports are soccer, dog racing, and polo.

12. Democracy has pros and cons.

13. The first survival skill to remember in the wilderness when you are lost is to remain calm.

14. When sewing a seam, there are three important steps to follow.

15. If a nuclear attack occurred, what would be its major effects?

16. Today, I want to talk about primary and secondary colors and how to use them effectively when doing pencil drawings.

17. Let's compare the Golf War with the Vietnam War.

18. Getting hired for a job usually involves a sequence of events starting with setting up your résumé.

19. How can we go about solving the problem of child abuse in our country today?

20. What are high school students like today versus 25 years ago?

Discuss the following concepts:

- Do any of the messages above imply a combination of patterns? If so, which ones?
- Why is it helpful as a listener to know the speaker's structural (organizational) pattern?
- What are words that cue someone to listen for a chronological pattern? For a procedural pattern? For a categorical pattern? For a comparative pattern? For a causative pattern?
- Do your friends use structural patterns when they talk? If so, when? Give some examples.
- Explain when you might use a structural pattern to tell something to a teacher. How might it help the teacher to listen to you better?

PATTERN VARIATIONS

PURPOSE

To recognize that patterns can vary based upon situational needs

●●●

LEARNING STRATEGY

The adolescent recognizes the speaker's pattern of organization.

Most topics can be organized in a variety of ways depending upon the need at the time. For example, given the broad topic of television, perhaps the structural pattern to listen for will be categorical (e.g., Let's discuss the kinds of programs that might be contributing to violence in this country) or comparative (e.g., Television today is very different than it was in the first decade it was invented).

For each of the following topics, have adolescents describe two or more structural patterns for which they could listen. Have them give examples of messages they might hear. For example, for "radio stations," a response could be "procedural—certain steps have to be followed when people buy and sell radio stations." Refer to the five structural patterns on page 92 when doing this activity and list the patterns where all students can see them.

1. radio stations
2. summer vacation from school
3. a baby brother or sister
4. how children should be raised
5. divorce
6. houseplants
7. a pet dog
8. automobiles
9. sports
10. military service

How did the structural pattern selected determine the example given? When do you need to be particularly aware of structural patterns while listening? When does it not really matter that you recognize a structural pattern while listening? If someone uses no obvious pattern, will you have trouble listening? Why or why not?

DEFINITIONS/ DISCUSSION OF *EXAMPLES* AND *ILLUSTRATIONS*

PURPOSE

To compare and contrast examples, illustrations, samples, and models

Many times during listening situations in the classroom, teachers will use examples and illustrations to clarify their messages. An erroneous assumption is that students know what an example and an illustration are. Explore first the definitions of *example* and *illustration*. Be certain to have a dictionary nearby during this activity.

Several other words in our language have nearly the same meanings (e.g., *sample* and *model*). What do these two words mean? Why do we have all these words that mean almost the same thing?

- Have each student share an *example* of something.
- Have each student share an *illustration* of something.
- Have each student share a *sample* of something.
- Have each student share a *model* of something.

Guide students in a discussion by asking the following questions:

- Could any of the *examples* also be considered *illustrations*? Why or why not?
- Could any *examples* be considered *samples*?
- Could any *models* also be considered *examples*, *samples*, or *illustrations*? Why or why not?
- Why do we use examples/samples/illustrations/models when we are communicating? How do they help us when we're listening?
- How are examples different from relevant details? Are any of their characteristics similar? How does this knowledge help a listener?

LEARNING STRATEGY

The adolescent comprehends how examples and illustrations relate to global ideas.

FROM GLOBAL IDEAS TO SIMPLE EXAMPLES: IDENTIFICATION

PURPOSE

To select and generate examples of items within a specific category

Have students select the items, if any, that are examples of each global idea presented. Since this is a listening activity, be certain information is delivered orally.

1. **Relative**
   Picnic
   Cousin
   Wedding

2. **Subject**
   Math
   Refrigerator
   Engine

   (Note: Be aware of divergent thinking. *Refrigeration* is a subject. *Engines* may also be a vocational subject. Students may not cue in to the subtle morphological endings.)

3. **Automobile**
   Harley-Davidson
   Ford
   Rolls Royce

4. **Government**
   Democracy
   President
   Communism

5. **Meal**
   Water
   Table
   Lunch

6. **Room**
   Kitchen
   Chimney
   Doghouse

7. **Wars**
   Korean
   Guns
   1812

8. **Organ**
   Skin
   Liver
   Fingernails

9. **Geometric Shape**
   Triangle
   Trapezoid
   Circumference

10. **Musical Instruments**
    Mute
    Bassoon
    Metronome

11. **Emotions**
    Jealousy
    Smile
    Anger

12. **Values**
    Money
    Honesty
    Loyalty

13. **Careers**
    Parenting
    Groundskeeping
    Teaching

●●●●

LEARNING STRATEGY

The adolescent comprehends how examples and illustrations relate to global ideas.

14 **Jobs**
Shopping
Driver
Waitress

15 **Postsecondary Schools**
Vocational-technical colleges
Universities
Kindergarten

16 **Appliances**
Washer
Photocopier
Toaster

17 **Machines**
Automobile
Computer
Stove

18 **Tools**
Ruler
Paintbrush
Hammer

19 **Jewelry**
Scarf
Watch
Earring

20 **Cosmetics**
Hand lotion
Mascara
Hydrogen peroxide

Have students suggest additional items that could be grouped under each of these global ideas.

Then discuss:

- Were some examples of global ideas more difficult to identify than others? Why?
- Was there ever disagreement as to whether an item was an example of a global idea? On which items did disagreement occur? How was the disagreement resolved?
- How could recognizing an example of a global idea help you while listening?
- How could getting a poor example (nonexample) of a global idea interfere with listening?

FROM GLOBAL IDEAS TO COMPLEX EXAMPLES: IDENTIFICATION

PURPOSE

To select an example of a global idea given a sentence context

Have students select the statements, if any, that are examples of the global ideas presented. Again, complete this exercise orally since this is a listening task, not a reading activity.

1. There were times when the settlers in this country weren't certain any of them would survive.
   a. In Jamestown, all but a handful died the first winter.
   b. People in Charleston arrived by boat.
   c. The Pilgrims were hearty people.

2. Education faces some serious problems.
   a. Most young children are eager to go to school.
   b. One out of four high school students drops out before graduating.
   c. More crimes against youth occur in high schools than anywhere else.

3. Inflation kept rising.
   a. The price of food doubled.
   b. The president of the country sold his car.
   c. Interest rates went up three points.

4. He was a cruel dictator.
   a. His top advisors were military generals.
   b. Anyone who spoke out against the dictator was imprisoned.
   c. More than two hundred women and children were murdered in the name of political freedom.

5. Reading is an excellent way to gather new ideas.
   a. I changed spark plugs in my car after reading how to do it, and I had never done it before.
   b. Reading at night without sufficient light can cause eye strain.
   c. Books can be checked out from the public library.

6. Sometimes decisions that we make are reversible.
   a. She started out at the vocational-technical college, but then dropped out of the program.
   b. He bought a dog, but then had to sell it when he rented an apartment that allowed no pets.
   c. He shot his friend, but then decided he did not want to hurt him.

●●●●

LEARNING STRATEGY

The adolescent comprehends how examples and illustrations relate to global ideas.

7 Having too much of something can be a mistake.

a. The little boy ate 12 candy bars after school and then began to feel sick.

b. She liked the shoes so much she bought them, even though they were a size too small.

c. She watched television from 7 p.m. until 11 and then remembered she had a test in math tomorrow.

8 Once I have solved part of the problem, I can usually get the rest immediately.

a. I worked and worked on the math problem, and finally decided to use a calculator.

b. After I found Sean's house, I remembered Kim's was two doors down.

c. The biggest problem I have is not eating so much.

9 A good friend will help us out any time of day or night.

a. When I ran out of gas on the freeway, I called up Abby and she brought me some.

b. Having friends takes too much time.

c. Nathan gets mad if anyone calls him after 8 o'clock at night because he doesn't want to miss any of his television shows.

10 The United States is turning into an information society.

a. Unemployment is high.

b. Computers are almost as commonplace as televisions.

c. The number of factory jobs is decreasing rather than increasing.

11 Some of our brightest and most creative people had trouble in school.

a. Clara Barton was an excellent nurse.

b. Orville and Wilbur Wright invented the airplane.

c. Thomas Edison never completed high school.

12 Grades in high school are no guarantee of future success.

a. I know someone who got terrible marks and is now a very good comedian.

b. High school students should study more.

c. I know someone who framed his high school diploma and hung it over his desk at work.

13 Some countries require that all young men spend some time in military service.
a. In Israel, everyone must enlist in the army for a period of time.
b. In the United States, there is an all-volunteer army.
c. Those in the National Guards go on active duty whenever called.

14 Petroleum is used in many products.
a. Petroleum is not used in steel beams.
b. Petroleum is used in plastic bags.
c. Petroleum is used in some artificial fabrics.

15 Some food has very little nutritional value.
a. Potato chips are almost totally carbohydrates.
b. Apples are full of vitamins and minerals.
c. Fresh vegetables are better for you than canned ones.

16 Drinking too much alcohol can be dangerous.
a. The unborn child of a drinking mother can develop fetal alcohol syndrome.
b. My friend can drink three cans of beer and not show it at all.
c. People who are drunk are more likely to have car accidents when driving.

17 It pays to smile and be friendly.
a. I told my mom she looked nice, and she took me out for pizza.
b. Smiling with your mouth full of food is not a good idea.
c. I smiled at the clerk and she let me return the shirt that had gotten ripped the first time I wore it.

18 A peninsula is a finger of land bound on three sides by water.
a. Florida is a peninsula.
b. Hawaii is a peninsula.
c. Upper Michigan is a peninsula.

19 There is no agreed-upon cure for the common cold.
a. Using first-aid cream may help.
b. Taking aspirin and drinking liquids may help.
c. Blowing your nose a lot may help.

20 Air travel is an extremely safe method of transportation.

a. Pilots must do an extensive amount of training before they get licensed.
b. Fewer people get killed per air mile than per land mile.
c. Air travel takes less time than any other form of transportation.

Discuss what made certain items examples of the global idea and other items nonexamples. Were any items controversial? What made them that way?

As you were listening, how did you pick out the nonexamples? (Point out that often the nonexamples were irrelevant to the global idea presented.)

FROM GLOBAL IDEAS TO EXAMPLES: GENERATION

PURPOSE

To generate numerous examples upon being given a global idea or category

Have each student generate an example (or sample, illustration, or model) after being presented with a global idea. With some ideas, such as *book*, it would be appropriate to talk about examples of books (e.g., *Moby Dick)* versus *model* books (e.g., the Bible) versus book *samples* (e.g., what a book salesperson would carry). Answers may be written first and then shared in group discussion. Have students closely listen to and monitor each other's responses. Are examples or relevant/irrelevant details being generated? (Note: The global ideas presented in the "From Global Ideas to Simple Examples: Identification" activity on page 96 may also be used for this task.)

1. Floor covering
2. Coin
3. Book
4. Musical group
5. Appliance
6. A good friend (What happens when you further qualify the idea [e.g., a good friend who doesn't go to this school]?)
7. A successful teacher
8. A disobedient child
9. An elderly, sick person
10. An excellent parent
11. A war the United States won
12. A southern (eastern, western, northern) state
13. A mathematical computation
14. A type of verb

●●●●

LEARNING STRATEGY

The adolescent demonstrates comprehension of how examples and illustrations relate to global ideas.

15 An author of poems

16 A great president

17 A useful class

18 An expensive gift

19 A way to spoil a child

20 A good meal

21 The best meal

22 The best band

23 The best actor/actress

24 The best month

25 The best job

Discuss with the students:

- Was it easier to generate examples for some global ideas than for others?
- Was it easier to listen to and monitor the accuracy of some examples than others? (Point out that familiarity with a topic makes a major difference in terms of relating to examples while listening.)
- What happened when a qualifying word such as *good* or *best* was added to a category? Did students agree on examples for such categories?
- How do judgmental words like *good* and *best* affect listening? If you strongly disagree with someone else's opinion concerning what is best, what cues might you give while you are listening? When might you want to hide your feelings in a disagreement situation?

REPETITION AND EXPLANATION OF DIRECTIONS

PURPOSE

To recall directions and demonstrate comprehension of how to follow those directions

Collect a wide variety of directions encountered in everyday situations. Read them orally (or tape-record them) and have students do the following:

1. repeat the directions;
2. tell the number of separate steps provided in the instructions; and
3. explain and/or summarize what they are to do.

Example: "Add one cup of water to the contents of this can. Heat thoroughly, but do not boil."

In addition to retelling the overt steps stated in the directions, discuss assumptions that the directions are making (e.g., some of the steps implicit in the example above are to open the can, to find an appropriate container, and to turn on the stove or microwave).

It is suggested that directions be delivered verbatim from these sources:

- cookbooks;
- food packaging labels;
- garment labels;
- household cleaning products;
- textbooks, particularly where student exercises are written;
- car owner booklets;
- drivers' instructional manuals;
- "How-to" books (home repair, woodworking, gardening, etc.);
- pharmaceutical products; and/or
- operating manuals for appliances/tools.

The following directions can also be used:

1. Overdue books are assessed at 50 cents per day. When the overdue charge reaches $15, the book is declared lost and a replacement fee of at least $40 is added to this maximum overdue charge. You would then owe the library $55.

●●●●●

LEARNING STRATEGY

The adolescent follows a sequence of instructions.

2. No lifeguard on duty. Swim at your own risk. Beach closes at 9 p.m. No glass containers allowed. No fires.

3. Caution: Staples have sharp points for easy penetration, so handle with care. Supervise children.

4. Load a paper roll on the paper holder. Rotate paper roll downward and insert end into the slot provided. Set the power "ON" and press the Paper Feed key.

5. Use this product only in well-ventilated area. Do not use or store near heat or flame.

6. Rub a paste of baking soda into rough skin areas on heels and balls of feet to smooth and soften.

7. Warning: May be hazardous to your health. If swallowed, drink at least 4 cups of water.

8. Take 1 to 2 tablets orally every 3 to 4 hours as needed.

9. Snap open small cap, remove and discard foil seal. Pull sheet out at an angle and snap off. Replace cover.

10. Skin should be clean and dry before applying bandage daily.

11. Take Highway 53 north, turn east at the intersection of Clyde Road and First Avenue. Take the first left turn. The store is the second building on the right.

12. Keep from heat and flame. Keep away from small children. Induce vomiting if ingested.

13. Add one cup boiling water. Add contents and stir until dissolved. Chill well before eating.

14 Before using, shake well and remove protective cap. Apply only to plastics, metal, or concrete. Do not breathe fumes. Keep away from small children.

15 To assemble, insert Tab A into Slot A and Tab B into Slot B. Apply glue to tabs before inserting if permanent decoration is desired.

16 For emergency, dial 911. Tell the dispatcher your exact location, including the community name, street number, and the type of help needed. Stay on the telephone.

17 Wet hair thoroughly before applying lotion. Apply liberally. Let penetrate for five to seven minutes. Rinse with warm water.

18 De-worm your animal every three months. Give one tablet one-half hour after a light meal. Use only for dogs.

19 Apply ointment to painful areas. Massage into skin. For external use only. Do not use internally.

20 For assistance, call toll free 1-800-123-4567 and ask for Room 3399.

Discuss any unfamiliar vocabulary contained within the directions. When would students be required to understand directions such as the ones listed above? Were any directions ambiguous? Why?

REFERENTIAL COMMUNICATION TASKS

PURPOSE

To improve comprehension of directions during a meaningful speaker-listener interchange

Few activities are more appropriate for listening to directions than referential communication activities (i.e., barrier games). Seat pairs of students across from each other with a screen (barrier) between them that allows them to see each other's faces but that prevents them from seeing material placed on the table. Designate one student as the sender of messages, the other as the receiver. Reverse roles periodically. The receiver may ask questions for clarification, if desired.

Many variations of barrier games can be derived. Descriptions of several alternatives follow:

1. **Transferring patterns: One step at a time**
   Beginning with two blank pieces of paper, one student (sender) draws a colored geometric shape somewhere on the paper and describes the shape, size, color, and location of the figure to the receiver. The receiver's (listener's) task is to reproduce the figure exactly as it is on the sender's paper. The listener may ask questions if directions are unclear or ambiguous. The number of figures can be gradually increased from 1 to 10 or more. Closely critique the precision of both the sender's message and the receiver's response.

2. **Transferring patterns: Multiple steps**
   The sender is provided a paper with a pattern already drawn on it or creates a complete drawing before sending any messages. When sending the message, the sender describes the complete pattern to be transferred, not isolated parts as in the previous task. The listener must listen to the complete message before beginning to reproduce the pattern.

   An example pattern can be found on page 108.

●●●●●
LEARNING STRATEGY
The adolescent follows a sequence of instructions.

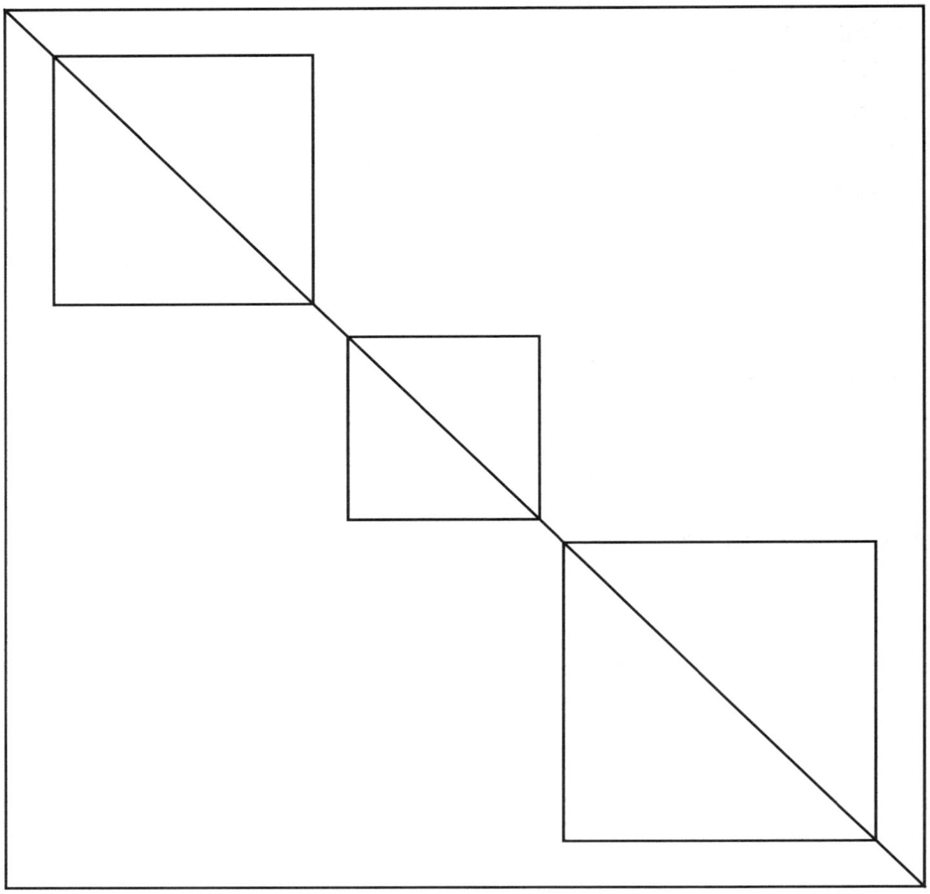

Sample directions:

Draw a diagonal line from the upper left corner to the lower right corner. Draw three squares bisected diagonally by the line. The lower right one is largest; the upper left one is medium sized; the one in the middle is smallest. The biggest square is about 1½ inches per side and the smallest is about 1 inch per side.

In this task, all directions need to be given at one time. Why? What would happen if only partial information was given? Have students discuss consequences of attempting the task before complete directions have been given. If they fail to grasp the rationale through discussion, have them experiment with giving partial instructions and discuss results. Chances are, students will experience numerous mistakes on their own without need of structuring them. The next page contains other patterns that could be transferred.

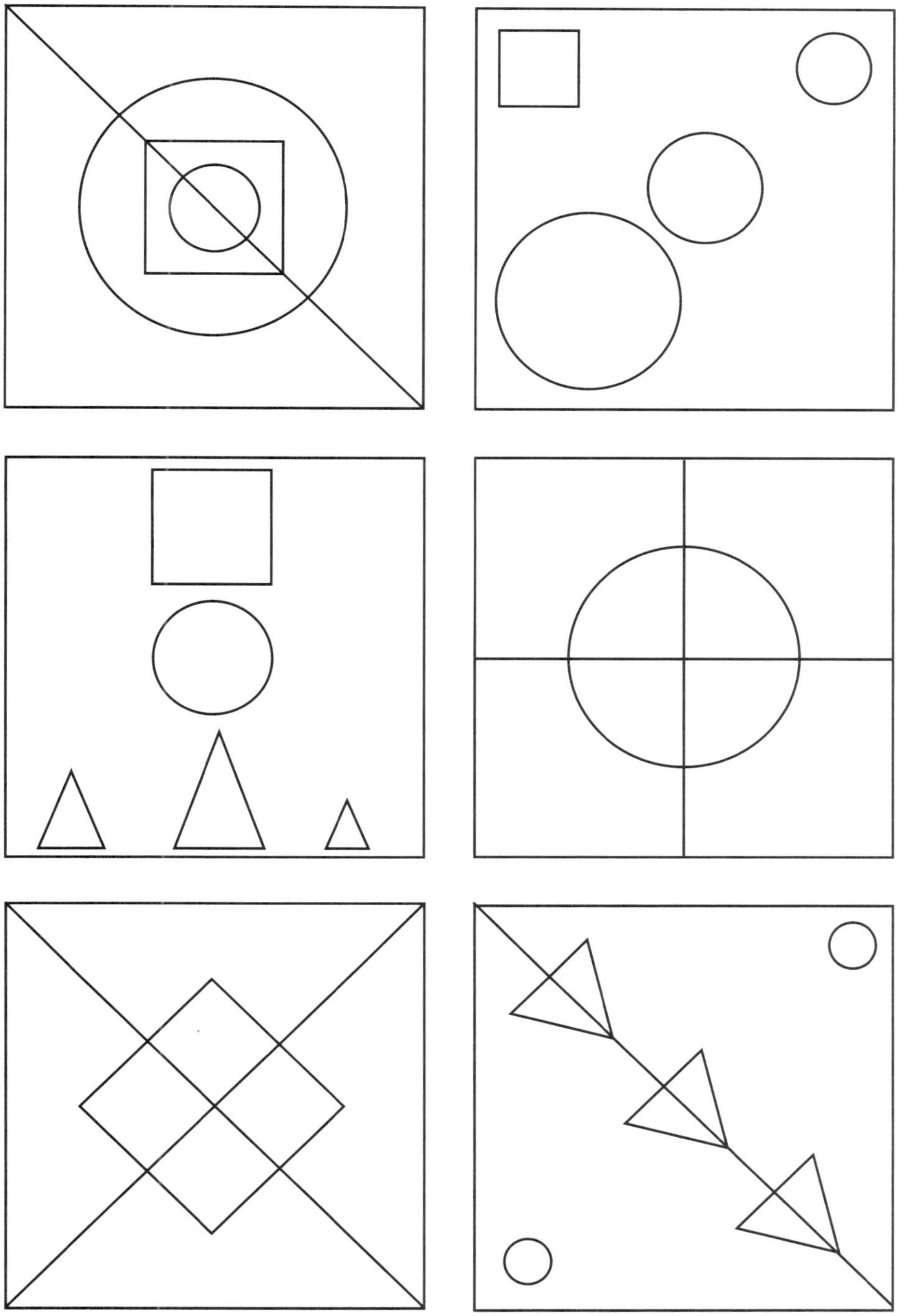

Color is a variable that can be added to increase the complexity of the task. The patterns on page 109 are reproduced in Appendix F for use during intervention sessions.

Once the students have learned the task with materials you have created, it is very simple for them to create their own patterns that, in turn, can be shared among groups of students.

(A variation for those students needing instruction in written language is to have them write the instructions, then read them to the receiver.)

3 **Spatial orientation**

While they are looking at identical street or road maps, the message sender describes a starting point and a route to the receiver. The receiver follows the sequence of directions and announces the final destination. At first, directions can be given and followed step by step. Later, as with the pattern-transfer activities, the entire sequence is given to the receiver at once, with no action permitted after each step of the directions.

For added variation, allow times when no questions are permitted. Does this make the task easier or harder? Why?

Many students may need simplified maps when beginning this activity. Local street maps can be enlarged and a selected small area designated. Allow "left-right" directions for students cognitively not ready for "north-south-east-west" directions. Push students to describe turns one would actually make if traveling to the destinations, dissuading them from descriptors like "top" and "bottom" of the map.

For those needing to create simplified maps, several models are provided in Appendix F. Remember, both the sender and the receiver need copies. The maps are also reproduced on pages 111–112.

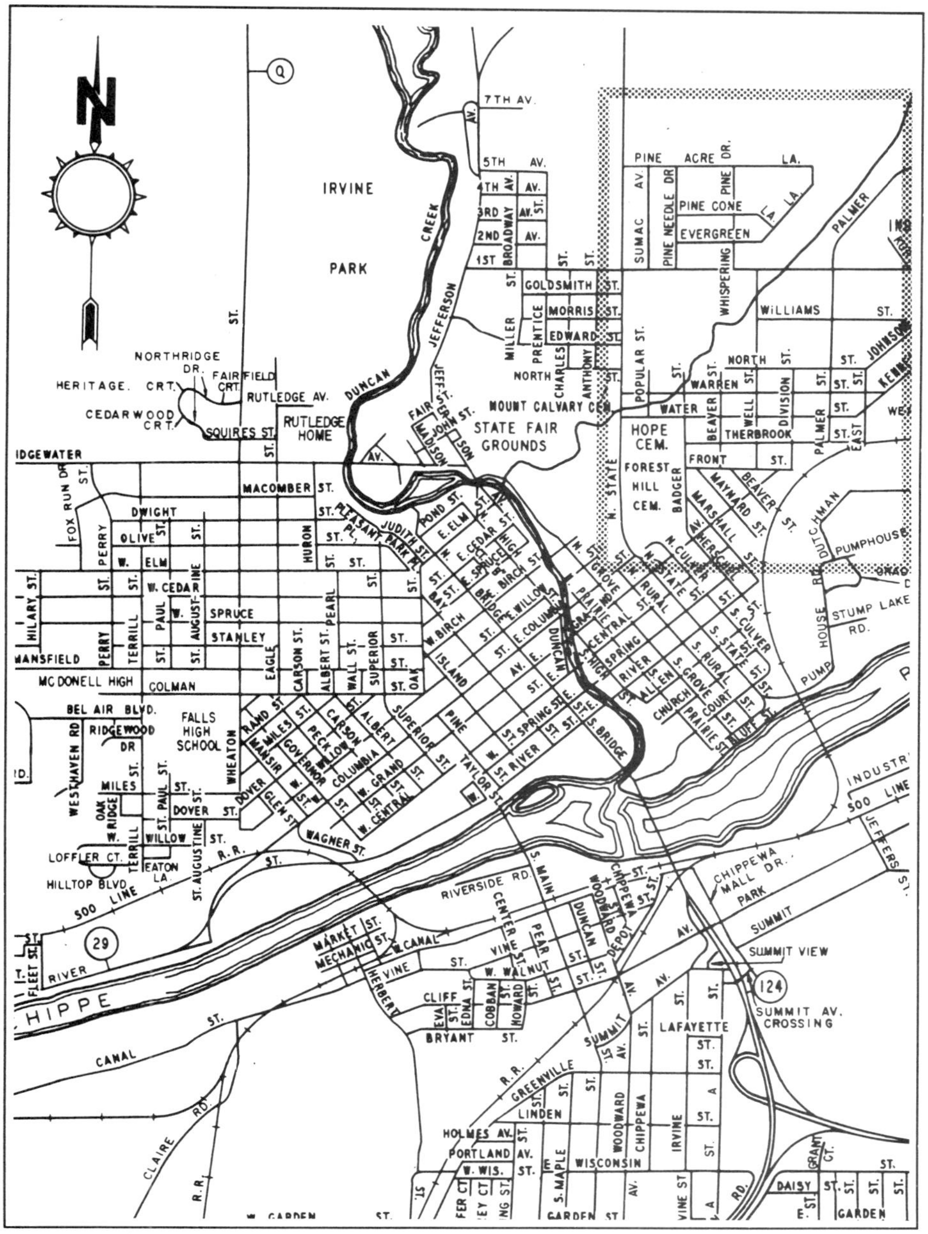

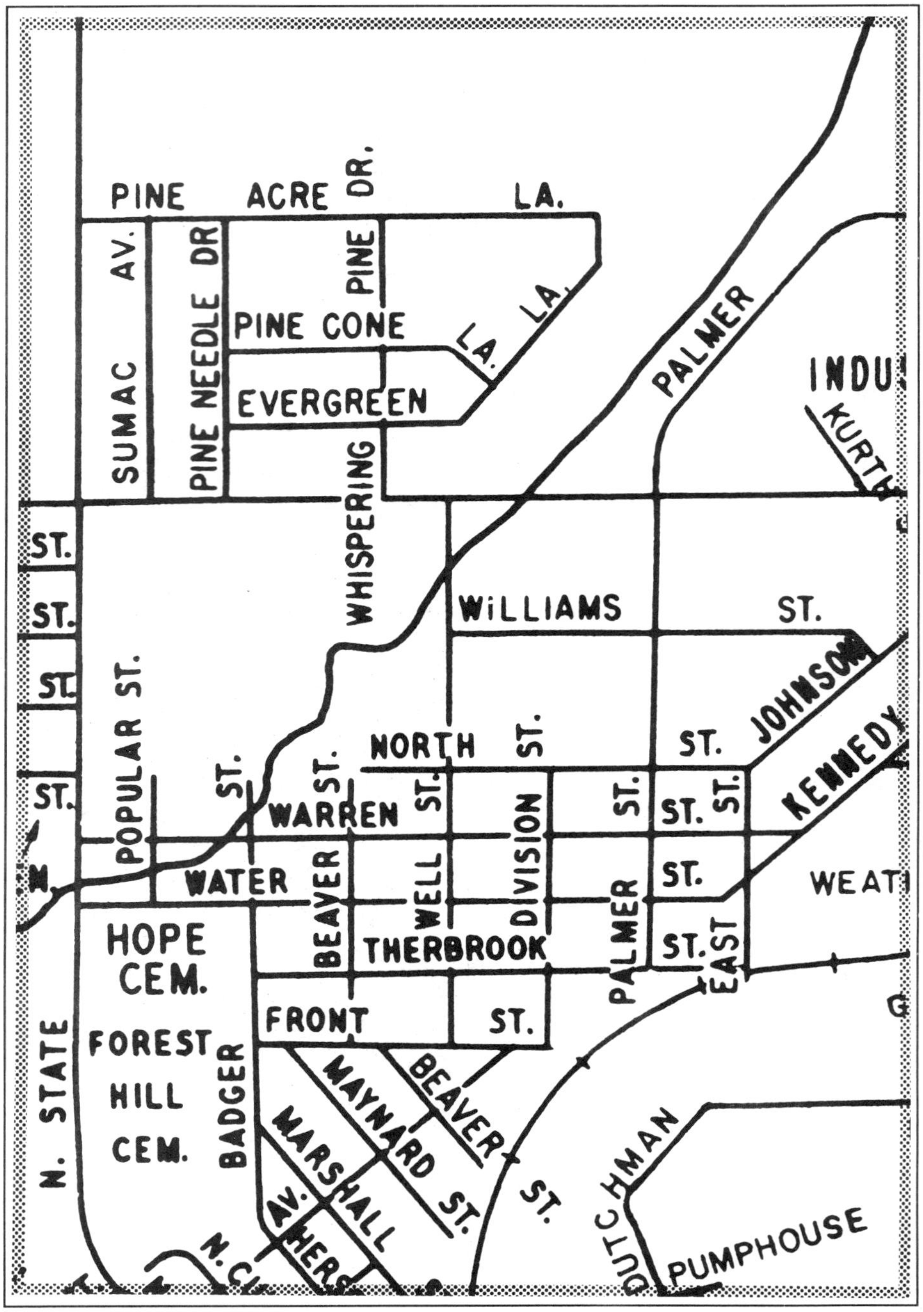
PINE ACRE DR. LA.
SUMAC AV.
PINE NEEDLE DR
PINE
PINE CONE
LA.
LA.
EVERGREEN
WHISPERING
PALMER
INDU
KURTH
ST.
ST.
ST.
ST.
WILLIAMS ST.
JOHNSON
KENNEDY
POPULAR ST.
ST.
ST.
NORTH ST.
ST.
WARREN
ST.
ST.
ST.
DIVISION
ST.
WATER
BEAVER
WELL
ST.
WEAT
HOPE CEM.
THERBROOK
PALMER
ST.
EAST
FRONT ST.
N. STATE
FOREST HILL CEM.
BADGER
MAYNARD ST.
BEAVER ST.
MARSHALL
AV.
DUTCHMAN
PUMPHOUSE

3

ACTIVITIES TO ENHANCE LISTENING STRATEGIES

EVALUATIVE (CRITICAL) LISTENING SKILLS

● Discrimination of facts from opinions

●● Detection of prejudice, propaganda, and bias

●●● Knowledge of criteria for judging statements and drawing inferences

●●●● Evaluation of arguments, or whether a statement is sufficient for the speaker's purpose

RESTATING FACTS AND OPINIONS

PURPOSE

To define *fact* and *opinion* and what differentiates a factual statement from an opinion statement

(Note: For some students, it may be more beneficial to complete the next activity first.)

LEARNING STRATEGY
The adolescent discriminates facts from opinions.

Have students generate definitions for *fact* and *opinion.*

Fact: Something that has been objectively verified. Something known with certainty.

Opinion: A belief or conclusion held with confidence. Judgment based on special knowledge.

In general, a fact can be proven while an opinion cannot be.

Encourage a diverse range of definitions by discussing answers to the following questions:

- What do we mean by *public opinion?*
- What is a *legal opinion?*
- What does it mean to say *after the fact?*
- Have students think of other contexts in which they have heard these words (e.g., in *fact,* you should go to the game).
- What are synonyms for *fact* (e.g., law, truth)?
- What are synonyms for *opinion* (e.g., *view, feeling, impression, conviction*)?
- What is a *poll?* Are the results of a poll fact or opinion?

Have students identify whether the following statements are facts or opinions. Read the statements aloud to students since this is a listening activity and students are practicing the discrimination of fact from opinion during oral communication. If a statement is a fact, request that it be made into an opinion. If a statement is an opinion, request that it be restated as a fact. Can all facts be transformed into opinions? Can all opinions be translated into facts? Why or why not? The first one is completed as an example.

1. All boys should play football. (Opinion) (Fact: Some boys play football.)
2. No one likes to return to school after vacation.
3. Some children have Roller blades.

4. I think that math is a difficult subject.
5. Few Americans live to be 100 years old.
6. Many chairs have four legs.
7. Parents should never spank children.
8. Students should always study for tests.
9. If you are on planet Earth, then the sun rises in the east.
10. If you hear a loud sound at night, you should call the police.
11. I hear someone at the door.
12. In reality, cats hate swimming.
13. Winter is the best season of the year.
14. The Coffee Cafe is the only good restaurant in town.
15. Plants need rain to grow.
16. When the weather is hot, everybody becomes grumpy.
17. July 4th is Independence Day in the United States.
18. Milwaukee is a city in Wisconsin.
19. Some roads are paved with blacktop.
20. All wheels are round.
21. The chili needs more salt.
22. Sometimes parents worry about the future of their children.
23. There is no place like home.
24. When I asked the poor man for money, he had none.
25. Nobody I know has an indoor pool at home.

Was it easier to transform facts into opinions, or vice versa? Did any general strategies emerge when going from fact to opinion? When going from opinion to fact? (Note: Be aware of students who restate one opinion for another [e.g., "Parents should spank children" for item number 7]. To become a fact, the verb frequently needs to change [e.g., "Parents could spank children," "Parents can spank children," "Some parents spank children"]. There is no one correct answer for the restatement portion of this activity.)

COMPARISON OF TRUE-FALSE WITH FACT-OPINION

PURPOSE

To discuss the relationship between true-false statements and fact-opinion statements

Many students have learned the concept of true-false, but become confused by fact-opinion. Bridging from the known concepts to the unknown, discuss whether the following generalization can be made:

(All) Facts are true.

(All) Opinions are false.

Why or why not?

Have students label as true or false the statements listed for the preceding activity, "Restating Facts and Opinions." Read the statements aloud to students since this is a listening activity and students are practicing the discrimination of fact from opinion during oral communication. Were all the listed facts true and all the opinions false?

Challenge students to state a false fact. Challenge students to state a true opinion. Would it hold true for everybody? Can it be done?

Point out examples of opinion statements that are made to sound factual:

The most important skill is wilderness survival.

People prefer the taste of our brand. (*All* people or *some* people?)

Ring around the collar is embarrassing.

Have students think of other examples they have heard.

Monitor discussions and comments made during sessions. Point out when statements intended to be factual are opinions. After modeling for awhile, encourage other students to help explain why an opinion cannot be taken as factual information, or vice versa.

●
LEARNING STRATEGY
The adolescent discriminates facts from opinions.

DETECTION OF EVIDENCE/ LACK OF EVIDENCE

PURPOSE

To use familiar reference tools to substantiate facts

LEARNING STRATEGY

The adolescent discriminates facts from opinions.

It was once "scientific fact" that the earth was flat. That fact has been proven false. What other facts of today, assumed true, might one day be proven false? Once a fact is found to be false, does it become an opinion? A fact can be proven by citing evidence that supports it. An opinion has not been substantiated by positive proof. Have students identify which of the following statements have been proven as fact. If they have been proven, where would students go to find the information (proof) (e.g., reference books, encyclopedias)? Read the statements aloud to students since this is a listening activity and students are practicing the discrimination of fact from opinion during oral communication.

1. A mile is farther than a kilometer.
2. On average, men weigh more than women.
3. Earth is the only planet with life on it.
4. The year 2000 marks the beginning of a new century.
5. All plants need sunlight to grow.
6. Traveling eastward, each time zone advances one hour.
7. Horses are mammals.
8. Baby girls begin talking earlier than boys.
9. Women live longer than men.
10. McDonald's makes better hamburgers than Burger King.
11. Seven-Up is caffeine free.
12. Airplanes travel faster than the speed of sound.
13. Taking vitamin C daily prevents the common cold.
14. Adding fluoride to drinking water prevents tooth decay.

15. Chicago has a higher unemployment rate than any other major U.S. city.

16. Lake Michigan will never recover from its polluted state.

17. Baltimore won the World Series in baseball in 1983.

18. Eggs are high in cholesterol.

19. The United States has not had one black president to date.

20. All breakfast cereals are made from some type of grain.

When students don't know whether a statement is a proven fact, what is a strategy for finding evidence to support or refute the statement? When evidence can't be readily found, does that mean the statement is always false?

DEFINING *PREJUDICE, PROPAGANDA,* AND *BIAS*

PURPOSE

To differentially describe and define the terms *prejudice, propaganda,* and *bias*

Ask students if they have ever heard the word *prejudice.* If so, who used the word and when? Explore the topic of prejudice by asking the following questions:

- Have you ever felt prejudice against yourself? When?
- As you listen to people talk, what are some of the things they might say that indicates prejudice (or lack of prejudice) against someone else?
- Have you ever felt prejudice toward others (e.g., beliefs about teachers, ideas about older people)?
- What is the relationship between the words *prejudice* and *opinion*?
- Looking around the room, do you notice prejudice against anyone (e.g., no access to the room for those in wheelchairs, all desks for right-handed persons)?
- Is prejudice always bad, or could it also be good?

Ask students if they have ever heard the word *propaganda.* How is this word the same as/different from *prejudice*? (Questions used above may be rephrased for *propaganda,* if desired.)

Ask students if they have ever heard the word *bias.* How is the word the same as/different from *prejudice* and *propaganda*? As you listen to people talk, how can you detect bias?

●●

LEARNING STRATEGY

The adolescent detects prejudice, propaganda, and bias.

IDENTIFYING LISTENER FILTERS

PURPOSE

To identify negative emotional reactions that interfere with listening effectiveness

Listeners are exposed to messages that contain prejudice, propaganda, and bias. The activity following this one ("Identifying Speaker Filters") will focus on message types. However, listeners frequently set up filters that are equally prejudiced, biased, and propaganda based (e.g., the student listener who has predecided that anyone with a bald head is stupid and not worth listening to). This activity is intended to identify those situations in which the listener, not the speaker, shows prejudice.

Where all students can see them, write these headings:

People

Subjects

Language

Voice

Have the students identify when they felt negative emotions during a listening situation to the extent that they no longer wanted to listen.

- Who was the speaker? (Identify by position rather than name, if it's more appropriate.)
- What was the person talking about?
- Did the speaker have a right to speak, to bring up the subject, to use the language?
- How did the speaker's voice sound?
- Is this as important in your life as you are making it right now (i.e., did you have a right to be prejudiced)?

Help students identify patterns to their own filters (e.g., the subject of math *always* turns off their listening; Mr. So-and-so is impossible to listen to; there are too many big words in the class to listen to; I can't stand to listen to anyone who yells; she's so ugly I won't listen to her). The longer students hold on to these filters, the longer they will listen ineffectively. In a classroom setting, ineffective listening can be academically disastrous. Prejudging other students based on clothing, hairstyle, or address can also be socially disadvantageous.

●●

LEARNING STRATEGY

The adolescent detects prejudice, propaganda, and bias.

IDENTIFYING SPEAKER FILTERS

PURPOSE

To detect prejudice, bias, and propaganda in speaker statements

Daily, each of us is exposed to speakers whose messages contain prejudice, bias, and propaganda. Such statements are not factual, but they are based on opinion. (Remember that opinions can be stated in a very factual-sounding way!)

Have students identify whether the statements below imply prejudice, propaganda, and/or bias. Then have students generate additional examples. As an assignment, have them listen to commercials on radio and television and identify prejudiced statements. If you have the good fortune of teaching this listening strategy during political elections, be certain to make use of campaign speeches, a potentially rich source of propaganda statements.

1. I listen better when I feel comfortable with the way the speaker looks.
2. When I argue with my friends, I wish I could go into their heads and straighten out their thinking.
3. Sixth-grade children are too old to make kites.
4. Old houses are a sign of poverty.
5. Men shouldn't be hired to work with young children.
6. We have always had this job done by a teacher.
7. I have never seen the sun rise in the north.
8. If elected, I will be responsive to all my constituents' needs.
9. Chocolate cake is my favorite dessert.
10. I wish new jeans did not cost so much.
11. It is awful to share a bedroom with a younger brother or sister.
12. Teachers are boring people.
13. Military service is good for young men and women.
14. Swimming is fun.

LEARNING STRATEGY

The adolescent detects prejudice, propaganda, and bias.

15. This new soap called "Dazzle" is absolutely the best cleaning product available today.

16. Cars require gasoline to run.

17. The government shouldn't be involved in feeding the hungry.

18. All high school graduates should pass the same minimal competency tests.

19. It's all right for girls to have pierced ears, but not boys.

20. Everybody should take multiple vitamin pills twice a day, in the morning and at night.

Discuss whether any of the statements above would detrimentally affect people seeking a job. Which ones (e.g., number 5)? Prejudice in hiring employees has been at least partially eliminated by the Equal Opportunity in Employment Act. However, the fact remains that certain jobs demand certain skills. In such instances, people without these qualifications who are not hired are not victims of prejudice. Have students think of jobs where prejudice might still exist. Have any of them felt the effects of prejudice when applying for a job?

SUPPLYING AN ENDING

PURPOSE

To determine what is inferred within a given situation

Have students discuss definitions for *inference*:

- predicting an outcome based on known information
- combining facts or opinions heard with what we already know and drawing a conclusion
- examining factual information and making a judgment

(Project STILE, 1979)

Have students listen to, then orally complete each sentence story. Have them explain/defend their answers in addition to telling the conclusion.

1. The baby was hungry, so Ellie went to the grocery store and bought ______________.
2. The morning of the picnic there was a cloudburst, so Jeff and Bob decided ______________.
3. Sean kept getting a busy signal on the phone when he called Hannah, so he thought ______________.
4. Mr. Gore did not show up in class this morning, so he must have ______________.
5. The comb wasn't in the bathroom where it usually was kept, so ______________.
6. It snowed all night, so the next morning, ______________.
7. John forgot to lock his car while it was parked on a busy city street, and when he returned to it, ______________.
8. The lights weren't on at Amy's house, so I presume ______________.
9. Tony has five stitches in his lip and his bike is smashed. I guess ______________.
10. The bottle of aspirin is empty and 3-year-old Mandy looks ill. We'd better ______________.

●●●
LEARNING STRATEGY
The adolescent evaluates criteria for judging statements/drawing inferences.

11. The car is sitting near the side of the road with its hood up. Since the driver is gone, I'll bet ______________.

12. Your mother just looked at your report card and seems angry. That means the report card was ______________.

13. Your dog is gone and you see the Humane Society van drive by, so you decide to ______________.

14. The pep rally was cancelled, so you should report to ______________.

15. You received a letter from the library and you have an overdue book in your locker. The letter probably says ______________.

16. The mail carrier is knocking at the door with a package in his hands. He needs ______________.

17. Your father is waiting at the door with money in his hand. He's smiling at you because ______________.

18. The fish aren't biting today, so Kevin decided to ______________.

19. The music is so loud, the principal might ______________.

20. The score was 10-2, with the winning team at bat in the last inning. They ______________.

A number of answers could complete the sentences above. Provided an answer is logically defended, it is acceptable. (Note: An excellent, and nearly endless, source for supplying conclusions is the *Choose Your Own Adventure* series [Bantam Books]. Students help determine the stories' outcomes by drawing conclusions about the action taking place every few paragraphs. Stories can be read to students, thus enhancing listening skills. At each decision point, students can draw a conclusion and explain their reasoning for making the choice they did.)

SUPPLYING A BEGINNING

PURPOSE

To infer what might have led to a given situation

The following list presents situation outcomes. Have students state what possible inferences could be drawn about events leading to each outcome. Usually there is more than one correct answer, provided the student can supply logical reasoning for a given response.

1. She walked out of the house with a raincoat and umbrella in hand. (Possible inferences: It looks like it's going to rain later in the day; she is returning someone else's rain gear; she is traveling somewhere where it might be raining.)
2. The dog scratched and scratched itself all day.
3. The child cried until he fell asleep.
4. He is 8 years old and weighs 150 pounds.
5. The day after Julie's party, Tracey was sick in bed.
6. Brian refuses to call Heather any more.
7. The mother frowned at the baby.
8. He married at age 18.
9. The potted plant lay broken on the floor.
10. A car doesn't start.
11. The computer disk does not fit in this computer.
12. John's feet were sore.
13. The ambulance is at the next-door neighbors' home.
14. A siren is sounding.
15. John's bike is in the river.
16. The store is closed today.

LEARNING STRATEGY

The adolescent evaluates criteria for judging statements/drawing inferences.

17. The stoplight has been red for 10 minutes.

18. All the motels in town have "no vacancy" signs lit.

19. Students from Mrs. Murphy's music class did not report to classes today.

20. Ninth-grade students will no longer be allowed to leave the building during lunch break.

As an additional activity, pair students or put them on teams. Have one student generate an outcome and the other(s) discuss possible events that could be inferred from that outcome.

MAKING JUDGMENTS

PURPOSE

To infer why we think particular situations are occurring

LEARNING STRATEGY

The adolescent evaluates criteria for judging statements/drawing inferences.

Judgments can involve making the best decision based upon information available and one's prior experience. Judgments are frequently made unconsciously as we attempt to explain why we think people are acting, or reacting, the way they are. Have students discuss possible judgments that could be made in or about the following situations. Read each one aloud since this is a listening activity and students are practicing the evaluation of criteria for judging statements/situations. Upon what is their judgment based? Again, more than one answer is feasible, provided rationalization of one's judgment can be made.

1. John was a senior in high school and failing three classes. Why? (Possible judgments: He is not motivated; he is a slow learner/cognitively disabled; he has many personal problems that are more important to resolve right now; he was put in classes too difficult for him.)
2. Heather has been fired within two months from every job she has ever held. Why?
3. His hair looks like it hasn't been washed for two weeks. Why?
4. He hasn't paid his rent for three months, yet he drives a new car. Why?
5. Her father died of lung cancer, and she smokes two packs a day. Why?
6. She'd like to switch jobs from clerking to word processing. Why?
7. Mary seems to be a good student but doesn't like going to school. Why?
8. Lisa never goes to parties she's invited to and then complains she has no friends. Why?
9. She is collecting welfare and not working right now. Why?
10. He never knows what kind of mood his father is going to be in. Why?
11. Someone I know spends every night at the bar. Why?

12. Sue lied to Jason when she said she wanted to go to the dance with him. Why?

13. The police officers grabbed Tom, hurried him out of the store, and made him get into their car. Why?

14. Mrs. Jones looks terrible this morning. Why?

15. She looks like she hasn't had anything to eat for weeks. Why?

16. He's a good auto mechanic but hasn't had a job for the last year. Why?

17. His dad has crashed every car he has ever owned. Why?

18. It seems like Julio's mom is always going to school and meeting with the teachers. Why?

19. She is always taking pills of one sort or another. Why?

20. The clerk yelled at the customer in the doorway. Why?

RECOGNIZING ERRORS IN ARGUMENTS

PURPOSE

To prepare persuasive arguments and to evaluate arguments proposed by others

The student who can ably recognize propaganda and bias will be well on the way to evaluating arguments. Discuss with students how arguments attempt to persuade or convince us of another point of view.

The goals of the speaker/persuader are either adoption (i.e., having the listener accept a new idea) or discontinuance (i.e., convincing the listener to stop doing something).

Persuaders commonly commit these errors:

- ***False reasoning***
  Something has existed in the past, and therefore it should continue in the future.
- ***Hasty generalization***
  Conclusions are reached on the basis of one case or a few.
- ***Hidden variable***
  One event followed by another in succession is held responsible (i.e., correlation is promoted as causation).

Have one group of students prepare persuasive arguments on one or more of the following topics. Have a second group note (1) whether any common errors were made, (2) whether the goal of the argument was adoption or discontinuance, and (3) whether they, as listeners, were persuaded by the argument.

1. John Goodlad, a noted educational researcher, has suggested that high school be completed by age 16.
2. The voting age should be lowered to age 15.
3. The federal government should supply more jobs for teenagers.
4. There should be a law that says each child in a family is entitled to a private bedroom.
5. There should be a soda (pop) machine located in the cafeteria.
6. Schools should provide personal computers for each student.

●●●●

LEARNING STRATEGY

The adolescent evaluates arguments.

7. Football should not be allowed as a school sport because of the injuries suffered by players.

8. Students should be allowed to smoke cigarettes in a designated area at school.

9. Students who do not meet minimum competency requirements should still be allowed to graduate.

10. Registration for the military should be required for 18-year-old females.

11. All books in the instructional media center should be censored for the good of the students.

12. A student with three missing assignments should be required to serve a detention.

13. Teenagers caught attending beer parties should still be allowed to participate in extracurricular activities.

14. Police officers should have blue flashing lights rather than red so they aren't confused with other emergency vehicles.

15. Drunken drivers should not lose their licenses on their first offenses.

16. Schools should be open during the summer as an option for students who want to graduate early.

17. Use of calculators should not be allowed during math classes.

18. The 55 mph speed limit on many highways should be changed to 65 mph during the daylight hours.

19. The United States should not interfere with Central American countries' domestic problems.

20. Oil drilling should increase along the California coast.

Depending upon the group's abilities, require students to find outside references/resources that support their arguments, if desired.

ANALYZING ARGUMENTS IN DAILY ENCOUNTERS

PURPOSE

To analyze an argument encountered during a daily living situation

Between sessions, have students note one or more situations in which they participated in an argument or found themselves listening to a persuasive speaker (e.g., their parents asking them to take out the garbage). Have students describe each situation, analyze the speaker's goal, determine whether common errors were made, and comment on whether they, as listeners, were persuaded. Let students critique each other's situations in addition to their own.

Have students prepare a persuasive argument for a situation in which they have frequently been the loser. Refer to information presented in Chapter 3 on confrontations. How are confrontations and arguments the same? How are they different? Does someone always need to win an argument? Role-play the persuasive argument each student has prepared. Evaluate its effectiveness.

●●●●

LEARNING STRATEGY

The adolescent evaluates arguments.

6 CONVERSATIONAL SPEECH STRATEGIES

CONVERSATIONAL SPEECH: AN ASSUMED SKILL

Unlike learning to swim or ride a bike, few of us consciously learned how to participate in a conversation. Perhaps that is why it is so difficult to teach someone else how to converse; we have never before had to define the general principles of conversation, nor be aware of the process. The normal developing communicator has acquired communicative maturity by age 13 (Wiig, 1982a), including the ability to change between an informal language code (i.e., peer register) and a more formal language code (i.e., adult register). The adolescent who is still acquiring basic conversational skills is penalized socially, and often academically as well. A history of oral communication failure and frustration is built up, and it influences all major aspects of the adolescent's life.

DEFINITION OF CONVERSATIONAL SPEECH

Goffman (1976) noted two different definitions of *conversation*. In one sense, it can refer to the casual talk that occurs in everyday settings; in another sense, it is the equivalent of spoken interaction. Although conversation is defined in terms of talk, it includes listening and nonverbal behaviors as well. Nonetheless, talk is seen to occupy a central place in the organization of conversation. A basic empirical finding about conversation, which can be seen by casual inspection of almost any fragment of conversation, is that talking by participants proceeds through a sequence of turns. Edmondson (1981) observed that the term *conversation* "is used loosely and non-technically to refer to any interactional stretch of talk involving at least two participants, and taking place in a non-formalized setting" (p. 6).

CONVERSATIONAL DEFICITS

Adolescents with language disorders frequently have deficits in conversation skills. Bergman (1987) noted that their speech is typically "simple, direct, imperative, and informal, rather than subtle, complex, elaborate, or polite" (p. 162). These students often are not adaptive to their listeners and rarely express support, compliment them, or consider their feelings (Bergman, 1987). Sometimes adolescents have the knowledge of social skill strategies but fail to generalize them for a variety of reasons (Ellis and Friend, 1991). This chapter contains strategies and activities of prime importance to adolescents with deficits in conversation skills.

RULES OF CONVERSATION

Considerable attention has been focused upon rules of conversation from the speaker's perspective, but equally important are the rules of conversation from the listener's perspective. There are also rules that both the speaker and listener share. Figure 6.1 summarizes the three sets of rules.

The rules for the speaker are based upon work by Grice (1975). An expansion of his rules includes these four conversational postulates:

QUANTITY

- Make your contribution as informative as possible.
- Do not be more informative than required.

QUALITY

- Do not say what you believe to be false.
- Do not say anything for which adequate evidence is lacking.

RELATION

- Be relevant.

MANNER

- Avoid ambiguity.
- Be brief.
- Be orderly.
- Be polite.

Of equal importance are the rules for the listener. The listener has tremendous power to influence the speaker by indicating agreement or disagreement, understanding, or confusion. (See Chapter 5 for additional information on listening.) Figure 6.1 is available in poster form (see page 450 for details).

FIGURE 6.1

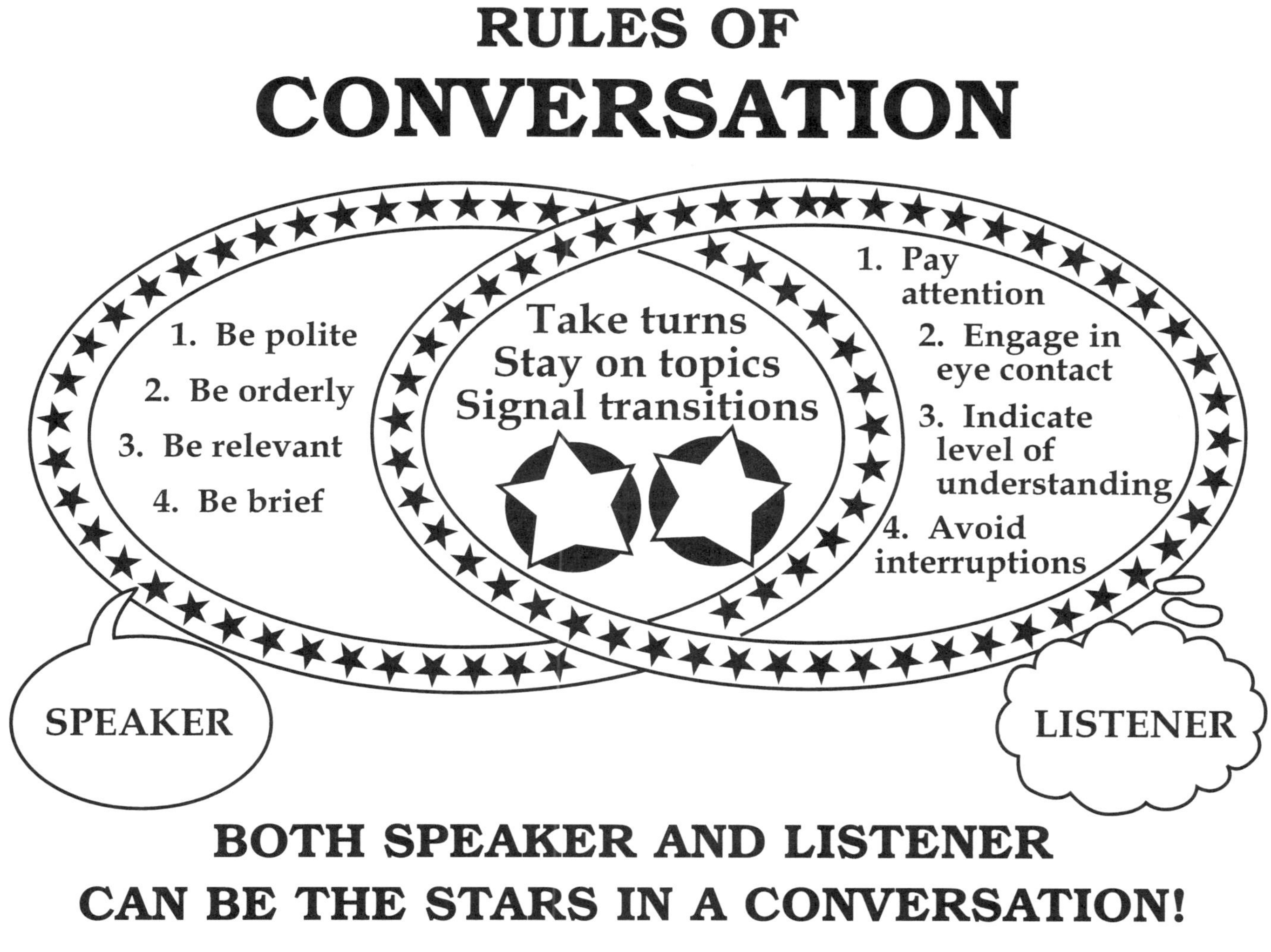

© 1983 THINKING PUBLICATIONS

ACTIVITIES TO ENHANCE CONVERSATIONAL SPEECH STRATEGIES

GENERAL CONVERSATIONAL SPEECH SKILLS

● Application of speaker rules

●● Application of listener rules

●●● Application of mutual speaker-listener rules

AWARENESS OF RULES

PURPOSE

To bring to a conscious level what conversational rules are and why we have them

It is difficult to apply a rule when it is out of sight and out of mind. Rules need to be clearly posted and discussed with students. Grice's (1975) list in poster form (see page 135), or an expanded list such as the one found on page 134, may be used. Post rules in a prominent location in the room so they can be easily scanned by all participants whenever needed.

Students need to recognize not only when they break a rule, but which one they have broken and what negative consequences will ensue. Meaningful and appropriate consequences will be as varied as the individuals applying speaker rules. Artificial or natural response cost could be used (e.g., losing points or privileges, paying a penny into a jackpot that can be "won" after one or more sessions of "perfect rule" conversational speech, or apologizing to the listener for breaking a rule). Although extrinsic consequences such as response cost might be used initially, guide adolescents toward use of conversational rules out of respect for the person(s) with whom they are talking.

Discuss with adolescents when they have been the "victims" of someone else not using conversational rules for speakers. How did they feel? What happens when rules are broken? What are the advantages of following conversational rules?

Ask adolescents to give examples of people with whom they enjoy talking. What is it about such people that makes conversation pleasant? Do they follow the rules? Discuss whether there are times when it is appropriate to break the rules. Under what conditions?

● LEARNING STRATEGY

The adolescent applies conversational rules for speakers across a variety of everyday communication situations.

PICTURE BOARD CONVERSATIONS

PURPOSE

To speak using relevant, orderly statements in a contrived conversational situation

Make a grid that measures approximately 24 inches square from a piece of cardboard or plywood, and divide it into 8 rows each way, yielding 64 squares.

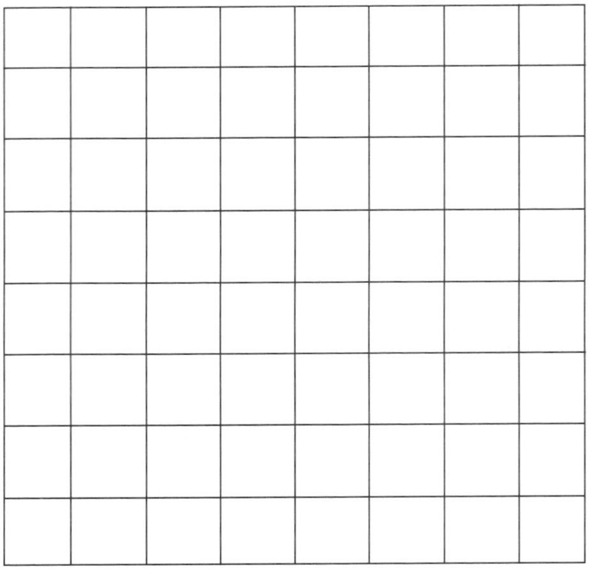

Find a wide assortment of pictures and lay one on each square of the grid. Department store catalogs are a great source and have appropriately small pictures of common, everyday items. Have a set of poker chips available for rewarding conversational speech. Weight poker chips so that white chips are worth 1 point, red chips are worth 5 points, and blue chips are worth 10 points.

Have each student, in turn, choose two pictures and describe them or tell a story involving them. Appoint a second student or all other students present to be listeners who ask questions and make appropriate comments to the speaker. Award the speaker with one white poker chip for minimal output, one red chip for an acceptable level of output, or one blue chip for exceptional performance. Although this might be a subjective judgment by the adult mediator based upon the individual's past performance, it should be based on how well the speaker applied rules of conversation, particularly those pertaining to being relevant or orderly. Similarly, reward the listener(s) with a white, red, or blue chip for minimal, acceptable, or exceptional performance. Students who are present may serve as judges of performance along with the professional.

LEARNING STRATEGY

The adolescent applies conversational rules for speakers across a variety of everyday communication situations.

Conversation proceeds around the group until all pictures are removed from the board. Conversational partners can remain constant throughout the game if pairs are being used, or for variety, these can change with each turn.

Determine the value of accumulated poker chips at the end of the game, if desired.

In a one-to-one session, the student and professional create the speaker-listener dyad.

CONVERSATIONAL STARTERS

PURPOSE

To participate in conversations as both speakers and listeners, given a specified topic

Transfer the following list of questions to index cards or use the cutouts in Appendix G. Keep the first 20 cards separated from the remaining cards. Have one student draw a card, pose the question to a selected partner (the primary speaker), and engage in a conversation focused on that question. Direct the student holding the card to remain primarily in the listener role by asking additional relevant questions. As the activity progresses, the speaker and listener have to assume roles to complete the conversations. Set a gradually increasing number of exchanges as a goal, but still remain sensitive to the rule of brevity. The ability for students to exchange approximately six to eight turns per topic sets the stage for many subsequent activities in this chapter. Use a poker chip system again as described in the previous activity ("Picture Board Conversations") if needed for motivation.

Initially, you may wish to participate in this activity directly to model appropriate conversational speech. If the activity is being done with a group of students, they may begin by taking turns observing and participating directly with you. As performance improves, direct pairs of students to engage in this activity simultaneously, spread throughout the room.

The term *conversational starters* and some of the following topic questions are derived from work by Peterson (1981). The appointed "listener" poses these questions to the designated "speaker." Each maintains the familiar role of student (and thus an informal register) unless otherwise indicated. The majority of the starters focus on the informing function of communication, one of the easier functions for students with language disorders, according to Wiig (1982a).

SPEAKER ROLE: STUDENT LISTENER ROLE: STUDENT

1. What is the most interesting thing you've done this week?
2. How would I look up the name of this school in the telephone book?
3. What was the funniest thing that ever happened at your home?
4. Who was the best teacher you ever had? Why?
5. How do you buy hunting and fishing licenses in this state?
6. How would I get to the best theater around here?

LEARNING STRATEGY

The adolescent applies conversational rules for speakers across a variety of everyday communication situations.

7. What clothes do you wish you could buy right now?
8. Where is a good place to eat around here? Why?
9. Who is your favorite singer or group? Why?
10. What happened on your favorite TV show the last time you saw it?
11. How do you get to your house from here?
12. What kind of job would you like to have some day?
13. What kinds of food do you like to eat?
14. If you could move to any place in the world, where would you go?
15. What do your parents do (for work)?
16. What are your brothers and sisters like?
17. What do you usually do during summer vacation?
18. What kind of jobs do you have to do at home?
19. If you could buy a car right now, what kind would you get?
20. What classes are you going to take next year?
    (Or for seniors, what are you going to be doing next year?)

SPEAKER ROLE: STUDENT

	LISTENER-ASSUMED ROLES	LISTENER-POSED QUESTION
1	A new student in school	I'm a new student here. What rules are there about being in the hallway, missing school, and things like that?
2	The school principal	How are your classes going?
3	The guidance counselor	What kind of job do you think you're interested in?

	LISTENER-ASSUMED ROLES	LISTENER-POSED QUESTION
4	The math teacher	What do you think would make this class a better one for you?
5	A parent	Who are you hanging around with most these days?
6	A school coach	Why aren't you going out for any sports this year?
7	A younger student	What teachers do you think I should avoid when I get to that school?
8	A school nurse	What can you tell me about the last physical examination you had?
9	A school psychologist	What kind of achievement tests do you remember taking in the last few years?
10	A friend of your parents	What kind of classes are you taking this year and how do you like them?

	SPEAKER - ASSUMED ROLES	LISTENER - ASSUMED ROLES	LISTENER-POSED QUESTION
1	A math teacher	A student	How can I make up the math test I will miss on Friday?
2	A principal or headmaster	A student	What do I have to do to get permission to be gone for a couple of days next week?
3	A baby sitter	A concerned parent	How will you go about contacting the fire department or police station if you need to?

	SPEAKER - ASSUMED ROLES	LISTENER - ASSUMED ROLES	LISTENER-POSED QUESTION
4	A customer in a restaurant	A waiter or waitress	What would you like to order to eat today?
5	A nurse	A sick person	How can I get rid of this cold?
6	A store owner	A young shopper	What can I buy for my mother that is under 10 dollars?
7	A customer	A store clerk	What kind of clothes are you looking for today?
8	A police officer	A motorist in the school parking lot, almost out of gas	How do I get to the closest gas station from here?
9	A patient	A doctor	How have you been feeling lately?
10	A parent	A principal	What do you think we should do about your son skipping school?
11	A parent of a small child	A young parent	What do you do when your child doesn't listen to you?
12	A dog owner	A potential dog owner	How much does it cost to take care of a dog? I don't know anything about the shots they need or how much food they eat.
13	A semi-truck driver who loves the job	A person interested in truck driving	What is it you like about truck driving?

	SPEAKER - ASSUMED ROLES	LISTENER - ASSUMED ROLES	LISTENER-POSED QUESTION
14	A probation officer	A juvenile offender	What happens if you catch me not going to school?
15	A grandfather, grandmother, or older person	A person interested in the past	What were things like when you were growing up?
16	A car owner	A curious child	How do you know when your car has a flat tire? How do you fix it?
17	A homeowner	A fellow homeowner	How can I find a good electrician and a plumber to fix some things in my home?
18	An older brother	A younger brother	How did you get your first date?
19	The manager of a fast-food restaurant	A person interviewing for a job	What kind of job openings do you have right now?
20	An experienced wilderness camper	A novice camper	If you were going on a camping trip and couldn't get to a grocery store in the next two weeks, what would you buy?

INITIATING CONVERSATION

PURPOSE

To initiate and/or maintain conversations that serve a variety of functions

This activity focuses upon appropriately initiating or maintaining a conversation in a variety of situations. In addition to an adolescent assuming the speaker role, a second student can assume the role of a listener and respond to the initiation as in the previous activity. This is optional. Judgments about the politeness and appropriateness of the stated context should be made by all observers and the participants themselves.

Appropriate responses that initiate or maintain conversation in various situations demand use of specific functions of communication as defined by Wells (1974) and popularized by Wiig (1982b, 1982c). They include:

- ritualizing;
- informing;
- controlling;
- feeling; and
- imagining.

Sample situations requiring these functions follow. Read the situations to the students. Then begin by modeling responses to these situations for the adolescents before having them take turns at assuming the speaker role. Situations include some formal and some informal register tasks. Formal register tasks usually involve talking with authority figures and individuals who are not well known to the adolescent. Informal register tasks usually involve talking with a friend, a sibling, and possibly a parent. Be sensitive to the ability of adolescents to switch registers during this activity.

1. You have just met a cousin your age whom you haven't seen for several years. He has come to visit you at your house with his parents. What will you say? (Ritualizing)

2. You are having problems understanding the math assignments and decide to let the teacher know. What will you say? (Informing)

3. You are admiring a T-shirt worn by your friend. You want to find out if you can borrow it sometime. What will you say? (Controlling)

4. Your brother is kicking his schoolbooks furiously around the room. What will you say? (Feeling)

LEARNING STRATEGY

The adolescent applies conversational rules for speakers across a variety of everyday communication situations.

5 You want to talk with your parents about what you could do for fun during spring break. What will you say? (Imagining)

Focus on those functions that are most problematic for the adolescent who has a language disorder. Situations emphasizing each of the functions follow:

RITUALIZING FUNCTION

1 Your new neighbors want you to feed their dog while they're gone. You go over to meet them and the dog. What will you say?

2 Your grandfather sent you a gift for your birthday and you see him for the first time since opening the present. What will you say?

3 You just slipped into your desk in homeroom and realize there is a new student sitting across from you. What could you say?

4 You answer the door and there stands a friend of your mother's. However, your mother is not home right now. What will you say?

5 Your friend has started talking with you after school about how awful the day was. However, you are concerned about getting to an after-school job on time. You politely want to get out of the conversation. What will you say?

6 You accidentally hit a ball through a window in a nearby house while playing with your friends. You go up to the house to talk with the people inside. What will you say?

7 Your brother's new friend comes over and you are in the same room together for a minute until your brother gets there. The friend is a year older than you, and you have never met. What will you say?

8 Your friend helped you finish a lot of homework last night. You see the friend first thing today and still feel grateful. What will you say?

9 Your mother is talking with you about chores that need to get done on the coming weekend, but you want to leave now to see your friends. What will you say?

10. You borrowed your friend's jacket and ripped the elbow out. Your friend is coming down the hallway toward you now. What will you say?

11. Your parents made a tentative promise that you would baby-sit children of old family friends. You need to call them to tell them you'll do it. What will you say?

12. There is a caller on the phone wondering if you or someone else in your family wants to buy magazines. You have just listened to the whole sales pitch and now want to say no. What will you say?

13. You helped a young child who fell off his bike. The bike is broken, and you must call the child's parents. What will you say?

14. Your mother asked you to phone the doctor's office to let them know that she is late but on her way. She will be there in 10 minutes. What will you say when you call?

15. You answer the phone and it's your dad's friend. Your father is sleeping and doesn't want to be disturbed. What will you say?

16. Someone calls you and asks for Donna. You think it must be a wrong number. They call back a second time. What will you say?

17. You decide to call in to a local radio station to request your favorite song and dedicate it to a friend. What will you say?

18. You and your hungry friends are sitting at your house. You have just finished dialing the nearest pizza restaurant. What will you say?

19. You wake up feeling terribly ill and decide to phone the school and let them know you will not be in today. What will you say?

20. Your friend is leaving on a trip tomorrow and you want to call him and wish him a good time. What will you say?

(Note: The last 10 items involve common telephone rituals. These items, as well as some of the first 10 items, necessitate using not only ritualized language but also the informing function. It is of prime importance in this activity that the student engage in a ritual such as greeting, leaving, thanking, apologizing, or a combination of these rituals.)

INFORMING FUNCTION

1. You need to let the school librarian know that you have lost a book. What will you say?

2. You want to tell your mother what clean clothes you need tomorrow and why. What will you say?

3. Your friend has been gone from English class the last two days, and you wonder whether she has remembered there is a test tomorrow. What will you say?

4. Your dentist wants to know what kind of dental work has been done in your mouth in the last couple of years. What will you say?

5. Your social studies teacher wants to know what is the most difficult kind of test for you to take. What will you say?

6. You want to tell your friend about the last movie you saw. What will you say?

7. Your mother wants to know if there are any clothes in your closet that are too small for you and that she can give away or put up for sale. What will you say?

8. Your friend is interested in finding out what you did last weekend. What will you say?

9. You just observed a middle-aged woman shoplifting and decide to tell a store clerk about it. What will you say?

10. A foreign exchange student wants to know how expensive it is to go to movies in America. The student also wants to know where the nearest theaters are and what times the shows play. What will you say?

11. A teacher wants to know how your family gets around most of the time (e.g., by car, bus, or subway). What will you say?

12. Your birthday is coming up, and you want to make sure that your family and friends know what you would like. What will you say?

13. Your parents want to know what kinds of curfews your other friends have right now. What will you say?

14. Your friend wants to know if you have ever been permitted to stay alone all night. What will you say?

15. You need to call the doctor's office and make an appointment for next week. What will you say?

16. The waitress wants to know how you want your hamburger cooked and what you want on it. What will you say?

17. Your new friend wants to know which sports you most enjoy watching and which you enjoy playing. What will you say?

18. The lifeguard wants to know how well you can swim and if you have ever had lessons. What will you say?

19. The school secretary needs to know what other schools you attended before this one, where they were, and how long you attended them. What will you say?

20. The doctor wants to know what people in your family have died from and at what ages. What will you say?

CONTROLLING FUNCTION

1. You approach your parents to see if they will take you to a concert at an arena 50 miles away. Your favorite group is playing. What will you say?

2. Your friend's house always has cookies in stock. You wish there were cookies at your house. You decide to talk to your mother about it. What will you say?

3. Your friend always seems to have more money than you do. You think perhaps you can start getting more money from your parents. What will you ask?

4. You want to go to a movie with a friend and already have a favorite film in mind. You are not certain your friend wants to go to that movie but decide to try asking anyway. What will you say?

5. You have an assignment due for a teacher on Friday. However, you need to be gone from school on both Thursday and Friday, so you want to suggest that you can turn in the assignment on Monday. What will you say?

6. You would like to stay overnight with a friend, but you're not certain your mother will approve because she needs you home at 8 a.m. tomorrow to baby-sit. What will you say?

7. You just hate to see your kid brother wear a sweater that's out of style. How will you suggest to him that he not wear it to school anymore?

8. The radio station your sister is playing is really starting to get on your nerves. You wonder if she will let you change it. What will you say?

9. You are about to head over to your friend's house. Whatever happens, you do not want your brother and his friends to go into your room while you are gone. You want to let your brother know before you leave. What will you say?

10. You want to stay with your aunt and uncle for a few days in the summer, but no offer has been made. What will you say?

11. Your mother bought you a new shirt, but you would like to take it back and exchange it for something you like better. What will you say?

12. Your parents would like you to come with them to visit your grandmother, but you would rather stay at home. What will you say?

13. You almost always end up walking over to your friend's house, and tonight you would rather have your friend come to your house instead. When you call your friend to suggest your plan, what will you say?

14. You would like to get your hair cut in a different way, but you're not certain your parents will like it. Besides, they know you just had your hair cut a few weeks ago. Can you arrange another haircut? What will you say?

15. You finished a science report, brought it to school, and then discovered the teacher had announced it was to be word processed or written in ink, not in pencil. You used a pencil. You would rather not recopy the whole assignment. What will you say?

16. You are taking a test in math class and do not understand one of the story problems. When you ask the teacher for some assistance, what will you say?

17. You have not finished your assigned chores around the home, but you would rather watch a TV show before you finish them. Can you get permission to sit down and watch TV for awhile? What will you say?

18. You forgot your English book at school, and you have an assignment to do. Can you borrow a book from a friend, even though that person needs to finish the same assignment? What will you say?

19. You want to stay out later than usual on Saturday night. How would you suggest this?

20. You are eating at a friend's house and the menu is chili. If there is anything you cannot stomach, it's chili. What will you say?

FEELING FUNCTION

1. You go to the school office because you feel so sick you don't think you can make it through another class. What will you say?

2. You find out from your friend that there is a surprise quiz today in science. You have not yet read any of this week's chapter. When you talk to your friend about how you feel, what will you say?

3. You are waiting in front of the movie theater for your friend. Finally, your friend saunters up more than a half-hour late because there was a good show on television. What will you say?

4. All of your friends are going to a concert next Friday night, but you cannot come up with enough money to go. When you talk to them about how you feel, what will you say?

5. You loaned some money to a friend last week, and now he seems to be avoiding you. He is coming down the hallway toward you, and you decide to ask about the money he owes. What will you say?

6. Your sister lost your favorite CD. When you let her know how you feel, what will you say?

7. You waited a long time for your own blow-dryer, and after a week, it is no longer working. When you take it back to the store and complain, what will you say?

8. You studied for the English test for two hours and still failed. When you let your friend know how you feel, what will you say?

9. Your mother has a friend you really don't like because that person treats you like a baby. When you talk to your mother about how you feel, what will you say?

10. It is the last day of school and you have two weeks of vacation stretched out in front of you. When you tell your good friend how you feel, what will you say?

11. You and a friend are watching TV late at night. You hear what might be a prowler outside the door. Several houses in your neighborhood have been broken into within the last few weeks. What will you say?

12. You get a C in math after thinking you were going to flunk the class. You want to let someone know how you feel. What will you say?

13. You like your mother a lot, but you wish she did not smoke. When you talk to her about how you feel, what will you say?

14. Everyone else says the jacket you are trying on looks great on you, but you don't think it does. You want to let someone else know what you are thinking. What will you say?

15. Adam is a teaser. Most days you can shrug off his teasing, but today it is really bothering you. What will you say?

16. You had a big fight this morning with your dad over what time you must be home tonight. He wanted you home an hour earlier than any of your friends had to be home. When you let a friend know how unreasonable you think your dad is being, what will you say?

17. One of your classmates was killed in a car accident. He had been drinking and drove into a tree. When you talk with a friend about how you feel, what will you say?

18. Next hour, you have to get up in front of class and give a report. You don't feel prepared. When you talk it over with a friend, what will you say?

19. You were just notified that you won a drawing. You have your choice of a home computer or $1000. When you let your best friend know how it feels to win a prize, what will you say?

20. You were looking forward to spending Saturday outside by the river with your friend. You wake up and it is pouring rain. When you call the friend and talk over your feelings about having to rearrange your plans, what will you say?

IMAGINING FUNCTION

1. You decide to talk to your friend about his cat and what it's like to own one because you think it might be fun to ask for one for your birthday. What will you say?

2. Your parents ask how you think your final grades will come out this marking period. What will you say?

3. You and your friend are talking about what kind of party would be fun to go to this Saturday night. What will you say?

4. You are talking with your friend about the kind of girls or boys you wish went to your school. What will you say?

5. Your friend wants to know what famous person you would choose for a date and what you would do. What will you say?

6. You and your friend are imagining what you would do if you were both rich. What will you say?

7. You and your friend are wondering what it would be like if kids could pick their own parents and who you would choose. What will you say?

8. You and your friends are talking about what it would be like to be married and if you ever want to be. What will you say?

9. You are talking with a high school dropout and wonder if that would be a good thing for you to do. What will you say?

10. You and your friends are wondering what it would be like to try some new drugs. What will you say?

11. You and your friend are talking about what it must be like to be an alcoholic. What will you say?

12. You and your friend are talking about whether you want your own kids some day. What will you say?

13. You and your friend are talking about what it might be like if a nuclear bomb were dropped on this country. What will you say?

14. You and your friend are discussing the possibility of four-day school weeks. What will you say?

15. You and your friends are deciding which three foods you would pick if you had to eat the same things for a month. What will you say?

16. You and your friend are thinking about how school would be if a new principal came who was much stricter. What will you say?

17. You and your friend are making an automobile wish list—what brand, model, color, and size you would purchase. What will you say?

18. You and your friend are imagining what it would be like not to have school and to have all your classes over cable TV at home. What will you say?

19. You are talking with your friends about how things would be if there were no parents. What will you say?

20. You are talking with a friend about the pros and cons of running away from home. What will you say?

AWARENESS OF RULES

PURPOSE

To bring to a conscious level what listener conversational rules are and why we have them

(Note: All activities listed under the previous strategy are also appropriate here when viewed from the perspective of the listener. See also Chapter 8, "Nonverbal Communication Strategies," and Chapter 5, "Listening Strategies.")

As with rules of conversation for the speaker, the listener needs to be aware of rules that apply to conversational speech. A number of rules for the listener rely on nonverbal communication (e.g., eye contact, giving feedback such as head nods and frowns).

Discuss all or some of the following questions:

- What happens to a conversation when nobody is listening?
- Have you ever taken the speaker role in a conversation and felt no one was listening? Describe the situation. How did you feel?
- Prisons use solitary confinement as one of the worst punishments possible. What makes it so punishing? (After all, the prisoners could talk all they wanted to.)
- How do you know when someone is really listening to you during a conversation?
- How do you let your friends know you're listening to them when they are talking?

●●

LEARNING STRATEGY

The adolescent demonstrates application of conversational rules for listening across a variety of everyday communication situations.

PAYING ATTENTION: CONSCIOUSNESS RAISING

PURPOSE

To raise listening to an active, conscious activity through dramatization

Have the students name body functions that we automatically and unconsciously perform, assuming no physical impairment is present.

Examples:

breathe

digest food

circulate blood

hear

see

We do not need to think about these body functions. Because we consider seeing and hearing as essentially automatic body responses, it is tempting to think looking and listening are automatic processes.

Have students look around the room and make a mental note of all the red objects they see. Then have them close their eyes and name all the blue objects in the room that they can think of. How many could they name? Why was it difficult to name blue objects, even though they had just scanned the room?

Just as we can form preset notions about what to look for, so can we make that mistake with our listening. Have students engage in this listening activity:

> You are driving the Humane Society truck. Three dogs are in the back of the truck. You pick up two more dogs, drive two miles north, and find a cat. You go another three miles and capture a dog, but two dogs escape while you're putting the new one on the truck. You go another five miles and find one of the escaped dogs and three baby kittens. How old is the driver?

What preset notions did the students have about the question to be asked (number of dogs, number of cats, total number of animals, total number of miles driven)?

> LISTENING IS NOT AN AUTOMATIC RESPONSE. IT TAKES CONSISTENT FOCUSED ATTENTION AND ONGOING AWARENESS.

●●

LEARNING STRATEGY

The adolescent demonstrates application of conversational rules for listening across a variety of everyday communication situations.

INDICATING LEVEL OF UNDERSTANDING

PURPOSE

To experience the use of positive and negative listener feedback, when it is used, and why

LEARNING STRATEGY

The adolescent demonstrates application of conversational rules for listening across a variety of everyday communication situations.

This activity is broken into three segments:

- Communicating "I Understand You"/"I Don't Understand You"
- Listening Triads
- Understanding Referents

COMMUNICATING "I UNDERSTAND YOU"/"I DON'T UNDERSTAND YOU"

Ask the students these questions:

- How do you know if your friends are understanding what you are saying to them?
- What do they say to you that indicates understanding?
- What are they doing with their body movements to indicate they understand you?
- How do you know when your friends are not understanding what you are saying?
- What do they say that indicates a lack of understanding?
- What are they doing with their body movements to indicate a lack of understanding?
- Did you ever pretend to understand someone when you really didn't? If so, why? What was the situation?

Using the situations in the activity "Conversational Starters" (see pages 140–144), have a pair(s) of students begin a conversation. However, before they begin, hand one student a card with a "+" or a "-" on it, or the word *positive* or *negative*. This student, when in the listener role, is to convey that he or she understands the speaker if holding the "+" card and is to convey a lack of understanding if holding the "-" card. Model for the students initially. Discuss whether the listener gave the speaker enough feedback to convey the message. Was the feedback so overwhelming that it was offensive to the speaker?

Now read the following situations to the students. Discuss how students would give feedback to the speaker to indicate their level of understanding. What would be said verbally? What would be done nonverbally? Role-play the situations, if desired.

POSITIVE FEEDBACK

1. A teacher is talking about something you really understand.
2. Your mother is talking about planning a special vacation.
3. Your friend is commenting on what a good time everyone had at the party.
4. You're talking with your dad on the phone, and he is telling you he thinks you deserve a bigger allowance.
5. You just finished getting a haircut, and you really like how it turned out.
6. After days of searching, you found a pair of running shoes that are the right size, the right color, and the right price.
7. You are talking with your grandmother on the telephone, and she announces she is soon making a trip to visit.
8. A special friend asks you to go out on Saturday night.
9. Your mother compliments you for picking up your room and getting your homework done.
10. A teacher just announced in class he will be giving one less test this grading period than he thought he would.

NEGATIVE FEEDBACK

1. You have no idea what the math teacher is telling you about solving equations.
2. You are talking with your mother on the phone. She tells you how to start the laundry, but you don't understand.
3. You are supposed to be doing an art project, but you don't understand it.

4. Your friend wants you to go out, but you want to stay home and watch a movie on TV.

5. Someone is accusing you of taking a pencil that you haven't even seen.

6. Your dad accuses you of leaving the lights on all night, but you think you turned them all off before you went to bed.

7. Your doctor is telling you that you need to take some pills, but you don't understand why.

8. You ordered a Coke and the waitress is asking if you want cream and sugar in it.

9. Your parents are questioning your time spent with a new friend. He is one of your favorite people and one of their least favorite, as you are finding out.

10. Your friend just called you and is very angry about your talking to his girlfriend today. You think there must be some mistake, because you did not even see that person today.

LISTENING TRIADS

Three people are needed for this activity. Inform one person ahead of time, unknown to the others, to engage in ineffective listening, including giving no eye contact to the person speaking and no feedback, positive or negative.

- Select who will be the speaker and who will be the listener.
- Arrange the seating so the speaker, listener, and informed person are sitting at a comfortable distance from each other.
- Direct the speaker to talk about his or her favorite things to do, see, etc. for one minute with the listener. This is repeated with the person who has been informed not to listen.
- Instruct the person who assumed the initial (uninformed) listener role to now be the speaker, but to choose only one of the two other people to speak with. (Invariably, normal communicators choose the listener who is apt to give more feedback.)

Compare the two listeners. How did they differ? Were they alike in any ways? How did the speaker feel when talking with the person who gave no feedback?

UNDERSTANDING REFERENTS

All speakers will use referents that the listener must decode. Pronouns are a key example. Once singular-plural masculine-feminine referents are set, all pronouns that follow can be understood until a topic switch is initiated. Adolescents with attention and listening deficits frequently miss the referent, or they have no strategy for equating two different labels for the same phenomenon (e.g., "national capital" and "Washington, D.C" are equivalent). Negative feedback that indicates "I don't understand" frequently results from not comprehending the vocabulary or a referent.

Given the following words, phrases, or sentences, have students identify the referent or possible referents when more than one might be feasible. Do the words used always have a specific referent? For example, how would one determine which state capital to name for item three below?

1. U.S. capital
2. largest city in North America
3. state capital
4. the principal
5. the senior high math teacher
6. the president of the United States
7. the largest ocean
8. the first month of the year
9. an important Christian holiday
10. the tallest senior
11. "It's the real thing"
12. white collar job

13 W.A.S.P.

14 metric unit of volume

15 The teachers were disappointed with their contract offers. They went on strike. Who are *they*?

16 Jamie's parents went on vacation. Vanna can't remember where they were going. I know Jamie has gone with them. Can you help watch their house while they are gone? Who are *they*?

17 Sean has five brothers. They all go to my school. All of them are really nice looking. He is the only kid I know with two home computers. Who is *he*?

18 Students ought to know better than to try to get teachers to change the dates of a test. After all, teachers are very busy people. They hurt themselves when they try to get special favors, since the test usually ends up harder. Who are *they*?

19 Brian talked with Tami for a long time on the phone. He thought about asking her to go to the dance but decided to do it tomorrow. Later that night, Jared called Tami and asked her to go to the dance. When he found out, he kicked himself for not asking sooner. Who is *he*?

20 Did you hear that Leslie got a bad shock when she was washing dishes and she reached over to turn up the TV? One has to be careful when mixing water and electricity. Who is *one*?

TOPIC MAINTENANCE

PURPOSE

To maintain a conversational topic when both participants have a primary objective

Have students form conversational dyads, or appoint one speaker and one listener and have others observe and critique their performance. Without the other students hearing, assign the speaker a major objective to be achieved during the conversation. The person assigned to be a listener will need to change roles as demanded by the objective. Make the listener aware of the role to be taken but do not inform him or her of the speaker's major objective. Instruct the listener to listen to the speaker and respond appropriately. Direct the speaker and listener to maintain the conversation until the speaker's objective is met.

LISTENER ROLE	MAJOR OBJECTIVE OF ASSIGNED SPEAKER
a friend of the student	1 To let your friend know you don't want to go out Saturday night
student's mother	2 To let your mother know you think you're getting a failing grade in English
student's brother	3 To let your brother know you don't want him to borrow your sweater
teacher	4 To let a teacher know you did not finish an assignment due today
student's boss	5 To let your boss know you need Friday night off

Discuss the following:

- Was the speaker able to achieve the desired objective? Were speaker rules applied? Did the listener use appropriate listener rules?

Now have the speaker reach the main objective when the listener also has a main objective. Roles do not need to be taken. Neither speaker nor listener should be aware of the other's assigned objective for the conversation. The following list can be mixed randomly. It is reproduced in Appendix G in the form of cards that can be cut apart. Discuss what happens when both conversational partners want to achieve their objectives immediately. Who determined which topic would be maintained first?

●●●
LEARNING STRATEGY
The adolescent demonstrates application of mutual speaker-listener rules across a variety of everyday communication situations.

MAIN OBJECTIVE OF ASSIGNED LISTENER		MAIN OBJECTIVE OF ASSIGNED SPEAKER
1	To talk about weekend plans	To ask if you can copy a page of homework
2	To talk about what fun you had going out to eat last night	To talk about how frustrated you are with your parents
3	To talk about the last time you were sick	To talk about what you would like to do this weekend if you could do anything in the world
4	To talk about a car driving experience you have had, or would like to have	To talk about what you're hungry for right now (or will be later today)
5	To talk about the best TV show you have seen recently	To talk about the worst movie you have ever seen
6	To talk about how it would feel to be an only child	To talk about how things have been going at school
7	To talk about a car accident you have seen or heard about	To talk about football—how well you like it or dislike it
8	To talk about what you would have done if you had not come to school today	To talk about the last new clothes that were bought for you
9	To talk about the kind of entertainment you like	To talk about how much you like or dislike being outside in the weather you're having right now
10	To talk about what you typically do on your birthday	To talk about what your family usually does on national holidays like July 4th or Thanksgiving
11	To talk about pets your family has owned or that you would like to own	To talk about the worst teacher you have ever had

MAIN OBJECTIVE OF ASSIGNED LISTENER	MAIN OBJECTIVE OF ASSIGNED SPEAKER
12 To talk about how much money you wish you had right now	To talk about a trip to a zoo you have taken or wish you could take
13 To talk about your least favorite season of the year	To talk about your favorite holiday
14 To talk about how it would feel if parents still arranged marriage partners for their children	To talk about motorcycles you have ridden or would like to ride
15 To talk about food that makes you gag	To talk about the kind of house you would like to live in some day
16 To talk about what radio station you listen to most of the time and why	To talk about what TV or cable channel you watch most and why
17 To talk about what cartoon character(s) you like best	To talk about the kinds of physical exercise you like to do best
18 To talk about what you hope gets changed/fixed soon in your house	To talk about how you wish your mother or father would change
19 To talk about what you would like to alter about your appearance	To tell someone about the hardest work you think you have ever done
20 To talk about how far behind (or ahead) you are with your homework	To talk about a favorite friend you had as a small child

TOPIC CHANGES

PURPOSE

To engage in topic changes using appropriate signaling devices

In the previous activity, students were asked to incorporate two objectives into one conversation. To do this necessitated at least one change in topic. How did this change occur? Were any verbal or nonverbal cues given to indicate a topic switch? If so, what were they? If no cues were given, chances are topic transitions were not signaled as clearly as they could have been. Discuss why it is important for listeners to know a speaker is switching topics. Can students recall any times when friends/parents/teachers changed topics and they didn't realize it? What happened? How did the students feel?

Repeat some of the conversations from the previous activity, paying attention to how topic switches or transitions are made. List verbal and nonverbal cues noted. Efficient communicators often signal transitions in very subtle ways. There are also occasions when very blatant, concrete signals are given that are acceptable to listeners. Examples include:

"This is changing topics, but . . ."

"This is a little off topic; however, . . ."

"That reminds me of . . ."

"Oh, I just remembered I wanted to tell you . . ."

"Before I forget, let me say . . ."

It is almost always acceptable to use these very obvious transition statements. They convey consideration for the listener's perspective.

Have students participate in the following conversations in which the speaker has two or more topics to share with the listener. (These are also reproduced in Appendix G for use during sessions.) Communication functions (i.e., ritualizing, informing, controlling, feeling, imagining) are interspersed. Pay attention to whether some functions are more difficult to switch between than others.

The listener should be unaware of the topics and follow appropriate listener rules. Encourage students in the speaker role to use straightforward strategies for switching topics if they get stuck. Provide an initial model for students. Switch speaker-listener roles for the students as the activity progresses. Critique topic changes following each conversation.

LEARNING STRATEGY

The adolescent demonstrates application of mutual speaker-listener rules across a variety of everyday communication situations.

MAIN OBJECTIVES OF SPEAKER

1. a. To ask for a ride home after tomorrow night's game
   b. To tell about the book that caught on fire during a science experiment

2. a. To tell about your fight with your father this morning and how you felt
   b. To suggest that the room would be more comfortable if windows could be opened to let in fresh air

3. a. To tell what you'd like to do during summer vacation
   b. To tell about your favorite actor

4. a. To tell about the hardest subject you are taking right now
   b. To talk about your favorite aunt, uncle, or cousin

5. a. To describe what your daily routine is before arriving at school
   b. To ask what kind of music your friend would like to listen to right now

6. a. To tell about the worst storm you ever lived through
   b. To ask if your friend would like something to drink

7. a. To explain how well you like the location of your locker at school
   b. To talk about what annoys you most at home

8. a. To talk about what your favorite song is right now
   b. To ask if your friend has ever had an eye exam

9. a. To ask what time it is
   b. To ask what homework your friend has to do tonight

10. a. To ask if there's anything exciting going on this weekend
    b. To tell about the last party you went to

11. a. To ask if your friend has ever gone to a wedding and what it was like (or what he or she thinks it would be like)
    b. To ask if your friend has ever gone camping and what it was like (or what he or she thinks it would be like)

12 a. To talk about what you think your family would do if there was a nuclear attack
b. To ask if your friend has ever considered joining the military after high school

13 a. To tell about the funniest teacher you know, or the one who tells the best jokes
b. To tell about a hotel that you have stayed at, or think would be fun to stay at

14 a. To tell about your parents' computer knowledge
b. To ask if your friend has a favorite computer game and why it is so much fun to play

15 a. To tell about the most expensive food you think you have ever eaten
b. To ask if your friend likes the weather today

16 a. To ask where your friend buys clothing most of the time
b. To talk about how much makeup you like to see girls wearing at school

17 a. To ask what part of the day your friend likes best
b. To describe your favorite way to study (e.g., noisy/quiet, sitting up/lying down)

18 a. To describe when you get yelled at most often at home
b. To describe something that you fear a great deal

19 a. To explain whether or not you feel bored at school
b. To ask if your friend would like to get something to eat

20 a. To ask your friend how much time it takes to get from home to school
b. To tell something you like about your friend's clothing or appearance today

TOPIC INTERRUPTIONS

PURPOSE

To experience topic interruptions and discuss their effect on conversational speech

Interruptions occur when listeners talk at the same time that speakers do. Interruptions often occur near the end of the speaker's turn when listeners misinterpret cues that signal the end of a turn.

In the "Topic Maintenance" activity (see page 163), both the speaker and the listener had a desired objective. Were any interruptions observed as both conversational partners attempted to maintain their specific topics?

For this activity, pair students or have two students role-play while the others observe. Give the speaker one or two main objectives for the conversation. The listener is unaware of the objective(s). (The speaker objectives are on the following pages and are also reprinted in Appendix G for use during sessions.) Use an initial topic unrelated to the objective(s) as the beginning point for the conversation. Both speaker and listener should be aware of the initial topic. Instruct the listener to continually interrupt the speaker in an attempt to return the conversation to the initial topic. However, speakers should remain unaware that the listener has been instructed to interrupt. Discuss the following with the students after completion of the activity:

- Was the task more difficult than the previous activities? Why or why not?
- How did it feel to be interrupted?
- How did it feel to be the one doing the interrupting?
- Are there any times when it is appropriate to interrupt the speaker? When?
- When you do interrupt, what can you say to excuse yourself (e.g., "I'm sorry, I didn't mean to interrupt"; "Excuse me, I thought you were finished")?

●●●

LEARNING STRATEGY

The adolescent demonstrates application of mutual speaker-listener rules across a variety of everyday communication situations.

	INITIAL TOPIC	MAIN OBJECTIVE(S) OF ASSIGNED SPEAKER	MAIN OBJECTIVE(S) OF ASSIGNED LISTENER
1	Places you would like to visit	To tell how mean your sister (or a friend) has been to you lately	Return to initial topic
2	Famous people you would like to meet	To express worry over passing math this year	Return to initial topic
3	Clothes you would like to buy	To ask if you can copy tomorrow's English assignment	Return to initial topic
4	Who is dating whom at school	To tell your friend he or she has to stop seeing someone and why	Return to initial topic
5	The best pizza to eat	To announce that your parents are out of town this weekend and talk about what to do while they're gone	Return to initial topic
6	The car you wish your family owned	To express disappointment in who won a recent game and to offer advice on what should have been changed	Return to initial topic
7	The best TV show you saw in the last week	To complain that you have to do more chores than your brother does	Return to initial topic
8	The musical group you'd most like to hear in concert	To ask if you can borrow some money to buy a candy bar	Return to initial topic
9	The worst class in school	To find out how much money your friend has to spend each week and where he or she gets it	Return to initial topic

	INITIAL TOPIC	MAIN OBJECTIVE(S) OF ASSIGNED SPEAKER	MAIN OBJECTIVE(S) OF ASSIGNED LISTENER
10	The next party you hope to go to	To talk about the last fight you had with your parent(s) or a friend	Return to initial topic
11	How parents should act when your friends come over	To find out where one of your teachers lives	Return to initial topic
12	Embarrassing things that have happened to you or to others	To ask when summer vacation begins and what your friend is doing	Return to initial topic
13	Grades you received that seemed unfair	To complain that you lost a quarter in a vending machine	Return to initial topic
14	Your favorite relative(s)	To find out who your friend thinks is the most popular boy or girl in school	Return to initial topic
15	Food you have eaten that tasted terrible	To find out whether your friend has a curfew imposed by a parent(s)	Return to initial topic
16	Things teachers do that you dislike	To ask what tomorrow's math assignment is and to tell your friend there's a black smudge on his or her face	Return to initial topic
17	How schools should be run	To tell about the best gift you ever received and to find out what kinds of gifts your friend likes	Return to initial topic

	INITIAL TOPIC	MAIN OBJECTIVE(S) OF ASSIGNED SPEAKER	MAIN OBJECTIVE(S) OF ASSIGNED LISTENER
18	The most fun times you have had with your family or friends	To ask what time it is and to announce you are late and have to go	Return to initial topic
19	Part-time jobs you wish you could have while in high school	To ask if you can borrow a comb and to complain that you have to be in by 10 p.m. this weekend	Return to initial topic
20	Your favorite hairstyles and who has them	To ask your friend what he or she is wearing to school tomorrow and to ask how much money he or she usually carries to school	Return to initial topic

THE CONVERSATION IDEA JAR: A SUMMATIVE ACTIVITY

PURPOSE

To expand rules of conversation to group discussions

Having explored thoroughly the rules for a two-person conversation, discuss what happens when three or more people attempt to converse:

- How are conversations between two people the same as conversations among three or more? What rules of conversation remain constant?

- How are conversations between two people different from conversations among three or more? What additional rules of conversation must be added?

Rees and Wollner (1982) identified several rules that specifically apply to turn taking in conversations involving more than two participants:

1. If the participants number more than two, it is not required that all take turns at speaking.
2. If two or more speakers start simultaneously, all but one should drop out.
3. Gaps between speakers' turns are brief or nonexistent.

"The Conversation Idea Jar" is intended as a summary activity in which students can apply previously learned rules for speakers and listeners as well as new rules that govern discourse among three or more people.

Ask students to list topics that they have always wanted to know about but haven't had the chance to talk about. Write these ideas on slips of paper and put the papers in a jar labeled "Idea Jar." Topics might include drugs, teenage pregnancy, runaways, parents, and teachers. If such broad topics are suggested, try to narrow them down to a specific question (e.g., "What does it feel like to be a teenage runaway?" "If you were a parent, how would you treat your children?" "What makes a 'good teacher' good and a 'bad teacher' bad?"). These ideas can simply accumulate in the jar until there is a session or partial session devoted to group conversation or discussion. Encourage students to add questions whenever topics come to their minds.

Initially, lead the group conversation or discussion. Keep questions open ended. Students who have been successful in conversational dyads may still need some special direction to pull them into verbal exchanges with more than one person at a time. After students have gained proficiency, appoint one of them to be the discussion leader. This student may need assistance in asking questions that are open-ended and thought provoking. Some groups will never

LEARNING STRATEGY

The adolescent demonstrates application of mutual speaker-listener rules across a variety of everyday communication situations.

arrive at the point of having discussion leaders. In such a case, continue to be the facilitator but involve students in critiquing their group conversations.

If an extrinsic reinforcement system is being used during this activity (e.g., poker chips or points), it would be desirable to phase it out, since expectations of secondary-level students include spontaneous participation in classroom discussions and successful interaction within a peer group.

Always allow 5–10 minutes at the end of this activity to summarize observations. How well were rules followed? Did everyone participate? Were some topics easier to discuss than others? Why? Did anyone dominate the conversation?

7 QUESTION-ASKING STRATEGIES

QUESTION ASKING

Use of basic question forms emerges during the preschool years. By the time children reach adolescence, the assumption is made that they know and use wh-question forms (i.e., who, what, where, when, why, how) and a variety of yes/no question forms, including tag questions. Older students may know how to ask questions, but they may ask in a way that offends the listener. If this is the case, their communication is considered impaired (Larson and McKinley, 1995).

The issue in this chapter is not to teach adolescents the syntactic form of questions but rather to ensure that adolescents ask questions in ways that do not alienate their listeners. The focus is on adolescents who know how to ask questions but not how to ask them appropriately. Very little research has been focused on teaching students to ask appropriate questions (Marzano et al., 1988). The activities in this chapter are based on the authors' experiences with adolescents.

PURPOSE OF QUESTIONS

Typically, questions are thought of as asking for information. Good questions focus attention on important information and then generate new information (Marzano et al., 1988). If students ask questions, they are actively involved in the activity within the classroom. Thus, question asking is a pragmatic and functional skill that will help students gain new information and question asking will indicate to teachers that students are actively involved in the learning activity. In Standard American English, questions also form the primary means by which polite requests are made (e.g., "Would you mind opening the door?" "May I leave early?"). Questions become an important way in which individuals control what is going on around them.

Questions also add variety to the language through remarks such as, "Wouldn't you know it? It's raining again today." Such questions do not expect a response per se from a listener but are rhetorical in nature.

ACTIVITIES TO ENHANCE QUESTION-ASKING STRATEGIES

GENERAL QUESTION-ASKING SKILLS

- ● Recognition of the functions of questions
- ●● Determination of how to ask the right question in the right way at the right time

NOT ALL QUESTIONS ASK A QUESTION

PURPOSE

To discriminate between questions that ask and questions that tell

Not all questions ask for information or require an oral response. Those that do not require a specific response are called *rhetorical questions.* Other questions request that something be done, and some actually give information rather than ask for it.

Have students generate examples of various question types (e.g., Will you please close the door? Can you be quieter? Do you believe how fast the day went? How much does that cost?). Point out the expectations for responses to the different question types (e.g., asking for information, requesting action, rhetorical). Define rhetorical questions (i.e., those that neither ask for information nor request action; they may emphasize ideas or feelings).

Read each of the following questions to the students and guide them in identifying which questions are primarily asking for information, which are primarily requesting action, and which are rhetorical:

1. Can you believe how angry her mom was?
2. How does it feel to be angry?
3. What did you do last weekend?
4. Isn't staying home all weekend boring?
5. Would you mind if we turned on the television?
6. Where do you live?
7. How can it possibly rain 20 days in a row?
8. Do you care if the light is flipped on?
9. Could you please feed my dog while I'm gone?
10. What kind of job would you like to have?
11. Who is the president of your country?
12. Why would anyone want to eat a dozen raw eggs?
13. What time is it?

LEARNING STRATEGY

The adolescent recognizes the various functions that questions serve in our language.

14. Would it be OK if this coupon were cut out of the paper?
15. Which school do you go to?
16. How do you suppose he expects us to get all our homework done?
17. Will you please hand me my jacket?
18. How would you like to move over?
19. Have you ever flown in an airplane?
20. Do you think this school year is ever going to end?

Pose these questions to the group for discussion:

- Could a question be considered a different type depending on the situation (i.e., could a question be rhetorical in one situation and interrogative in another)?
- What might the consequence be if a rhetorical question is answered with an informative response?

Encourage students to be specific in their responses by giving example situations.

EVERYDAY EXAMPLES

PURPOSE

To recognize the function of questions in everyday situations and to respond appropriately

LEARNING STRATEGY

The adolescent recognizes the various functions that questions serve in our language.

Duplicate one "Everyday Questions" activity form (found in Appendix H) for each student. Require a homework assignment that asks students to collect examples of each of the question functions (those that ask information, those that request action, those that emphasize an idea [rhetorical]) in the three situations listed on the activity form (in the classroom, at home, and with peers). Instruct students to record this information on the "Everyday Questions" activity form. An example of a completed activity form follows:

SITUATION	ASK INFORMATION	REQUEST ACTION	EMPHASIZE AN IDEA (RHETORICAL)
IN THE CLASSROOM	*How many problems do we have to do?*	*Would you loan me a pencil?*	*Do you believe Mr. Cook is making us take the test again?*
AT HOME	*When will the laundry get washed?*	*May I have the butter, please?*	*How many times do I have to ask you to quiet down?*
WITH PEERS	*Who is going out for pizza on Friday?*	*Could you hold my books while I open my locker?*	*Would you quit taking my CDs?*

Upon completion, direct adolescents in a discussion addressing the following questions:

- Were all the questions responded to appropriately? If not, what problems resulted?
- How do you know if a question is rhetorical or if the speaker expects an answer? Are there any specific words that provide clues to the function of the question?

ASKING IN THE RIGHT WAY: REQUESTS

PURPOSE

To phrase question-form requests in a pragmatically appropriate manner

Requests considered polite in Standard American English are phrased frequently in question form. The underlying message in these questions is to inform the listener that you would like something done. "Will you please stop arguing with your sister?" means "Please stop arguing!" Young children may take advantage of such a situation by responding "no" to the request phrased as a question. By adolescence, the listener expects that question-form requests imply a statement of action, not an either/or option.

Any request can be posed politely in a question form. A variety of polite question-form request starters exist. They include:

"Can you please...?"

"Will you please...?"

"Would you mind...?"

"Would it be all right if...?"

"How would you like to...?"

"What if...?"

"Do you mind if...?"

Have students generate additional examples of request starters. Then, using the following list of statements, ask adolescents to generate two or more ways that each statement could be turned into a polite request using a question form.

1. Take out the garbage.
2. Feed the dog.
3. Get the newspaper from the front step.
4. Mail these letters.
5. Get out of my face.
6. Stop bugging John.
7. Back off.
8. Hang up the phone.

●●

LEARNING STRATEGY

The adolescent determines how to ask the right question in the right way at the right time.

9. Go to bed.
10. Do your homework.
11. Put your clothes away.
12. Leave me alone.
13. Get out of my way.
14. Move over.
15. Sit down.
16. I want that chair.
17. I want a glass of water.
18. I want something to eat.
19. I want to go home.
20. I want to borrow your comb.

Encourage each adolescent to contribute one more statement that another student rephrases as a polite request. Generate a discussion of when direct statements would be used as opposed to polite requests. Include discussing the advantages of using polite request forms, how one's familiarity with another person affects the decision to use a direct statement versus a polite request, and how students feel when someone orders them to do something rather than making a polite request. Ask what effect a demand has on their willingness to fulfill the request.

ASKING IN THE RIGHT WAY: STRANGERS AND AUTHORITY FIGURES

PURPOSE

To phrase questions one would typically ask a stranger or authority figure in a pragmatically appropriate manner

●●
LEARNING STRATEGY
The adolescent determines how to ask the right question in the right way at the right time.

When talking with authority figures or strangers, a formal code or register is more appropriate than the usual question-asking behavior used with familiar peers and adults. This is true whether the question is to make a request or to ask for information.

Given the following situations, have students determine whether they need to ask a question for information or to make a request. Then read the question choices to the group and direct them to select the best question listed for the situations.

1. You are seated at the bus stop and want to know if the stranger next to you will watch your backpack while you make a phone call.

   Will you ask a question to get information or to make a request?

   - "Wanna watch my backpack?"
   - "Hey, will you watch this for a minute?"
   - "Would you mind watching my backpack while I make a phone call?"
   - "You gonna be sitting here for awhile?"

2. You are in an unfamiliar grocery store and want to find pancake syrup as quickly as possible because your family is waiting in the car.

   Will you ask a question to get information or to make a request?

   - "Could you please direct me to the pancake syrup?"
   - "Hey, where's the pancake syrup anyway?"
   - "You got any pancake syrup in this store?"
   - "Why's the pancake syrup in this aisle?"

3. You are trying to find the phone number for Rollie Thomas in Boston and have just called the information operator.

   Will you ask a question to get information or to make a request?

   - "Give me the number for Rollie Thomas in Boston."

- "You got Rollie Thomas from Boston's phone number?"
- "What's Thomas, T-H-O-M-A-S, Rollie's phone number?"
- "Could you give me the telephone number for Rollie Thomas, T-H-O-M-A-S, in Boston?"

4. You are at a good friend's party and want to know if anyone would mind if you turned down the music.

   Will you ask a question to get information or to make a request?

   - "Do you all want to go deaf, or what?"
   - "Would you mind if I turned down the music a little?"
   - "Can you stand the volume lower?"
   - "Do you want the neighbors to call the police?"

5. You are at a gas station and would like to use the restroom, but you need to obtain the key from the attendant first.

   Will you ask a question to get information or to make a request?

   - "Hey, where's the restroom key?"
   - "Why's the restroom locked?"
   - "May I please have the restroom key?"
   - "Can you gimme that key?"

6. You need to travel to Montreal and decide to check on the bus rates.

   Will you ask a question to get information or to make a request?

   - "Would you please tell me the bus fare between here and Montreal?"
   - "How do I get to Montreal by bus?"
   - "Do buses go to Montreal?"
   - "You know any bus routes to Montreal?"

7. You are eating out at a restaurant when you notice your fork is dirty.

Will you ask a question to get information or to make a request?

- "Don't you wash your forks around here, or what?"
- "Would you please bring me a clean fork?"
- "Why don't you wash your forks?"
- "Is this the fork you expect me to use?"

8. You are driving in an unfamiliar city, trying to find the baseball stadium. You are really late and the game is about to begin. You notice a police officer standing on the sidewalk and think he might be able to help you.

Will you ask a question to get information or to make a request?

- "Where's the ball game at?"
- "How on earth do you find the stadium in this place?"
- "Has this city ever heard of putting up signs to find the stadium?"
- "Can you please tell me how to get to the baseball stadium?"

9. You are in study hall at school and would like to talk with your friend, Larissa, about a group project you are doing together for English class. The study hall rules dictate that talking must have prior approval of the adult supervisor.

Will you ask a question to get information or to make a request?

- "May I please talk with Larissa about our group project for English?"
- "Can I talk to Larissa?"
- "Will you let me talk to Larissa?"
- "How about if Larissa and I talk about our English project?"

10 You are feeling sick and would like to leave your history class.

Will you ask a question to get information or to make a request?

- "Would you believe I'm sick?"
- "Can I please be excused?"
- "May I please leave because I'm feeling sick?"
- "Can I get out of here for awhile?"

Discuss why some choices are better than others. Do the "better choices" have any commonalities (e.g., the better choices provide more information than the other options, as in the first question in #9 and the third question in #10, which both provide reasons for the request)?

After discussing the best (i.e., most pragmatically appropriate) questions, continue with the following situations. Ask students to generate their own question(s), but first have them identify what function the question will serve.

11 The two adults next to you at the movie are being obnoxious. They are talking so loudly you can't hear.

12 You want to get to Third Street. You are certain the bus you are on doesn't go directly to Third Street, but you don't know where to get off to transfer.

13 You think you recognize a person, Mr. Lopez, who once lived next door to you. You haven't seen for him for years, so you're not positive it's him. You decide to talk to the man to find out who he is.

14 You're at a party standing next to a girl you've never met. You decide to start a conversation by finding out about this girl.

15 The person next to you on the bus has a radio and you don't. You would like to know who won the Milwaukee Bucks-Chicago Bulls basketball game.

16 You want to ask the principal's secretary for the date that summer vacation begins.

17. Your cousin is being held by the police in a juvenile detention center for shoplifting. You would like to visit him and need to ask permission of the security guard.

18. A job posted for a local grocery store sounds perfect, except you don't know how many hours a week the job will be. You have gone to talk with the store manager.

19. You are in a large department store and desperately need to find the restroom. You decide to find out your options.

20. You need to have a vision exam because you've been having problems reading road signs. You have just dialed a local optometrist to find out how much an exam will cost.

ASKING IN THE RIGHT WAY: INFORMATION SEEKING

PURPOSE

To phrase information questions in a pragmatically appropriate manner

Several problems can emerge when students ask for information. They may ask in an abrasive manner and/or they may ask a question that is too broad or too specific to communicate what they really want to know. These problems can become particularly troublesome when asking teachers for information during or after class.

Equally problematic can be the total absence of asking questions when it would be appropriate to ask them. Failure to ask questions can be due to factors such as past negative experiences in question asking, not knowing what questions to ask, or a lack of confidence in asking questions.

NONABRASIVE QUESTION ASKING

This activity focuses primarily on asking informational questions related to academic concerns. It also focuses on common informational questions adolescents might ask their friends.

Demonstrate an abrasive request and then define the term *abrasive*. Discuss with students factors that contribute to an abrasive-sounding question as opposed to a nonabrasive question. Abrasiveness is primarily affected by the tone of voice one uses. Try asking the following questions using two different voice qualities, one pleasant sounding and one abrasive sounding. Model the first pair or two and have students discriminate which questions are not pragmatically appropriate in the classroom due to tone of voice:

(Polite sounding) Do we have to do all the problems on page 10?
(Abrasive sounding) Do we have to do *all* the problems on page 10?

(Abrasive sounding) *Why* can't we have the test on Friday?
(Polite sounding) Why can't we have the test on Friday?

(Polite sounding) Do I have to word process this paper?
(Abrasive sounding) Do I *have* to word process this paper?

(Polite sounding) When can our group have a turn?
(Abrasive sounding) When can *our* group have a turn?

(Abrasive sounding) *Where's* the worksheet I'm supposed to do?
(Polite sounding) Where's the worksheet I'm supposed to do?

●●
LEARNING STRATEGY

The adolescent determines how to ask the right question in the right way at the right time.

Explain to students that individuals are more inclined to answer a question if the person asking it does not sound abrasive, irritating, challenging, or disrespectful.

KNOWING WHEN TO ASK QUESTIONS

Information questions should be asked of teachers when something is not clear. In most cases, asking questions is viewed as a sign that students are paying attention. Discuss this concept with students and ask them to identify exceptions (e.g., asking for information to be repeated a third and fourth time). The following are examples of situations in which information may not be clear in a classroom setting and might require a question for clarification:

- The meaning of a word is unknown.
- It is unclear whether the speaker is stating a fact or an opinion.
- There seem to be things the teacher meant indirectly but did not say.
- An assignment is confusing.
- The content and format of an upcoming quiz or test are unknown.

Facilitate a discussion of other instances requiring question asking for clarification. With the group, identify common but unspoken rules for question asking in a classroom or large-group setting (e.g., a common rule is to wait until the teacher or the speaker pauses, then ask questions). Students who lack the confidence and skills to ask a question in front of the whole class should be encouraged to ask questions of teachers before or after class. Whenever possible, alert classroom educators to the fact that the student being seen in intervention has a goal of appropriate question-asking behavior. Most often, the classroom educator will be willing to facilitate the process by cueing the student in the classroom (e.g., "Candace, do you have any questions?"). If rapport with teachers permits, counsel them not to give negative feedback to students that would discourage future question asking, particularly for those students who tend not to ask questions.

SPECIFIC QUESTION ASKING IN THE CLASSROOM

Questions may be either too general or too specific. An example of a question that is too general is, "What did you say our assignment is?" when the student knows the answer except for one or two specific details. An example of a question that is too specific is, "Will the test have true-false questions?" when what the student wants to know is all of the types of questions that will be on the test. Questions are considered too general or too specific in relationship to the actual information the student is attempting to gain. Thus, students must (1) identify what it is that is unclear to them, (2) determine how to ask a polite-sounding question to gain the desired information, and (3) determine when to ask the question.

Read the following situations to the group. Direct students to generate pragmatically appropriate questions for each situation given. First discuss what needs to be asked, then role-play asking the question. As students ask the questions, they should use a tone of voice that does not irritate the listener(s).

1. You know the math assignment is on page 20, but you don't know which problems to do. Ask the math teacher.

2. You have just read the sentence, "Put the clutch in before engaging the gear shift." You don't understand what the gear shift is. Ask the driver education teacher.

3. You want to know what kind of history test to expect next Wednesday. Ask the history teacher.

4. You're not certain how you are doing in English class and are worried about failing. Ask the English teacher.

5. You know you're supposed to write a five-page paper on the weather for science class. The teacher has explained it at least twice, and you still don't know exactly what to do. One time the teacher said to use three outside references, and the second time he didn't say how many references you had to use. Ask the science teacher.

6. You are supposed to write a short poem for English. You're not certain what the teacher means by "short." You have a poem written that is seven lines long. Ask the English teacher.

7. Your art assignment is to find a common "something" to bring to class for a special project. You thought she said a "leaf," but you're not certain. Ask the art teacher.

8. In world history class, the teacher said there were three important dates to remember: 1776, 1812, and you didn't catch the third one. Ask the history teacher.

9. In world history class, the teacher said there were three important dates to remember for your test and you have four dates recorded in your notes. Ask the history teacher.

10. You originally had two assignments due on Friday in math. Now one is due on Friday and the other can be turned in on Monday, but you don't know which is which. Ask the math teacher.

11. In comparing English worksheets with a friend, you notice that your answer for number 10 was counted wrong, and your friend's answer was the same and was counted correct. Ask the English teacher about this.

12. You have a younger brother who has been sick at home for the last two school days. You stop by his math class to collect his make-up work. Ask the math teacher.

13. You need to leave class early for a doctor's appointment. Usually, the assignment is given near the end of the class period. Ask the teacher.

14. You need to be absent from school two days next week. You think there might be a conflict because one of the days might be when you're supposed to give your report for social studies. You're not really sure what day your report is scheduled. Ask the teacher.

15. You tripped on a step at school early in the morning and twisted your ankle. You think it might have a slight sprain. In physical education class, the teacher wants you to play basketball. When you start playing, your ankle hurts much more, and you think you'd better stop. Ask the physical education teacher.

16 You know your friend lives several miles north of where you do, but you don't know exactly where or the best way to get there. Ask your friend.

17 You have nothing planned for the weekend and are afraid it's going to be a long, boring two days. Your best friend will be away, and you wonder about asking another friend about her (his) plans. Ask your friend.

18 You and your friend are in the same classes. You didn't understand the English teacher today when she was talking about different verbs. You thought she said something that sounded like "infinite" verb. Ask your friend.

19 A good friend of yours is having a birthday tomorrow. You are invited to go to a birthday dinner at a restaurant with your friend's family, but you don't know where or when. Ask your friend.

20 You want to get a haircut this weekend. You really like the way Jesse's hair looks and wonder who cut it. Ask Jesse.

ASKING THE RIGHT QUESTIONS: INTERVIEWS

PURPOSE

To phrase questions in a pragmatically appropriate manner during interview situations

Job interviews are particularly conspicuous occasions for inappropriate questioning and can prove disastrous for the adolescent. The adolescent's ability to ask clear, relevant questions can be a key factor in an employer's decision to proceed with hiring.

During this activity, role-play a job interview situation. Play the role of the potential employer while students take turns playing the role of an interviewee. Before role-playing, discuss the following key issues that need to be discussed during an interview:

- What responsibilities does this job entail?
- Who is the immediate supervisor?
- What is the salary?
- What are the hours?
- When does the job begin?
- Where is the location of the job?

Encourage adolescents to think of other issues they might want to know about when interviewing for a job. If these issues listed are not addressed by the employer in role-playing, direct the adolescent to ask for the information as part of the interview process.

Some questions are best avoided during the initial job interview and may actually harm the adolescent's chance of being hired. Have students think of questions that might be potential "turn offs" to employers. Discuss those questions that are likely to be abrasive to the employer—in terms of the question content or the way in which the question is asked, or both. Such questions may include these:

- "Do you really expect me to work on weekends?"
- "When can I get a raise?"
- "Can I get a longer paid vacation?"
- "Can I read a magazine if there aren't any customers around?"

●●
LEARNING STRATEGY
The adolescent determines how to ask the right question in the right way at the right time.

- "Do I have to stay here 'til closing time even if nobody's here?"
- "Do the customers really care if the floor is washed?"
- "I'm not really very good at math, so could someone else give the customers their change?"

In turn, engage each student in an interview. Have key questions recorded clearly within everyone's sight. Instruct students who are not participating in the interview to tally key questions as they occur. If possible, audiotape or videotape the interviews. Play them back and critique them as a group. At the end of each interview, vote on the question, "Would you hire this adolescent if you were an employer?"

While conducting the interviews, gradually decrease the number of key issues addressed to increase the number of questions the adolescent will need to ask (to a maximum of three or four). Possible interview situations include the following:

ROLES

	ADULT INTERVIEWER	JOB POSITION
1	Restaurant manager	Dishwasher
2	Newspaper circulation manager	Newspaper carrier
3	Parent of a two-year-old	Baby sitter
4	Grocery store manager	Carry-out person
5	Gift store manager	Shelf stocker
6	Car wash (drive-through) manager	Towel drier
7	Pharmacist	Drug store clerk
8	Parks director	Gardener
9	Recreation manager	Lifeguard
10	Head waiter/waitress at restaurant	Waiter/Waitress

8 NONVERBAL COMMUNICATION STRATEGIES

NONVERBAL COMMUNICATION: AN IGNORED SKILL

Great differences often exist between the meaning we think we communicated and the meaning actually perceived. Nonverbal, not verbal, factors are the major determinants of meaning in the interpersonal context. Birdwhistell (1970) asserts that only 30–35 percent of the social meaning of a conversation is carried by words. Mehrabian (1968) estimates 93 percent of the total impact of a message is due to nonverbal factors. Furthermore, Fridlund (1994) explains how emotions are universally recognized from facial expressions. "Happiness, surprise, fear, anger, contempt, disgust, and sadness—these seven emotions, plus or minus two, are recognized from facial expressions by all human beings, regardless of their cultural background" (Fridlund, 1994, p. 192).

DEFINITION

Nonverbal is commonly used to describe all human communication events that transcend spoken or written words (Knapp, 1978; Knapp and Hall, 1992).

There are five categories of nonverbal communication study described by Knapp and Hall (1992):

- body motion or kinesic behavior, including gestures (i.e., emblems, illustrators, affect displays, regulators, and adaptors), posture, touching behavior, facial expressions, and eye behavior.
- physical appearance of the communicator, including artifacts (e.g., perfume, clothes, eyeglasses);
- paralanguage, including voice quality and vocalizations;
- proxemics, or use and perception of social and personal space; and
- the communication environment, or those elements that impinge on the human relationship but are not a direct part of it (e.g., the furniture, lighting, temperature; perceptions of time and timing).

Only the categories of kinesic behavior and proxemics will be considered in this chapter.

FUNCTIONS OF NONVERBAL COMMUNICATION

Nonverbal communication may serve the following purposes (Ekman, 1965; Knapp and Hall, 1992):

- **Repetition**
  Nonverbal communication repeats what was said verbally.
- **Contradiction**
  Nonverbal behavior contradicts what was said verbally.
- **Substitution**
  Nonverbal behavior substitutes for verbal behavior.
- **Complementation**
  Nonverbal behavior modifies or elaborates upon verbal messages.
- **Accentuation**
  Nonverbal behavior accents parts of the verbal message, much like underlining written words.
- **Regulation**
  Nonverbal behavior regulates the communicative flow between the interactants.

DEVELOPMENT OF NONVERBAL BEHAVIOR

Gates conducted a facial expression recognition study in 1923, and its findings have not been seriously challenged since then (Knapp, 1978). Laughter has been found to be identified by age 3, pain by age 5–6, anger by age 7, fear by age 9–10, and surprise by age 11. However, even by age 14, most did not yet recognize scorn.

Interaction distance (proxemics) seems to stabilize and closely reflect adult norms around third grade (Jones and Aiello, 1973). Young boys have been found to maintain 1.2–1.6 times the amount of space that females occupy during play (Harper and Sanders, 1975).

Gazing patterns during childhood have received very little attention. The two studies available (Ashear and Snortum, 1971; Levine and Sutton-Smith, 1973) disagree on whether there is a gradually increasing or decreasing trend in gazing behavior up to adolescence (Knapp, 1978). Adolescence represents a nadir for eye gazing (Knapp, 1978; Knapp and Hall, 1992).

Cultural guidelines for physical attractiveness are established by age 6 (Cavior and Lombardi, 1973). Peer popularity and physical attractiveness are highly correlated for students in elementary and secondary schools (Cavior and Donecki, 1973). Juvenile delinquents are rated lower on attractiveness (Cavior and Howard, 1973). Teachers tend to see attractive children as more intelligent, socially adept, and higher in educational potential even when unattractive children have similar academic performance records.

Females consistently score higher on tests of nonverbal sensitivity than do males. This is true from grade school through the middle twenties (Knapp, 1978). Decoding nonverbal cues has been found to be a gradually increasing skill from kindergarten until ages 20–30, at which time there is a leveling off (Dimitrovsky, 1964). In students, neither I.Q., Scholastic Aptitude Test (SAT) scores, class rank, nor scores on vocabulary tests have been found to have a significant relationship to nonverbal ability (Knapp, 1978).

Listener responses such as "mm-hmm" and head nods have been found to be nearly absent through fifth grade. By eighth grade, a dramatic increase in these listener responses is found (Dittman, 1972). Before that point, adults probably cannot expect much overt evidence that children are listening to them. In general, persons who learn to become good senders of nonverbal communication are also good receivers (Knapp, 1978).

TERRITORIAL ENCROACHMENTS

Violations of expectations about space and distance usually produce disruptive effects on interpersonal communication. Lyman and Scott (1967) have identified three types of territorial encroachments:

- **Violation**
  The unwarranted use of another's territory. This may be done with the eyes (e.g., staring at someone trying to eat in a restaurant), with the voice (e.g., talking too loudly in a library), or with the body (e.g., taking up two seats in a crowded bus; sitting too close to a stranger when there is plenty of room to spread out).
- **Invasion**
  The attempt to take over someone else's territory (e.g., armed invasion of another country; the act of a wife who turns her husband's den into a sewing room).
- **Contamination**
  The defilement of another's territory by what we leave behind (e.g., personal papers left in a desk or locker that was to be cleaned out for the next person).

1 ACTIVITIES TO ENHANCE NONVERBAL COMMUNICATION STRATEGIES

GENERAL NONVERBAL COMMUNICATION SKILLS

● Recognition of nonverbal communication pervasiveness and utility

●● Recognition of nonverbal communication effects on receivers

THE "COMMUNICATE NOTHING" ASSIGNMENT

PURPOSE

To illustrate how our bodies communicate continuously, even when nothing is said

Tell a student to stand up in front of you and/or the group. The assignment is "simple": Communicate nothing (i.e., do not say or do anything). Say to the student, "I'd like you to stand up and make sure you communicate nothing to us (me) for the next minute. Whatever you do, don't communicate."

After 20 seconds to a minute, have the individual sit down. Discuss:

- What was communicated?
- How do you think ____*(name)*____ felt? How do you know that? What clues did ____*(name)*____ give?
- Is it ever possible to communicate nothing?
- Have you ever attempted to communicate nothing at home or at school when you were feeling angry or depressed, but did not want to talk about it? Were you successful? What happened to your body language? Could you smile even when you felt really angry?

LEARNING STRATEGY

The adolescent demonstrates an awareness that the body always communicates, even when no words are spoken.

BODY LANGUAGE: PERCEPTIONS ABOUT RELATIONSHIPS

PURPOSE

To read body language and experience how it influences our perceptions of people

LEARNING STRATEGY

The adolescent demonstrates an awareness that the body always communicates, even when no words are spoken.

Collect pictures that illustrate two or more people. (This could be done as an assignment for students.) Have students divide the pictures into these categories:

- friends;
- enemies;
- neutral/indifferent; and
- cannot judge.

Discuss:

- What cues in the pictures determined how to sort the pictures? Why were some pictures not possible to judge?
- What other categories would be helpful to create?
- What other organizational systems could be used when sorting the pictures (e.g., happy/unhappy/neutral; intelligence above average/below average)?
- On what nonverbal cues are judgments being made when using other categories?
- Whom do you select as friends? Whom do you avoid? Whom would you choose to help with your homework? Why? Upon what nonverbal cues are decisions based?

In lieu of collecting pictures, participate in the activity by acting like a friend, an enemy, and an indifferent person. No words should be used. Have the student identify which category is being portrayed. This activity would also be appropriate for students who need a concrete experience before the picture-sorting task.

An additional task is to select two students and instruct one of them not to say anything, but to communicate friendliness, hostility, or indifference to the other student. Have observers decide what was communicated. Check with students:

- What message were you sending?
- What message did you want to send?
- Did the two messages (i.e., what you sent and what you wanted to send) match?

Note: Save the pictures collected for use in the "Distance Messages" activity (see page 227).

ALL TIED UP

PURPOSE

To recognize the utility of nonverbal communication by experiencing the absence of it

Find a paper bag that is large enough for both hands but small enough so that movement of the hands within the bag is limited. Tie the bag around a student's wrists. Require that the adolescent explain something without the use of gestures. If gestures are attempted, others will be alerted by the sound of the paper bag rustling. Have students take turns using the bag and explaining something (see the following tasks), or pair students and supply one bag to each dyad.

The following explanation tasks could be used:

1. How do you get from this school (or present location) to your home?
2. How do you get from this room to the gymnasium?
3. How is the game of football played?
4. How do you make toast?
5. How would you teach a child to bat a ball?
6. How is the furniture arranged in your living room at home?
7. How many rooms are in your house and how are they laid out?
8. Explain how you went about getting dressed this morning.
9. Explain how you would drive a car/ride a motorcycle.
10. Explain how you play your favorite video arcade game.

Discuss:

- Was it more difficult or less difficult to communicate with others when gestures were restricted? Why?
- What would have been easier to describe or explain if you could have used your hands?
- How did you change what you said based on not being able to use your hands?

LEARNING STRATEGY

The adolescent demonstrates an awareness that the body always communicates, even when no words are spoken.

TV STAR OBSERVATION

PURPOSE

To recognize how distinctive patterns of nonverbal communication contribute to one's identity

This activity can be an outside-of-class assignment while working on nonverbal communication skills.

Have students pick out a television star from a show they watch frequently and observe that person for a week or two. Instruct students to not reveal whom they are observing to anyone else. During the observation period, students should notice the following nonverbal communication characteristics of their selected TV stars:

- gestures used;
- body posture or stance;
- dress;
- facial expressions; and
- other mannerisms.

At the end of the observation period, have students share data and try to guess the stars. The sharing can be done through pantomime and/or verbal description (written or oral). Was it possible to guess everyone's star based only on the nonverbal data that was pantomimed or described? For those stars who were identified, what nonverbal clues were most important in determining the star? How have their distinctive nonverbal communication skills aided their careers?

LEARNING STRATEGY

The adolescent demonstrates an awareness that the body always communicates, even when no words are spoken.

SILENT MOVIES

PURPOSE

To determine meaning through observation of nonverbal communication

LEARNING STRATEGY

The adolescent demonstrates an awareness that the body always communicates, even when no words are spoken.

Find a short action movie or an action program on videotape. Turn off the sound and have students watch only the nonverbal cues. Discuss what might be going on based only on the action and background or contextual cues. Can students interpret what is going on? Can they determine the plot when only nonverbal information is used?

Watch the movie a second time, with sound. How accurately did the students interpret what they saw? Would it be possible to understand what is happening on TV if they could not hear any sound?

When movies were first made, they were silent. How do those first silent movies differ from our present movies? (If students have never seen a silent movie, try to obtain one. Frequently, they can be videotaped off the air, copyright permitting, by media personnel if such staff members are available.)

A variation of this activity is to use a foreign film without footnotes or to cover up the footnote area to prevent reading. Now students have both nonverbal and vocal (paralanguage) cues. Can students identify the plot? Was it easier to understand the silent movie or the movie that had some vocal cues?

RECOGNITION OF NONVERBAL COMMUNICATION THAT IRRITATES

PURPOSE

To discuss examples and effects of nonsupportive nonverbal communication

Discuss the three territorial encroachments listed in the opening of this chapter (i.e., violation, invasion, contamination). Have students generate examples of times when they have felt their space had been violated, invaded, or contaminated.

Explore with the students:

- What was your reaction?
- How did you feel?
- What did you want to say or do to the person who encroached on your territory?

If students have a difficult time generating examples, plot a violation, invasion, or contamination of their space to illustrate (e.g., attempt to sit too close to a student and then stare at the student while at that distance). Have them think of other students or teachers who exhibit occasional nonverbal communication that irritates them or others (e.g., the person who cracks knuckles in an otherwise quiet room).

Ask these types of questions:

- What do your parents do that encroaches on your territory?
- What do you do that encroaches on your parents' territory?
- What have been the consequences of such actions?

Then brainstorm what other types of nonverbal communication behaviors have been irritating to students (e.g., certain gestures, certain facial expressions). Discuss:

- Did the sender intend the message to be irritating? How did you know?
- Does it make any difference whether the intent was to irritate (i.e., did it have the same effect on the receiver)?

●●

LEARNING STRATEGY

The adolescent recalls the effects of nonverbal communication.

RECOGNITION OF NONVERBAL COMMUNICATION THAT SUPPORTS

PURPOSE

To discuss examples and effects of supportive nonverbal communication

Have students think of times when nonverbal communication has felt supportive (e.g., a smile from a parent, teacher, or friend; a pat on the back). Ask these questions:

- What do you like other people to do to let you know you are OK (e.g., smile, wink, touch)?
- What have you ever communicated nonverbally to others to let them know you like them?
- How can you tell if someone likes you or doesn't like you (when that person has not said a word to you)?

●●

LEARNING STRATEGY

The adolescent recalls the effects of nonverbal communication.

2 ACTIVITIES TO ENHANCE NONVERBAL COMMUNICATION STRATEGIES

KINESIC BEHAVIOR SKILLS

● Maintenance of eye contact/gazing behavior

●● Interpretation and expression of facial expression

●●● Use and understanding of body movements/gestures

GAZING AND DISTANCES

PURPOSE

To experience differences in eye contact due to differences in distance between participants

Eye contact is not always reliably distinguished from gazing at the area surrounding the eyes. Thus the phrase *mutual gazing* will be used to mean eye contact. In gazing, the eyes of the participants do not need to engage. In mutual gazing, the eyes of the participants do engage. Gazing and mutual gazing seem to increase as the distance increases between two people communicating with each other. There is usually less mutual gazing when two people are close together, especially if they are not well acquainted (Knapp, 1978; Knapp and Hall, 1992).

Set up a conversational pair. Direct the pair to talk for at least one minute. (Use topics suggested in many of the activities in Chapter 6, "Conversational Speech Strategies.") Assign a student to time the amount of gazing directed by Student A toward Student B, another person to time the amount of gazing directed by Student B toward Student A, and a third person to time the amount of mutual gazing ("eye contact"). If this many "timers" are not available, have conversational partners each time their own gazing by clicking on and off a stopwatch, or you can time mutual gazing. Begin with a distance of 5 feet between the conversational partners. Record all gazing times. Repeat the minute conversation with a distance of 10 feet. Time the gazing and mutual gazing as before and record. Repeat the conversation a third time with a distance of 2 feet. Time and record gazing.

Compare results. Under which condition did the most gazing and mutual gazing occur? Did it follow the rules explained in the opening paragraph of this activity? Kendon (1967) has found that people tend to look away when having difficulty encoding their language. Was that observed?

Average gazing and mutual gazing patterns reported by two studies are as follows:

	Gazing During Talking	Gazing During Listening	Mutual Gaze	Average Length of Mutual Gaze
Nielsen (1962)	38%*	62%	Not analyzed	Not Analyzed
Argyle and Ingham (1972)	41%	75%	31%	1.18 sec.

* Percentages reflect the amount of time spent gazing relative to total interaction time.

How closely did the times recorded match average gazing patterns as described above?

● LEARNING STRATEGY
The adolescent engages in socially appropriate eye contact during oral communication.

VARIABLES THAT INFLUENCE GAZING

PURPOSE

To discuss what gazing behavior can communicate to others and to explore figurative expressions that refer to gazing

Situations that result in more or less gazing behavior are summarized below (Knapp, 1978; Knapp and Hall, 1992). To facilitate discussion, write the following information where everyone can see it or provide printed copies by duplicating the page pertaining to this activity in Appendix I.

More gazing is predicted when

- you are female.
- you are physically distant from your partner.
- you are discussing easy, impersonal topics.
- you have nothing else to look at.
- you are interested in your partner's reaction.
- you like/love your partner.
- you are of a lower status than your partner. (This may be reversed for interactants who are from Asian or Native American cultures, in which looking at an elder or an authority figure can be regarded as a sign of disrespect.)
- you are trying to dominate or influence your partner.
- you are listening rather than talking. (This may be reversed for interactants who are African-American. LaFrance and Mayo [1976] found that African-Americans gazed more while speaking, while Caucasians gazed more while listening.)

Less gazing is predicted when

- you are male.
- you are physically close.
- you are discussing difficult, intimate topics.
- you have other relevant objects, people, events, or backgrounds to look at.
- you are not interested in your partner's reaction.
- you perceive yourself as a higher-status person than your partner. (Note the caveat mentioned previously.)

LEARNING STRATEGY

The adolescent engages in socially appropriate eye contact during oral communication.

- you have a mental disorder like schizophrenia.
- you are embarrassed, ashamed, sad, submissive, or trying to hide something.
- you are talking rather than listening. (Note the caveat mentioned previously.)

Discuss situations in which students have engaged in more or less gazing behavior. Have students ever been in a situation where someone gazes too much (i.e., to the point of feeling uncomfortable)? How did they feel? If students cannot report an experience, appoint a "starer" who gazes continually. How does the recipient feel? Have students experiment with too much gazing outside of the intervention session. Report results.

Many idiomatic expressions that involve eyes exist. What does it mean, for example, to say "he was making eyes at her"? (According to Knapp [1978], sources have confirmed an increase in eye behavior between two people who are seeking a more intimate relationship.) Discuss what it means to say:

- "She's all eyes."
- "Eyeball the situation."
- "We see eye to eye."

Can students think of other figurative expressions?

RECOGNIZING MEANINGS OF FACIAL EXPRESSIONS

PURPOSE

To interpret basic facial expressions by using contextual clues

Depending upon the source, anywhere from 6 to 10 basic classes of meaning can be communicated by facial expression (Knapp, 1978). They include:

happiness	disgust
surprise	contempt
fear	interest
anger	bewilderment
sadness	determination

Establish definitions with the students for each of the terms above, particularly for those listed in the right-hand column.

Point out that to interpret facial expressions correctly, gazing is necessary. Without gazing and mutual gazing, facial communication becomes impossible. Correct interpretation of facial expression is also augmented by noting the accompanying gestural and postural communication and by knowing the context in which the expression occurs.

With students, first model and then practice facial expressions for each of the meanings listed. To aid students initially, provide an imaginary context in which the expression could occur (e.g., "Now as you watch my face, imagine that I am opening a huge present on my birthday").

Obtain a series of photographs that illustrate various facial meanings. These may be clipped from magazines, but several excellent books include ready-made sequences of pictures or examples of expressions:

Ekman, P., Friesen, W., and Ellsworth, P. (1972). *Emotion in the Human Face: Guidelines for Research and an Integration of the Findings.* New York: Pergamon Press.

Fridlund, A.J. (1994). *Human Facial Expression: An Evolutionary View.* San Diego, CA: Academic Press.

Izard, C. (1971). *The Face of Emotion.* New York: Appleton-Century-Crofts.

Leathers, D. (1976). *Nonverbal Communication Systems.* Boston: Allyn and Bacon. (This text includes pictures and a description of the *Facial Meaning Sensitivity Test.*)

●● LEARNING STRATEGY

The adolescent appropriately decodes (interprets) and encodes (expresses) facial expressions.

Have students identify the emotions portrayed in the photographic collection. Do they agree? Could some pictures be interpreted in several ways?

To help decide facial expressions, provide assistance by calling attention to detail. Such details have been outlined for six emotions that seem to be the foundation for most expressions: surprise, fear, disgust, anger, happiness, and sadness (Ekman, Friesen, and Tomkins, 1971).

Share the following information with students. It is also printed in Appendix J for convenience.

SURPRISE

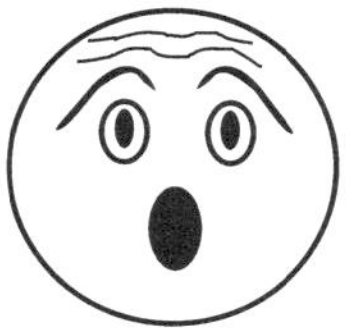

- Eyebrows are raised, curved, and high.
- Skin below the brow is stretched.
- Forehead has horizontal wrinkles all the way across.
- Eyelids are wide open; the sclera (white of the eye) shows above and below the iris.
- Jaw drops; lips and teeth are parted, but with no tension or stretching of the mouth.

FEAR

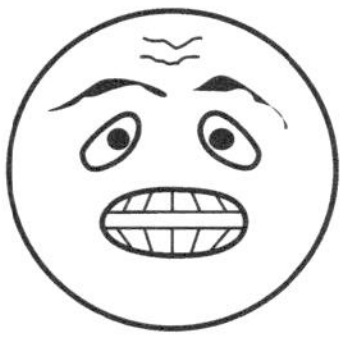

- Brows are raised and drawn together.
- Forehead has wrinkles in the center area only.
- Upper eyelids are raised; lower eyelids are tensed and drawn up.
- Mouth opens; lips are tense or stretched and drawn back.

DISGUST

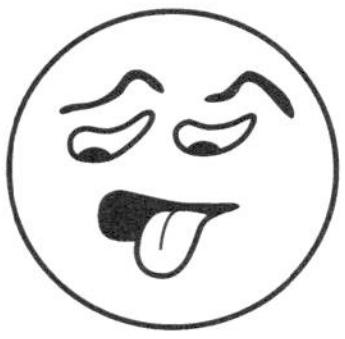

- Upper lip is raised; lower lip is raised and pushed up to the upper lip, or lowered and protruded slightly.
- Nose is wrinkled.

- Cheeks are raised.
- Brow is lowered; upper eyelids are lowered.

ANGER

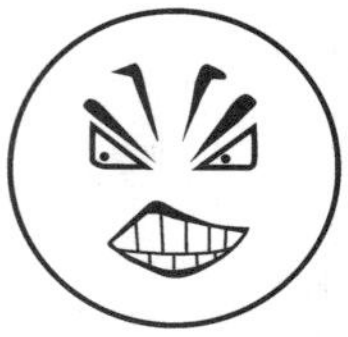

- Brows are lowered and drawn together; vertical lines appear between the brows.
- Eyes have a hard stare and may appear to bulge.
- Lips are either pressed together firmly or open, as if shouting.

HAPPINESS

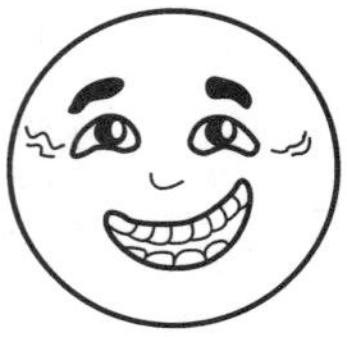

- Corners of the lips are drawn back and up (i.e., forming a smile).
- Cheeks are raised.
- Wrinkles extend down the nose to the outer edges beyond the lip corners.
- "Crow's foot" wrinkles go outward from the corners of the eyes.

SADNESS

- Inner corners of the eyebrows are drawn up.
- Inner corners of the upper eyelids are raised.
- Corners of the lips are down; the lips may be trembling.

Discuss with students how seeing facial expressions of the speaker aids understanding of the message. How is this different from talking with someone on a phone when the parties can't see each other? Point out how electronic mail (E-mail) users invented "smileys" or "emotions" (Sanderson, 1993) to fill in the missing facial expressions during communication. Some common smileys (meant to be viewed by tilting one's head 90 degrees to the left) are these:

:–)	:–(	:–|	:–,	:–J
said smiling	said frowning	disgusted	smirk	said tongue-in-cheek

EXPRESSING MEANING BY FACIAL EXPRESSION

PURPOSE

To express basic emotions by varying facial features

Assign a student to choose one of the six foundational emotions discussed in the previous activity (surprise, fear, disgust, anger, happiness, sadness) and communicate that emotion through facial expression. Can the other students accurately interpret the chosen emotion? Use the details listed in the previous activity to guide accurate encoding. Were all the details evident in the student's facial expression?

If possible, videotape students or take Polaroid pictures as they are engaged in making various facial expressions. Can they interpret meaning on subsequent days? Can one student or group of students accurately interpret emotions communicated by a different group of students (e.g., can students in Period 1 understand the emotions portrayed by students in Period 2, even though they did not observe each other while videotapes or photographs were being made)?

Using the same methodology, have students encode more difficult emotions facially, such as interest/lack of interest (boredom), understanding/bewilderment, and determination. Can facial details be outlined for these emotions? Attempt to specify several details of the eyes, brow, nose, and/or lips that are common to each emotion.

●●

LEARNING STRATEGY

The adolescent appropriately decodes (interprets) and encodes (expresses) facial expressions.

ENCODING AND DECODING EMBLEMS

PURPOSE

To interpret and express common gestures used in daily communication

Emblems are nonverbal acts that have a specific verbal translation known by most members of a communicating group; they can substitute for spoken language. Johnson, Ekman, and Friesen (1975) have identified American emblems that have been verified. To qualify as verified emblems, at least 70 percent of the encoders had to perform the action in a similar way, and at least 70 percent of the decoders had to match the emblem and the meaning and judge it to be used naturally in everyday communication (e.g., gestures used primarily for games like charades were not considered natural). Common emblems (e.g., yes, no, come here, be quiet, good-bye, I don't know) are able to be encoded and decoded by age 7 (Michael and Willis, 1968, 1969).

Have students take turns encoding and decoding the following emblems taken from Johnson, Ekman, and Friesen's (1975) work. When encoding, instruct the student to communicate the message without talking. When decoding, direct the student to tell the meaning of the emblem just observed. The following emblems could be put on separate index cards, then handpicked at random by students. They are reproduced in Appendix K for use during sessions. As each student takes his or her turn encoding, guide the other students to decode that emblem.

COMMANDS

1. Sit down beside me
2. Be silent/Hush
3. Come here
4. I can't hear you
5. Wait/Hold it
6. I warn you
7. Get lost (may be decoded as "Get out" or "Go away")
8. Follow me
9. Time to go (may be decoded as "What time is it?")
10. Stop

●●●

LEARNING STRATEGY

The adolescent uses and understands a range of gestures while communicating.

11. Go the other way (may be decoded as "No, not that way")
12. Got a cigarette? (may be decoded as "I want to smoke")
13. Look!
14. Take it away (may be decoded as "Go away" or "Get out of here")
15. Stay here

PHYSICAL STATE

1. I'm hot/It's hot (may be decoded as "hard work" or "close shave")
2. Hard work (may be decoded as "I'm hot" or "close shave")
3. Close shave (may be decoded as "I'm hot" or "hard work")
4. I'm cold/It's cold
5. I'm full (of food)
6. I've got a headache
7. I've got a toothache
8. I've got an earache
9. Tastes good
10. I am smart
11. How could I be so dumb?

INSULTS

1. To hell with you/Rejection
2. He's crazy/He's stupid
3. Shame on you

REPLIES

1. OK
2. No/I disagree
3. I don't know
4. Yes/I agree (may be decoded as "I like it")
5. Absolutely no! (may be decoded as "No way")
6. I dislike it
7. I promise (may be decoded as "Cross my heart")
8. Absolutely yes!
9. Hard to think about this/Thinking (may be decoded as "puzzlement")
10. I doubt it

AFFECT

1. I'm angry
2. I'm disgusted (may be decoded as "Something stinks")
3. I'm surprised
4. Whoopee/Hooray!

GREETINGS

1. Hello/Good-bye

UNCLASSIFIED

1. Me
2. You
3. Hitchhiking

4. Counting
5. Gossip (may be decoded as "talk, talk, talk")
6. Fighting
7. Peace/Victory
8. Good luck
9. Money
10. It's far away (may be decoded as "over there")
11. Suicide by gun (may be decoded as "shoot myself")
12. Finished (may be decoded as "That's enough")

Discuss the following with students:

- What other emblems not verified by Johnson, Ekman, and Friesen do you use? Do you think 70 percent or more of the people decoding the emblem could do so successfully?
- Observe friends, teachers, and parents for a day or two. What additional emblems did you notice?

The origins of 20 common gestures, many of them emblems, are explained in detail by Morris, Collett, Marsh, and O'Shaughnessy (1979) in their book, *Gestures: Their Origins and Distribution.* Most of the gestures were in use in Europe when Columbus set sail and can still be seen around the United States today (Morris et al., 1979). Some of the gestures that have persisted more than 500 years include the fingertips kiss, the cheek screw, the forearm jerk, and the chin flick. Discuss whether any of these emblems are used locally and, if so, what they mean.

ILLUSTRATORS: LINKING WITH SPEECH

PURPOSE

To discriminate when verbal and nonverbal messages match and when they fail to match

Illustrators are those nonverbal acts intimately linked to spoken discourse. Speech behavior and movement behavior are synchronized. Condon and Ogston (1966) have found that people suffering from various pathologies will manifest "out of sync" behavior in which there is a mismatch between the verbal and nonverbal messages being communicated.

Illustrate a mismatched message (e.g., scratching your head and looking confused while saying, "Yes, I understand. I know perfectly well what you mean"). Discuss why the message was mismatched. What was the nonverbal behavior communicating? What was the oral message communicating?

Discuss how we purposely mismatch messages on occasion to circumvent "speech taboos." For example, if a waiter in a restaurant is asked whether an entree is worth ordering, he may say, "It's OK" but grimace at the same time. The restaurant may forbid him to say anything negative about the food, but his facial expression gives him away. Guide students to trust the nonverbal message more than the spoken message when interacting with others.

Have students send matched or mismatched messages. Direct other students to observe, decode the nonverbal message, and decide if a match or mismatch has occurred. When messages are mismatched, discuss why the nonverbal behavior did not support the verbal behavior. How could the nonverbal behavior be changed to match the verbal message? How could the verbal behavior be changed to match the nonverbal message? Are there times when you would want to keep the mismatch because of "speech taboos"? The following verbal and nonverbal messages could be put on separate index cards for use in this activity. They are also reproduced in Appendix L.

SPOKEN MESSAGE *Examples:*	NONVERBAL MESSAGE
I hate doing math.	Matched
I can't stand it when my brother borrows my clothes without asking. I get so mad at him.	Mismatched (e.g., smiling)

●●●
LEARNING STRATEGY

The adolescent uses and understands a range of gestures while communicating.

	SPOKEN MESSAGE	NONVERBAL MESSAGE
1	I really like the new English teacher. She's nice to me and lets me get assignments in late.	Matched
2	I'm really not very comfortable. I ate a whole pizza by myself an hour ago.	Matched
3	I would like everyone to remain seated. It should be just a few more minutes to wait. I'm as impatient as you are.	Mismatched
4	The new math teacher is OK. You'd do all right in her class next year.	Mismatched
5	My aunt is so disgusting. She comes to our house and eats all our food and never brings any. She's already so fat she wouldn't have to eat for a month.	Mismatched
6	I wish we didn't have a test tomorrow. I'm really scared I'm going to flunk it.	Matched
7	I have a friend who never comes to see me any more. I really miss seeing her and wonder if I've done something to make her mad.	Mismatched
8	I'm so angry at my dad. He promised to buy me new shoes, and now he says he won't because I got home late last night.	Mismatched
9	I really like her new haircut. I wish I could get mine to look that way.	Matched
10	The class is so boring. I recommend you don't take it next year. You'd be sorry.	Mismatched
11	He said to take the second right turn to get to his house, but that took me down to the edge of the river. I was so lost and confused.	Matched
12	My brother always beats me at computer games, but I'll show him. I've really been practicing, and I'm going to beat him.	Mismatched

	SPOKEN MESSAGE	NONVERBAL MESSAGE
13	Mr. Roberts, the math teacher, always winks at Sue because he knows she has the answer. She's such a teacher's pet it's disgusting.	Matched
14	Mr. Smith's dog just had puppies. He's going to be gone this weekend and asked me to look in on them every day. I'm really interested in seeing the little puppies.	Mismatched
15	The grocery store window was broken yesterday, and they called my mom to see if I did it. I was with my friends near the store the night before, and they thought we did it. I can't believe they accused us.	Matched
16	My grandmother just went into the hospital. She has terminal cancer, and they don't think she's going to live much longer. She's the only adult who cares about me.	Mismatched
17	Mr. Jones said he'd give us two weeks to write our reports, and now he says he wants them Friday. I can't stand it when he does that.	Mismatched
18	I hate it when teachers tell us what to do and how to act even when we're not in their classes. They're so mean to us.	Mismatched
19	My mom just got a letter from her sister. She's coming to visit us for the whole month of December. Were we surprised! We don't even like her that much.	Matched
20	I keep getting strange phone calls. As soon as I answer the phone, the person hangs up. It happens all the time, especially late at night. I'm getting scared.	Matched

REGULATORS: NONVERBAL CONTROL

PURPOSE

To study how nonverbal communication affects turn taking during conversational speech

Regulators are nonverbal acts that maintain and regulate the back-and-forth nature of speaking and listening between two interactants. They tell the speaker to continue, repeat, elaborate, hurry up, become more interesting, give others a chance to talk, and so forth (Knapp, 1978; Knapp and Hall, 1992). Regulators also play a prominent role in initiating and terminating conversations.

For example, if head nods occur frequently in rapid succession, what is the message? ("Hurry up and finish!") What do slow, deliberate head nods that follow points made by the speaker mean? ("Keep talking," "I understand," "I like what you're saying!")

Speakers engage in two turn-taking behaviors. Discuss this information with students:

1. **Turn yielding**
   When speakers are finished, they want to give up their turn and expect the other person to start talking. This may be marked nonverbally by an extended unfilled pause, illustrative gestures that come to rest, body tenseness that relaxes, or gazing at the other person. If the listener does not perceive the turn yielding, the speaker conveys more explicit cues (e.g., touching the other person, raising and holding the eyebrows in expectation, saying "Well?").

2. **Turn maintaining**
   When speakers do not wish to yield their turn, one or more of these behaviors is likely to be seen: gestures will not come to a rest at the end of an utterance, voice loudness increases, filled pauses (e.g., "uh," "er," "um") increase and unfilled pauses decrease, and sometimes there is a light touching of the other person as if to say, "Hold on a bit longer. Then you can talk."

Listeners initiate two types of turn-taking behavior. Discuss this information with students:

1. **Turn requesting**
   When listeners do not have the floor and want to talk, they exhibit one or more behaviors. The most common is an upraised index finger, which almost seems to create a conversational "hole" in the speaker's stream of words (Knapp, 1978). There may be an audible inspiration of breath and a straightening and tightening of posture.

●●●

LEARNING STRATEGY

The adolescent uses and understands a range of gestures while communicating.

2. **Turn denying**

   When listeners receive turn-yielding cues from the speaker, they do not always want to talk. To communicate this, they exhibit one or more behaviors: maintain a relaxed listening pose, maintain silence, or gaze intently at something in the surrounding environment. More often, listeners exhibit behaviors that show continuing involvement in the content of the speaker's words but deny that a turn is being sought (e.g., smiling, head nodding, completing a sentence started by the speaker, briefly requesting clarification of the speaker's remarks, showing approval by appropriately placed "mm-hmm's" and "yeahs").

Using conversation topics listed for various activities in Chapter 6, set up speaker-listener pairs. Have students consciously and deliberately engage in the following turn-taking behaviors as much as possible during the conversation:

SPEAKER	LISTENER
Turn yielding	Turn requesting
Turn yielding	Turn denying
Turn maintaining	Turn requesting
Turn maintaining	Turn denying

Explore the following questions:

- Which combination(s) was/were most comfortable? Why?
- What happened when the speaker was yielding the turn while the listener was denying the turn?
- Which combination(s) felt competitive?
- Which combination(s) resulted in the most interruptions?
- How did you know if the speaker was trying to yield or maintain a turn? What cues were given verbally or nonverbally?
- How did you know if the listener was trying to request or deny a turn? What cues were given verbally or nonverbally?

ADAPTOR BEHAVIOR

PURPOSE

To identify adaptor behaviors and potentially isolate any that adolescents want to change

Behavioral adaptations are made in response to certain learning situations. Generally, people are not aware of nonverbal adaptors, but spoken feedback can heighten our sensitivity (e.g., when someone tells us, "Stop chewing your fingernails!"). Adaptors are associated generally with negative feelings. Self-adaptors increase as a person's psychological discomfort and anxiety increase (Ekman and Friesen, 1972). They can include picking and scratching, rubbing, covering one's eyes or mouth, and self-grooming behaviors.

Adaptor behaviors can be a source of distraction during interaction if excessively used (e.g., pushing up one's glasses repeatedly; tapping fingers on a desk). We all use adaptors in public some of the time. The issue is how frequently and whether they are interfering with communication.

To illustrate interference, talk with the students and continually clear your throat. Ask them to identify what the adaptor behavior was. Were they able to ignore the adaptor and focus on your spoken message?

Discuss with students others they know who use adaptors that are distracting to them during communication. Are all adaptors equally distressing or distracting to each person?

As the adult mediator, share any behavioral adaptations you have or have had in the past (e.g., you used to crack your knuckles). If the group psychologically can handle it, discuss adaptors used by students in the room. Is there an advantage to using fewer adaptors? Would any student like to reduce a particular adaptor? What strategy might be used to do this?

●●●

LEARNING STRATEGY

The adolescent uses and understands a range of gestures while communicating.

3

ACTIVITIES TO ENHANCE NONVERBAL COMMUNICATION STRATEGIES

PROXEMIC BEHAVIOR SKILLS

● Perception of space during communication

●● Use of space to communicate

COMFORTABLE CONVERSATIONAL DISTANCE

PURPOSE

To determine comfortable physical distance during conversational speech

Each of us seeks a comfortable distance during conversational speech. This distance will vary depending upon age, sex, cultural and ethnic background, setting, attitudes, emotions, topics, physical characteristics, personality, and our relationship with the other person (Knapp, 1978; Knapp and Hall, 1992).

Have students pair off, or appoint a speaker and listener while others observe. Place them 10 feet apart. Instruct them to talk about events at school and, while doing so, to move closer to each other until they reach a comfortable distance. Measure the distance. Repeat this process with one or more students and yourself. Measure the final, comfortable distance.

Compare measurement results. Were all the final distances equal? If not, what were some of the variables that caused it to change?

Have students determine into which distance zone(s), as identified by Hall (1969), their measurements fell:

1	Intimate Distance:	From body contact to 12–18 inches
2	Personal Distance:	Close—1½ to 2½ feet Far—2½ to 4 feet
3	Social Distance:	Close—4–7 feet Far—7–12 feet
4	Public Distance:	Close—12–25 feet Far—25+ feet

Did all students' measurements fall into the same zone? Give examples of when each of the distance zones would be used (e.g., close social distance used between a store clerk and customer; far social distance used between a receptionist and a client). Give examples of violations of distance zones.

What are possible consequences of violating distance zones?

LEARNING STRATEGY

The adolescent appropriately interprets and engages in shifts of distance between people as they interact with each other.

SPATIAL INTRUSIONS

PURPOSE

To discuss intrusions on space, particularly as the density of people increases

An opening activity in this chapter made reference to territorial encroachments. We each have a spatial distance we like to maintain from others. Unless we permit someone to enter that space surrounding our body, we feel intruded upon, violated, and perhaps outraged. If, for example, you climb on a city bus that is deserted except for one passenger and proceed to sit right next to that person, he or she will feel an intrusion. Nonverbally and/or verbally, you will have sent some messages. What will your messages be saying? Have students generate other examples of spatial intrusions.

As the density of people increases, we become forced to let other people intrude upon space we normally do not share. Consider sharing a crowded bus or subway, or waiting in a long line (queue) or a full elevator. Frequently, people are forced into the intimate distance zone without wanting to be there.

Discuss with students:

- How do you nonverbally communicate to someone else, "I know we're in intimate contact with each other, but I don't want to be here any more than you do"? What do you do with your eyes, hands, body?
- What would involve spatial intrusions in situations of high density where people are already crowded together?
- People in large metropolitan areas are often accused of being unfriendly—of not looking at other people or smiling. Why might this accusation be made, based upon what you know about each person's need for space? How do intrusions of that space occur? Do you think it's fair to call people in high-density areas unfriendly?
- Frequently, highly populated areas have a greater incidence of crime. Do you think lack of space contributes to the crime problem? Why or why not? What could be done to solve the problem?

LEARNING STRATEGY

The adolescent appropriately interprets and engages in shifts of distance between people as they interact with each other.

DISTANCE MESSAGES

PURPOSE

To perceive relationships among people based on physical distance and messages that are implied by that distance

In the activity "Body Language: Perceptions About Relationships" (see page 200), students were asked to categorize the pictures according to selected criteria (i.e., "friends," "enemies," "neutral/indifferent," "cannot judge"). Use the pictures gathered for this activity again for the following activity. Divide the pictures according to the above categories or others established earlier. After the pictures are grouped, have students study them for distance between people. How close or far apart are they positioned in the pictures? Are there any commonalities in the distances within a category (e.g., those standing at an intimate or close personal distance tend to be judged as friends more often than those standing at a social distance)?

Discuss how far students might stand from their receivers when communicating messages in the following situations. Distances may be reported either as number of feet apart or as those classified by Hall (1969) (i.e., intimate, personal, social, public). What does speaker/listener distance communicate in each of these situations? In the last tasks in this activity, students are asked to judge appropriate distances used by others.

1. You're asking a teacher about today's assignment. You have stayed after class to talk to her. How far apart will you stand?
2. You are yelling at your brother for losing a CD. How far apart will you be?
3. You are asking the school secretary if you can use the office phone. How far apart will you be?
4. You have gone up to the teacher's desk during a test to quietly ask a question. How far apart will you be?
5. You want to get your friend's attention in a crowded, noisy room. Right now he is on the other side of the room. When you say your friend's name, how far apart will you be?
6. Your mother is outside. She is wanted on the phone. When you let her know she has a call, how far apart will you be?
7. Your mother is outside. She doesn't hear very well. She is wanted on the phone. When you let her know she has a call, how far apart will you be?

●●
LEARNING STRATEGY
The adolescent uses space appropriately and effectively to communicate specific messages.

8. You go to your friend's house on Saturday to talk, only to discover he or she has the flu. You are not interested in becoming sick. You talk for just a few minutes. How far apart will you be?

9. The person with a locker next to yours is not someone you enjoy being around. He tries to start up a conversation. How far apart will you be?

10. You are asking your parent for permission to stay overnight with a friend. How far apart will you be?

11. You are telling a friend how much fun you have together and how much you like being with him or her. How far apart will you be?

12. You are reading a book to a 3-year-old. How far apart will you be?

13. You are walking down the street and ask a stranger directions to the nearest bus line. How far apart will you be?

14. You see a small child ahead of you on the sidewalk who is about to run out into a busy street to chase a ball. You try to stop the child by yelling, "Stop!" How far apart will you be?

15. A teacher is telling a student not to act that way in his classroom again. How far apart should they be?

16. A stranger has approached a girl by a bus stop to ask where the nearest McDonald's is. How far apart should they be?

17. Two students are talking about a third student. They are saying some rather unpleasant things within earshot of many other people. How far apart should they be?

18. A young man is asking a young woman if she would like to go to a movie. He really likes her but isn't certain she likes him. How far apart should they be?

19. A young man is trying to tell a young woman he no longer wants to date her. They have been going out for several months. How far apart should they be?

20. A mother is telling her young child never to hit his brother again. How far apart should they be?

DISTANCE GIVEAWAY

PURPOSE

To determine the content of a message through observation of physical distance

This activity requires three or more participants. Give each participant five red poker chips, five blue chips, five white chips, and written instructions that include one of the following:

You want all blue chips.

Give away red and white chips.

You want all red chips.

Give away blue and white chips.

You want red and blue chips.

Give away white chips.

Participants should not be aware of anyone else's instructions except their own. Instruct the adolescents that they may not use any spoken messages during this activity. Explain that they are to communicate their messages through nonverbal communication, primarily physical distance. They can be told that the activity is one of obtaining chips they want and giving others away. At your cue, give them several minutes to trade chips nonverbally. Direct participants to stand up for this activity so they are free to move around the room, since physical distance is one of the behaviors that will be discussed later.

After several minutes have elapsed, when it is clear that nobody wants white chips and everyone is avoiding them physically, end the exchange.

Guide students to determine what each other's instructions said. Did anyone want white chips? What nonverbal communication behaviors were noticed that sent the message "I do not want white chips" to the receiver? Discuss whether physical distance increased or decreased when participants were avoiding the white chips. If it increased, can students think of other examples when physical distance is used to communicate the message "I am avoiding you" or "I don't want you around" (e.g., walking down a different hall to avoid meeting someone we dislike; sending people to prisons)? Does greater physical distance always mean we are trying to avoid someone or something? Think of examples when being farther away does not necessarily mean "I'm avoiding you" (e.g., grown children who move away from home; a parent who needs to travel a great deal for his or her job).

●●
LEARNING STRATEGY
The adolescent uses space appropriately and effectively to communicate specific messages.

9

STUDY-SKILL STRATEGIES

STUDY SKILLS—LEARNING STRATEGIES

The major concerns, within the school setting, of adolescents with language disorders are academically related. While underlying cognitive or communicative problems may exist, students often perceive their problems as not meeting the "immediate" requirements of a course. Frequently, their requests for help are attempts to survive the upcoming exam or to finish tomorrow's assignment. In an effort to meet these needs, this chapter presents study-skill instruction as strategies for learning. Study skills can be learned and applied to all curriculum areas and all grade levels; they are also critical for lifelong learning.

Consistent with the philosophy of mediating "how to think" rather than "what to think," this method of teaching study skills lies within a "strategies for learning" format rather than following a tutorial approach. Guiding students in "how to learn" encourages them to become responsible for their own learning and therefore facilitates independent learning. Learning strategies give students the tools they need to improve their own learning abilities (Paul, 1995). Applied to the workplace, learning strategies can ensure success, and in the home setting they can help students cope with demands (Gall, Gall, Jacobsen, and Bullock, 1990). As the national dropout rate continues to rise and higher national standards are at the forefront of education, the need to include strategies for learning and studying is apparent.

EFFECTIVE STRATEGY USE

Hayes (1981, 1989) maintains that nearly everyone uses strategies for learning; the differences in the ways people perform in learning situations depends more on differences in their learning strategies than in their ability. Some learners make better and more extensive use of strategies than do others. Some use ineffective strategies and continue to do so because they do not know any alternative strategies. Effective strategy users have a repertoire of strategies and access particular strategies with flexibility (Jones, Palincsar, Ogle, and Carr, 1987). They know when to use a specific strategy and when to abandon it and select another. All types of students are able to learn strategies if provided with effective instruction (Brown, Campione, and Day, 1981; Holley and Danserau, 1984; Jones, Palincsar, Ogle, and Carr, 1987).

COGNITIVE PREREQUISITES

This approach to study-skill instruction requires metacognitive reflection; students reflect on their own thinking processes and learning strategies, and they reflect on how to use strategies to effectively facilitate their own learning. Gall, Gall, Jacobsen, and Bullock (1990) describe three metacognitive processes that are important to strategy learning:

1. knowledge of one's learning process (e.g., "I fall asleep during lectures");
2. selection of an appropriate strategy for a particular task; and
3. monitoring use of a strategy (e.g., "Will repeating this to myself help me to remember this information?").

IMPLEMENTING STUDY-SKILL INSTRUCTION

The way in which strategies are taught to students with disabilities significantly affects the degree to which students will change as learners (Schumaker and Deshler (1994/95). Seidenberg (1988) and Schumaker and Deshler (1994/95) suggest these steps to teaching strategies:

1. Introduce the strategy.
2. Explain why the strategy is relevant.
3. Describe the strategy, including steps to implement it.

4. Model use of the strategy—think aloud the steps.
5. Guide students in applying the strategy to low-difficulty materials; provide multiple opportunities.
6. Encourage students to self-evaluate their performance (and provide individualized feedback as well).
7. Guide the students in practicing on curricular materials (and provide more feedback).

These steps should be referred to as each of the study-skill strategies in this chapter are developed.

Additionally, Deshler and Schumaker (1986), who developed a learning strategies curriculum for students with learning disabilities at the University of Kansas, described three steps to ensure that transfer of a learning strategy occurs:

1. provide orientation—develop awareness of the context in which the skill can be used;
2. activate the strategy—apply the strategy to a variety of situations; and
3. encourage maintenance of the strategy—promote skill use through periodic checks.

These three steps are implemented in a mediational style of teaching in this chapter by (1) allowing students to generate examples of when the strategy might have been used in the past, how it was used, and whether its use was successful; (2) providing opportunities for applying the strategy (particularly by using current assignments to provide relevant opportunities); and (3) having students discuss where else the strategy might be used, not only in an academic setting but also at home or in the community or workplace.

Jones, Palincsar, Ogle, and Carr (1987) suggest assessing the student's use of learning strategies by having the student think aloud while attempting a learning task. This allows the educator to determine if the student is using a strategy and what the strategy is. Students who are reluctant to share strategies aloud can be interviewed and asked what advice they would give a younger student who wants to learn a similar task.

DELIVERING INSTRUCTION

Some schools infuse a study-skill component within the basic curricular areas (e.g., English courses might include note-taking skills). If this is the case, the professional is encouraged to reinforce the skills taught elsewhere within the curriculum. Students with language disorders often need more time for application, more feedback and support for successful use of the strategies, and more examples of where else to apply the strategies. The consistency in study-skill instruction will be helpful to the students. The professional should supplement what is taught elsewhere by adding new strategies, helping students explore their own learning styles and strategies, and offering guidance and support when students are not motivated to apply strategies.

Study attitudes and motivation should not be overlooked in this chapter, as students may have appropriate study strategies but not apply them effectively. (Refer to Chapter 2 for ideas to improve overall student motivation.) However, as stated earlier, students are often eager to learn new strategies because they desire to "survive" their current courses or assignments.

STUDY STRATEGIES

The following study strategies are presented in this chapter as a framework for study-skill instruction:

- recognition of learning style;
- efficient use of time;
- memory strategies;
- text organization;
- color coding of text and notes; and
- test-taking strategies.

Background information describing each of the strategies follows in the next six sections.

RECOGNITION OF LEARNING STYLE

In interviews of 80 high- and low-achieving students, high-achieving students reported arranging their physical setting to make learning easier more often than did low-achieving students (Zimmerman and Pons, 1986). Research on high-ability students also indicates that high levels of achievement result from allowing students to pursue topics of personal interest in their preferred styles of learning (Baum, Renzulli, and Hebert, 1994b). In a national study examining ways to reverse the cycle of underachievement, Baum, Renzulli, and Hebert (1994a) found that students may underachieve because of poor self-regulating strategies, but once allowed to pursue a self-determined goal in their preferred style of learning, they are more willing to discuss the learning strategies that caused the underachievement. Dunn, Dunn, and Price (1989) have shown that students with strong learning style characteristics achieve more successfully when the instructional conditions complement students' learning styles.

Learning styles within classrooms are as diverse and varied as the students themselves. While educators have recognized these varied styles, students have traditionally been expected to conform to the status quo. However, a growing body of information is available to educators regarding diagnosis and identification of learning styles and techniques for classroom implementation (Armstrong, 1987, 1993a, 1993b; Dunn, Beaudry, and Klavas, 1989; Dunn, Dunn, and Price, 1989; Gardner, 1993; Renzulli and Smith, 1978; Sternberg, 1994). These researchers/educators employ varying definitions of learning styles. For example, Armstrong (1993a) views a person's learning style as multiple intelligences put to work. Gardner (1993) sees each person as having learning style capacity in seven intelligence areas. Sternberg (1994) and Dunn, Beaudry, and Klavas (1989) define learning style as a preferred way of using abilities; the preferences are not good or bad, just different. This chapter explores the latter definition of learning style. In doing so, the authors would caution that you verify the students' "preferences" match the best conditions under which to study. For example, do students who prefer reclining in a soft chair to study also learn best that way? If not, effort should be spent explaining that "preferences" should align with the most efficient, effective conditions under which to study. Activities in this chapter encourage student awareness of personal learning patterns, preferences, or methods for effective learning. This awareness ideally translates into more efficient use of time—especially study time.

Dunn, Dunn, and Price (1989) have identified elements of learning style. They recommend that students identify preferences in the following areas:

1. Environmental
   - sound—quiet versus noisy background
   - light—bright versus dim light
   - temperature—environment warm versus cool
   - design—relaxed, casual design versus hard chair/table design
2. Emotional
   - motivation—eager to learn versus unenthusiastic
   - persistence—working to complete a task versus short attention span
   - responsibility/conformity—responsible versus irresponsible
   - structure—requiring well-defined limits versus little structure and supervision
3. Sociological
   - learning best—occurs alone versus in a pair (with an adult [a parent or a teacher], with a peer, or with a sibling) versus in a team versus varied
4. Physical
   - auditory strength versus visual strength versus tactual strength
   - perceptual strength versus kinesthetic strength
   - intake—requiring snacks, drinks while studying
   - time—studying best at certain time of day (e.g., morning, late morning, afternoon)
   - mobility—requiring mobility versus stationary position during studying

This chapter discusses how the professional can guide students in exploring these elements. Students' awareness of the best conditions under which their own learning takes place encourages them to be realistic during their study times. Arranging their study environments can make learning easier.

EFFICIENT USE OF TIME

Many students, but particularly students with learning problems, experience frustration keeping pace with daily classroom assignments, projects, extracurricular commitments, and home duties. This is evidenced by the all-too-frequent excuse students give regarding past-due assignments and projects: "I didn't have time to do it." That comment is most likely an indication of their difficulties with time management. Procrastination is a persistent issue with these students, often because they don't know how to break the task into manageable units and other times because they fear failure with the task. This chapter presents strategies for task analysis and time management.

MEMORY STRATEGIES

Memory strategies are activities people consciously perform to store information in long-term memory and to retrieve it (Marzano et al., 1988). Memory deficits are characteristic of students who have language disorders. Yet, on a daily basis, students are faced with memorizing large amounts of information, including spelling words, lists, procedures, dates, and facts. Without effective strategies for memorizing and recalling information, adolescents with language disorders are at an extreme disadvantage.

By adolescence, students are able to engage in metamemory discussions (i.e., discussions of memory knowledge and strategy use). Rafoth, Leal, and DeFabo (1993) report a distinct progression of independent strategy use by children. Rehearsal strategies (i.e., rote repetition) are displayed at age 6, semantic organizational strategies by age 10, and elaboration strategies (creating visual or verbal connections that add meaning to the material) by adolescence or later.

Daily Communication presents seven memory strategies for students whose recall techniques are not serving their needs. Some of the memory strategies assume that students have developed the underlying cognitive base for relating new information to old information and for classifying and categorizing ideas. Memory strategies are presented within the context of the problem or information needing memorization. Each strategy is introduced with an appropriate awareness activity. In all memory strategy activities, the group is involved in a discussion of strategies that could improve recall of given information. Often group members may have developed more appropriate techniques than those listed.

Information regarding memory functions and types of memory are also included within memory strategy activities. Teaching memory strategies as isolated skills is not recommended. However, facilitating memory strategies in relevant contexts using, for example, content area material (e.g., memorization of procedures for biology, dates for world history, vocabulary terms for English) has proven beneficial. Memory strategies support not only academic success, but also success in the home and workplace settings.

TEXT ORGANIZATION

By the time students have reached adolescence and especially middle school, the expectation is that they will acquire a good portion of their knowledge by reading, especially through text. *Text*, in this chapter, refers to all forms of required reading, such as textbooks, magazines, teacher handouts, and reference books. The student's task is to decipher the text's organization to learn effectively.

The organization of each type of text varies. However, most contain some of these predictable parts: table of contents, index, glossary, bibliography, chapter titles, and sometimes appendices. Within text, authors use headings, subheadings, and other structural elements to help students follow the material. These elements highlight and organize the information presented. For example, a chapter title cues students about what to expect, giving them a mental set about what the chapter includes. Students need to know how to use this mental set to help assimilate the information in the chapter (Gall, Gall, Jacobsen, and Bullock, 1990).

Too often, the organization of text and the methods for using that organization seem so obvious to experienced adult readers that they assume adolescents know how to use text efficiently. This chapter's activities facilitate understanding of the organizational structure of text. They do not, however, address understanding of text structure known as "story grammar." Identification of story grammar elements (e.g., setting, characters, problem, resolution) has been shown to improve reading comprehension of narrative text but is not addressed in this chapter on study strategies.

COLOR CODING OF TEXT AND NOTES

A well-known study strategy with which most students and adults are familiar is color coding—the highlighting of main ideas and relevant details in reading materials or student notes. There are various perceptual systems used for coding information, such as underlining, circling, and marking with asterisks, all whose main purpose is to separate the parts from the whole, making important information "stand out." Color coding is a visually apparent system. It's an efficient study tool, and it's easy to learn.

Underlining or highlighting important elements of text or notes while reading stimulates active reading and active searching for important content. Research has shown that highlighting information is effective in improving test-taking performance when relevant information is highlighted (Fowler and Barker, 1974; Schnell and Rocchio, 1975). The critical step in color coding is deciding which information is important enough to highlight; color coding will not be effective if students choose information that is irrelevant to the task (Gall, Gall, Jacobsen, and Bullock, 1990). Without instruction in identifying relevant elements of texts or notes, students who have language disorders frequently color or mark information continuously, with little or no differentiation between important points and supporting, less important details. While color coding as a strategy assumes students have underlying classification skills in separating parts from wholes and main ideas from supporting ideas, the activities in this chapter facilitate identification of relevant information.

TEST-TAKING STRATEGIES

The majority of classes in which students who have language disorders participate will most likely require examinations to indicate concept mastery. Not only are adolescents expected to listen, sort relevant from irrelevant information, take notes effectively, and manage study time efficiently, but they are also expected to communicate their mastery of class information satisfactorily via performance on written examinations.

Observation of students' test-taking strategies suggests that some of the following occur in relation to test taking:

1. inadequate preparation gives way to cramming;
2. material studied is not included on the exam;
3. material studied is not relevant;
4. the student experiences "blocking" (inability to retrieve information studied);
5. time runs out before the exam is finished; or
6. test vocabulary terms are misunderstood or misinterpreted.

Tutoring students to survive exams is not advocated. Rather, a systematic, planned approach to preparing for and taking exams is recommended as a way to improve students' mastery and communication of class objectives. Study strategies discussed throughout this chapter will ultimately benefit students at test time, but specific strategies are also included to address test taking.

ACTIVITIES TO ENHANCE STUDY-SKILL STRATEGIES

● Recognition of personal learning style

●● Description of ideal study environments

●●● Analysis of time use

●●●● Efficient management of time

●●●●● Use of strategies for remembering information

●●●●●● Effective use of text

●●●●●●● Use of color coding as a strategy

●●●●●●●● Improvement of test performance

EXPLORATION OF SELF: LEARNING STYLE

PURPOSE

To explore personal learning styles and patterns

Duplicate the "Learning Style Questionnaire" form found in Appendix M (adapted from *Language Disorders in Older Students* by Larson and McKinley [1995]), one per student and one for yourself. This questionnaire considers the learning style elements described by Dunn, Dunn, and Price (1989) (refer to page 235).

Inform students that this is not a test and that there are no right or wrong answers. Emphasize the importance of considering how learning "best" occurs. For example, a student might like to play music while studying, but in reality learning "best" occurs for this student in a quiet environment. (The reverse might also be true.) To help students determine preferred learning styles, direct them to think of an activity in which success is of great importance to them (e.g., studying for the written portion of the driver's license exam). Tell them to write this important subject on their questionnaires and to anticipate studying for this subject when they consider their learning style preferences.

Direct students to complete the questionnaire. Read the directions and questions to the students. Rephrase questions or answer students' questions if necessary as you progress through the questionnaire. Guide students in knowing when to rank items versus when to check items. Emphasize that students should answer as honestly as possible.

Be sure to also complete the questionnaire yourself, as this information will be important in a later activity that includes discussing matches and mismatches of teaching and learning styles.

Once students have completed their questionnaires, have them share their learning style self-studies with the group or privately with you. Guide students to use the information obtained from the self-studies throughout this chapter.

● LEARNING STRATEGY

The adolescent recognizes his or her personal learning styles.

CLASSROOM LEARNING STYLE PATTERNS

PURPOSE

To become aware of diverse learning styles of classmates

A survey of learning styles within your classroom could further students' awareness of the diverse learning preferences among their peers. Assign each student a preference element to survey. Have students generate questions to ask their classmates. Direct students to tally the data on a blank "Learning Style Questionnaire" form (duplicate from Appendix M).

Create overhead transparencies of the "Learning Style Questionnaire" form. Have students share their survey results, and tabulate the results on the displayed transparencies. (Save these transparencies for use in the "Ideal School Study" activity on page 242.) Discuss the patterns observed:

- Were there any surprises?
- Are any two students' identified preferences identical?

LEARNING STRATEGY

The adolescent recognizes his or her personal learning styles.

IDEAL HOME STUDY

PURPOSE

To create an ideal study environment at home

Based on information from each student's completed "Learning Style Questionnaire" form, guide them to analyze their ideal study setting at home. Have them add this information to the "Ideal Studying at Home" form in Appendix N. Then direct students to analyze how they currently structure their study environments and add this information to the form as well.

Are any "ideals" in conflict with what is possible in their home settings? Encourage students to consider constraints that exist within their homes. Given these constraints, what changes can or can't be made? Present the following example to the students:

> Kristin realizes that she studies best in a quiet environment with a comfortable, casual design. The most productive learning for her might occur when sitting comfortably on the couch, provided that the room is quiet. However, Kristin has a sibling who plays her boom box in the same room in which Kristin is studying. Therefore, she will need to find another comfortable place to study or ask her sibling to move or wear headphones.

Present other situations to the students, such as the following, and have them decide how the constraint could be overcome:

> Monroe knows he needs an adult to set well-defined limits to help him get an assignment done. His mother usually reminds him to study at night, but now she has a night job. Monroe will need to set his own limits. What are his options?

> Marcus checked "drink liquids" on his learning style questionnaire because he likes to sip Coke when he's thinking. He knows that caffeine makes him less attentive to the task. How else can he fill his need to "drink liquids" while studying?

Encourage the students to compare their current study environments to their "ideal" study environments. Have students complete their "Ideal Studying at Home" forms by placing an X in the "Make a Change" column if the element can be changed at home and then completing the statement referring to changes they will make. Challenge them to make as many changes in their study environments as possible and discuss the reasons for these changes. Encourage them to share and discuss their "Learning Style Questionnaire" and "Ideal Studying at Home" forms with their parents or caregivers.

●●
LEARNING STRATEGY
The adolescent will describe an "ideal" study environment.

IDEAL SCHOOL STUDY

PURPOSE

To create an ideal study environment at school

Present the transparencies from the "Classroom Learning Style Patterns" activity (see page 240). Using the tabulated information, extrapolate the ideal study classroom environment for students in the group.

Critique the present classroom environment:

- What changes would students recommend be made in your room? In study hall? In other study areas at school?
- Which possibilities are realistic?
- What changes might students make in their own learning behaviors?

Sternberg (1994) recognizes that mismatches occur between the way a student thinks and learns and the way an educator teaches the course. The mismatch can place students at a disadvantage, since Sternberg has found that students whose learning styles more closely match those of their teachers receive better grades. Explore this concept with students.

Share your own learning-style analysis with students. Then discuss the following:

- Does your learning style match your teaching style?
- What mismatches exist between your teaching style (i.e., how the class is taught) and the students' learning styles?
- Which learning styles are being accommodated in the classroom? Which are not? Which additional learning styles could be accommodated in the classroom?

Discuss strategies students might use to adjust to other classroom environments and teaching styles that do not accommodate their learning styles.

●●
LEARNING STRATEGY
The adolescent will describe an "ideal" study environment.

ANALYSIS OF TIME USAGE

PURPOSE

To become aware of group time usage

●●●
LEARNING STRATEGY
The adolescent will analyze present use of time.

A common approach to analyzing how one's time is spent is to track the use of time for a day or a week. Since adolescents most often have multiple ongoing activities in a day or in a week, expecting a weeklong recording of time use may be unrealistic and may add to an already frustrating situation. Monitoring and recording time use in one day is realistic and tends to be enlightening to students.

Begin this activity by analyzing a class period in a school day, preferably the time period in progress. Appoint a pair of students to measure the time use. Instruct one to use a stopwatch or clock to track time and the other to record the activity. Calculate the minutes spent getting to the class, waiting for all students to arrive, taking attendance, gathering materials for class, accomplishing actual instruction, completing "off-topic" discussions, putting materials away, etc. As a variation to this activity, videotape a segment of a class period, then calculate the use of time as a group.

Analyze the time use during your next class session. As a group, discuss the following:

- How was each minute used? Was each minute used effectively?
- What percentage of time could have been managed better? What could be done to make better use of class time?

Have students imagine that every well-spent minute in a day is worth $1. Would they carefully plan how they would spend their time, considering there are 1,440 minutes in a day?

The following fantasy, adapted from Bragstad and Stumpf (1982), stimulates students' thinking about the merits of time management:

> Imagine that a friend deposits $1,440 into your bank account each morning. You have 24 hours in which to spend the money, with no balance carried over from day to day. Any money that you fail to use will be cancelled at the end of that day. What would you do? Would you carefully plan how to spend $1,440 each day or would you spend the money impulsively? No doubt you would want to use all of it. (p. 37)

Bragstad and Stumpf go on to explain that students have a daily account in a bank called "Time." Each day they are given 1,440 minutes of time to use. Whatever they have not invested well is lost forever. They cannot go back to make up or to reuse time from the past and cannot draw against tomorrow's deposit. Only today's minutes may be used.

Given this explanation, how would students spend their time? Would they plan better use of their time?

WHERE DOES THE TIME GO?

PURPOSE

To evaluate the student's present use of time

LEARNING STRATEGY

The adolescent will analyze present use of time.

Once the students are familiar with measuring time use, distribute a schedule for recording time-use data for a day. A sample time schedule is provided in Appendix O. Direct students to complete this schedule on a typical day.

TIME	ACTIVITY	MINUTES
7:00–7:30	*get up, shower, get dressed*	*30*
7:30–7:45	*eat breakfast*	*15*
7:45–7:55	*wait for the bus*	*10*
7:55–8:15	*get on bus, ride to school*	*20*
8:25–9:15	*attend 1st period class*	*50*
9:15–9:20	*go to next class*	*5*
9:20–10:10	*attend 2nd period class*	*50*

When completed, the total minutes should equal 24 hours. Time unaccounted for would indicate free time. Guide students in completing the time schedule by categorizing their activities and totaling the number of minutes for each category. An example follows:

ACTIVITY CATEGORY	MINUTES PER DAY	TOTAL MINUTES PER DAY
sleeping	*480*	*480*
getting ready	*30*	*30*
eating	*15, 30, 30, 30*	*105*
going to and from classes	*20, 20, 5, 5, 5, 5, 5, 5*	*70*
sitting in class	*50, 50, 50, 50, 50, 50, 50*	*350*
studying	*15, 20, 60*	*105*
doing chores/duties	*60, 25, 25*	*105*
waiting for bus	*15, 15*	*30*

Total minutes in a day 1,440

Minus total minutes accounted for *1270*

Total minutes free time *170*

Direct students to subtract the total time accounted for from 1,440 minutes to determine their free time in a day. Multiply that number times 5 to calculate free time in a schoolweek. Contrast and compare the variety of time usage among students.

Discuss the following:

- What percent of the day was spent on free-time activities? On necessary activities such as eating or dressing? On study time?
- How do the data compare to what the students believed to be true regarding their management of time? What changes could take place regarding use of time?
- Tell each student to identify the blocks of free time in his or her schedule. The authors acknowledge that free time is important. It's a time to relax—a time each day that is free of obligations, a time just for ourselves. This free time also provides flexibility. On days when there is much to be accomplished, free time can provide the scheduling flexibility needed to prevent forgoing necessary activities such as sleeping, daily chores, etc.

Repeat this activity as necessary for assessing use of time. Challenge students to compare improvements made in the management of their schedules over time.

MANAGING TIME

PURPOSE

To discuss and develop time management and planning strategies

●●●●
LEARNING STRATEGY
The adolescent will manage his or her time efficiently.

Distribute 10 blank three-by-five-inch index cards to each student. Ask students to write 10 assignments (one per card), including the subject area and date due, that they have completed or are to complete within the next few weeks. The following are example assignments:

> Math—pp. 243–244, problems 1–25, due tomorrow
>
> Science—answer questions 5–10, end of chapter 6, by tomorrow
>
> Health—worksheet due in 2 days
>
> Physical Education—study for basketball exam next Thursday
>
> Social Studies—oral report on the Civil War due in 1 week
>
> English—book report due in 4 days
>
> Reading—read *Sounder*, pp. 39–78, for tomorrow
>
> Science—endangered species project due in two weeks

Shuffle and place the index cards face down on a table or desk. Direct students to take turns drawing two cards each. After reading the assignments, discuss how students would manage their week to complete the assignments on time. Challenge students to estimate the amount of time each activity might take and discuss variations in student responses.

- What causes activities to take more or less time for each of us?
- Do assignments with many problems necessarily mean the assignment will be harder?
- Do more problems mean the assignment will take more time? Given two algebra problems or 50 simple addition problems, which would take longer?
- Should assignments requiring the most time be done first or last?

Discuss various approaches to completing assignments. For example, doing smaller assignments first might reduce the number of activities to be completed but may not leave enough time to complete a more time-intensive project. On the other hand, using short blocks of study time (15 minutes, 5 minutes, etc.) may help get the shorter assignments out of the way. What kinds of assignments would students consider to be priorities? How can they determine which tasks are priorities?

Continue the process of having students draw cards, now drawing three more and then four more. Have them describe the specific times in their daily schedules when these assignments could be completed.

For long-term projects, discuss how the project could be dissected into smaller tasks and when each task could be completed. Demonstrate how to plan a larger project by working back from the due date.

Emphasize the consequences for not planning time effectively. Assignments that are completed five minutes before class present more opportunity for error (due to work under pressure) and less opportunity for checking one's own work. Making more errors may necessitate making corrections later, which will require time that could have been spent freely or used to complete other assignments. The cycle itself devours time—especially free time.

Extend this activity by scheduling the assignments on a monthly calendar plan (see the "Organizational Plans" activity on page 251 and Appendix P for a blank form). Simplify this activity by having students use their time schedules completed in the "Where Does the Time Go?" activity.

Save the assignment cards for use in the "Expecting the Unexpected" activity on page 249.

EXPECTING THE UNEXPECTED

PURPOSE

To discuss and develop flexibility in the management of time

This activity requires use of the assignment cards prepared in the "Managing Time" activity, page 247.

Have each student complete a projected time schedule (see Appendix O) for the day. Then, as a group, generate commonly used excuses for late work or incomplete activities. Write these excuses where everyone can see them. The following are examples:

- Your mother informs you of Aunt May's birthday party tonight.
- Your brother is ill; you'll have to wash dishes tonight.
- You have a doctor's appointment after school.
- Your grandmother is stopping by tonight.
- You took a nap and overslept.
- You have to go to a funeral tonight.
- You had an unexpected shopping trip for new shoes.
- You had a computer meeting after school.
- Your school basketball team won the conference game; the regional game is tomorrow night. Tonight you need to help make signs for it.
- You lost a filling and must see the dentist this afternoon.
- You need to stop to pick up groceries for your mom on the way home.
- Your father wants the garage cleaned now!
- Your science teacher requires you to watch a two-hour Jacques Cousteau special tonight.
- Your parents need you to help clean the house.
- You feel ill most of the night.
- A friend calls on the telephone and you talk for a hour.

●●●●
LEARNING STRATEGY
The adolescent will manage his or her time efficiently.

Given the students' projected schedules for the day, have them each choose an assignment card and describe when in their day they will complete their respective assignments. Then, present an unexpected schedule change (i.e., the excuses generated and listed). Guide students in estimating the amount of time the interruption (i.e., unexpected schedule change) might take. What effect will the schedule change have on the students' schedules? How will they adjust their schedules to accommodate the assignments needing completion?

Challenge students to generate at least two alternatives for adjusting to the change. Are there small blocks of free time, such as a bus ride, time between classes, etc., that can be used more efficiently when a schedule is "tight"?

ORGANIZATIONAL PLANS

PURPOSE

To discuss and choose a plan for organizing time

Students have found the following time-management plans to be helpful in developing efficient study habits. A blank form for each system can be found in Appendices P, Q, and R. Introduce these management systems to students. Then discuss as a group or individually with each student which options might meet students' individual needs. Students often need to use a combination of these options to manage their time efficiently.

Students may also develop their own systems for managing and organizing time (e.g., assignment notebooks, appointment books) that are just as efficient as the following. They should be allowed to adapt these systems or others to meet their needs. The authors advocate that the student become the "responsible party" in managing time and in choosing a plan that will work. The authors strongly recommend that each student use an organizational notebook or folder that includes his or her chosen time-management plan.

MONTHLY CALENDAR

SUNDAY	MONDAY	TUESDAY	WEDNESDAY	THURSDAY	FRIDAY	SATURDAY
	1	2	3	4	5 *dentist 5:00*	6
7	8	9 *exam Soc. St.*	10	11 *B.B. practice*	12 *B.B. practice*	13
14	15 *B.B. practice*	16 *B.B. practice*	17 *science project due*	18 *B.B. practice*	19 *B.B. practice*	20
21	22 *B.B. practice*	23 *B.B. practice*	24	25 *B.B. practice*	26 *school play* *B.B. practice*	27
28	29	30	31			

The monthly calendar allows students to see the gestalt of monthly events, projects, assignments, and exams. It allows students to plan for upcoming exams, reports, etc. The calendar might be kept inside an organizational folder

●●●●
LEARNING STRATEGY

The adolescent will manage his or her time efficiently.

or a notebook that the student carries to all classes. Model the process of jotting exam dates and project deadlines on this calendar for a week or two. Then frequently monitor the students' use of this calendar, providing feedback for as long as necessary to develop a consistent and habitual system for recording schedule information.

WEEKLY ASSIGNMENT SCHEDULE

WEEKLY ASSIGNMENT SCHEDULE

Name ____________ Week of ____________

Subject ____________

Teacher ____________

MONDAY	TUESDAY	WEDNESDAY	THURSDAY	FRIDAY

The weekly assignment schedule requires students to enter assignments due each day. A separate assignment schedule is completed for each course or class each week. The schedule should be placed in an organizational notebook or folder the student carries to each class.

"TO DO" LISTS

(adapted from Bragstad and Stumpf, 1982, 1987)

The "to do" list encourages students to establish priorities. To set priorities, students should identify activities that interfere with accomplishing their tasks (e.g., watching TV) and consider the priority of such activities in relation to the other tasks they want to accomplish.

To complete the list, students first write tasks to be accomplished on the back of the "to do" list. Then they decide if the task is an A—a must do immediately task, a B—an important task but one that could wait a little while, or a C—a task that could be postponed or not done at all. Tell students to list each task in the appropriate columns on the "to do" list. All A activities should be completed before B and C activities.

Students can check off tasks as they are accomplished. This list helps students organize activities that are most important so they receive the most time and attention. The "to do" list can also be maintained on a daily or weekly basis.

"TO DO" LIST		
A (MOST IMPORTANT)	**B**	**C** (LEAST IMPORTANT)

"TO DO" LIST					
	MONDAY	**TUESDAY**	**WEDNESDAY**	**THURSDAY**	**FRIDAY**
A					
B					
C					

MEMORY CAPACITY

PURPOSE

To identify the types of memory, the human capacity for remembering, and the causes of forgetting

LEARNING STRATEGY

The adolescent will use a variety of strategies for remembering information.

Adolescents should be made aware of the capacity of memory and the variables that determine that capacity. Discuss information regarding memory research such as the following.

TYPES OF MEMORY

Several types of memory have been described in research literature:

Sensory Memory

Sensory memory holds images for a quarter of a second (Hayes, 1981, 1989). It has large capacity but retains messages for a brief duration (Parente, 1992). Messages, received through our sensory system, are stored for very short periods of time and then lost unless attention is called to them. For example, in a cafeteria setting, many voices surround the students; all enter their sensory memories. Students may have no idea what the voices are saying unless they consciously pay attention to them. Giving attention to a message transfers it to short-term memory, where it can be kept by repeating or rehearsing the message. Without rehearsal, however, this message is lost within a few seconds.

By the age of 6 years, children spontaneously display application of rehearsal memory strategies. They begin rehearsing three or four items at a time (Rafoth, Leal, and DeFabo, 1993).

Short-Term Memory

Short-term memory holds seven (plus or minus two) numbers, letters, or "chunks" for a short period of time (approximately 15 seconds) until the importance of each is determined (Miller, 1956). The determination needs to be made quickly, because short-term memory has limited capacity and the continual influx of new information deletes anything not consciously held (Hayes, 1989; Sylwester, 1995).

The capacity of short-term memory is limited to a half dozen "chunks" (or units) of familiar information (Sylwester, 1995). Combining smaller bits of information into larger units by identifying similarities, differences, and patterns can increase short-term memory capacity.

Long-Term Memory

Long-term memory holds large quantities of information for an extended time. Long-term memory can hold factual, label-and-location information (e.g., the name of your dog) or automatic skills or procedure sequences (e.g., how to ride a bike or use the computer keyboard) (Sylwester, 1995). Information can be held in long-term memory for years and years. Its capacity is unknown (Parente, 1992).

REMEMBERING INFORMATION

Effective studying is, in essence, the process of transferring information from short-term memory to long-term memory (Gall, Gall, Jacobsen, and Bullock, 1990). Transferring information from short-term memory to long-term memory requires more than "rehearsal" strategies; it requires categorizing information, asking questions about it, making associations, or creating images.

Chi (1978) compared the memory performance of young children (average age 10 years) with college students on a short-term memory task for remembering long strings of numbers. It did not surprise Chi to see that the college students performed better than the younger children by remembering an average of eight numbers per trial (the younger children remembered only six). Using these same groups of college students and young children, Chi also examined their performance in remembering chess pieces arranged meaningfully on a chess board. The younger children remembered 9 pieces on average, while the college students remembered only 5½. The younger students were well-versed in playing chess, and the college students did not play the game. Chi's research illustrated that memory is not just the ability to store information, but that the ability to remember also depends on previous knowledge or information previously acquired.

Research has defined *memory* as a thinking strategy because the greater the extent of thinking about something, the more likely it will be remembered (Jenkins, 1975). Researchers have also shown that it doesn't take much to trigger a strong memory, but it may take a lot of effort to recall a weak memory (Sylwester, 1995). Our brain is efficient at recalling and using memories that have important personal meaning and less efficient at remembering important but context-free facts and skills (which is most like the memory required in academic situations).

FORGETTING INFORMATION

Information stored in long-term memory can be forgotten for a number of reasons (Devine, 1981):

- **Decay Through Disuse**
  Learning is lost with the passage of time.

- **Interference Effects**
  Proactive interference occurs when things learned earlier interfere with things learned later (learning how to drive a five-speed auto is complicated by your memory of driving a car with an automatic transmission); retroactive interference occurs when things learned later interfere with things learned earlier (after learning your gym locker combination, you forget your street locker combination).

- **Motivated Forgetting**
  Some information is forgotten because learners choose to forget it (e.g., because the information is unpleasant or painful).

- **Processing Breakdown**
  The information has not been rehearsed enough to place it into long-term memory, not enough cues are available to locate the information in long-term memory, or the coding system is ambiguous.

Reviewing, overlearning, and frequently using information can reduce the effects of interference. Memory strategies included in this chapter address interference effects and processing breakdowns.

Present the following items to students. Challenge them to determine the type of memory that would store the information and how strong the memory might be:

1. the names of the months in a year;
2. the meaning of a new word;
3. how it feels to have a toothache;
4. background noises in a classroom;
5. your own phone number;
6. how to write;
7. an animal sound at the zoo;

8. the kinds of cars you saw on your way to school;
9. your name;
10. the singing of a bird;
11. a foreign word;
12. the address of a friend;
13. the color of your eyes;
14. how to operate a car;
15. how to peel a banana;
16. how it feels to touch a hot burner;
17. the names of plants in your home;
18. the name of a new person in your class;
19. how to speak English; and
20. the procedure for dividing numbers.

Following in this chapter are activities to facilitate use of several memory strategies. When deciding which memory strategy to apply, knowing how a student will eventually need to remember and use the information is helpful (Gall, Gall, Jacobsen, and Bullock, 1990). For example, a student might apply a rehearsal strategy to remembering specific terms for biology if the test requires matching terms and definitions. If the biology test requires an essay describing steps in a procedure, the student might apply a mnemonic memory strategy. Discuss this concept as a group.

Remind students that a single strategy can be used to remember information or a combination of strategies can also improve performance on a memory task (Kaniel, 1995).

AWARENESS OF MEMORY USE

PURPOSE

To develop an awareness of personal memory strengths and weaknesses and to discuss the effects that attitude, interest, and biological factors can have on memory

Students should be made aware of strategies that can improve their concentration and attention, thus improving their memory of information. Parente (1992) suggests the following strategies for improving concentration and attention:

- **Control Your Diet**
  Stimulants, especially caffeine products, tend to hinder learning, though they might improve physical performance.
- **Control Internal Distractions**
  Both physical and emotional distractions can reduce concentration.
- **Eliminate External Distractions**
  Both visual and auditory distractions can impede concentration.
- **Create Incentives and Motivations**
  Give yourself a reason to concentrate.
- **Establish Personal Relevance**
  Identify how knowing this information will help you personally.

Pair students. Have each pair generate two lists, one of items in and out of school that are difficult to remember, and the other of things that are easy to remember. The following lists are examples:

LIST 1 (DIFFICULT TO REMEMBER)	LIST 2 (EASY TO REMEMBER)
names/faces	song lyrics
dates	my name
homework assignments	names of family members
telephone numbers	the directions to school
completing chores at home	bringing the CD player for the class trip

Have pairs share their lists with the group. Can any conclusions can be drawn about the kinds of things that are easy or difficult to remember? Did the partners agree on what is easy to remember versus what is difficult to remember?

●●●●●

LEARNING STRATEGY

The adolescent will use a variety of strategies for remembering information.

Encourage students to identify the factors that affect their memories of particular items. What parts do motivation, interest, and attitude play in their concentration? Have students generate strategies that might motivate them to remember things on their "difficult" lists.

What other factors can students physically change to improve their attention and concentration?

(Save the lists generated in this activity for discussion during subsequent activities.)

CHUNKING STRATEGY
(ADAPTED FROM HAYES, 1981)

PURPOSE

To heighten awareness of chunking as a strategy for short-term memory

Memory of seven items (plus or minus two) appears to maximize the capacity of short-term memory. To remember more than seven items requires grouping or "chunking" items into larger units. *Chunking* increases the amount of information that can be remembered. For example, if attempting to remember these 10 shopping items—glass cleaner, wrapping paper, Band-Aids, paper plates, balloons, birthday card, carpet powder, ribbon, lemon oil, and toothpaste—a chunking strategy could be used by grouping the supplies into three categories: birthday party supplies, cleaning supplies, and health supplies. The categories tend to trigger the memory of the items and the memory task is reduced to remembering three units rather than 10 items.

Present the following list to students to memorize for 15 seconds:

CIAVHFFMGMCPM

Remove the list and have students write what they remember. Repeat this activity with the following list:

CIA VHF FM GMC PM

- Which list was easier to remember?
- How are the first list and the second list similar and how they are different? What effect does chunking have on memory?
- What effect does memorizing information with some meaning have on the student's ability to recall it?

●●●●●
LEARNING STRATEGY
The adolescent will use a variety of strategies for remembering information.

REHEARSAL STRATEGY

PURPOSE

To discuss rehearsal as a strategy for remembering

When using a *rehearsal strategy,* an individual links information by simply repeating it over and over until it is remembered. This strategy might also be referred to as *verbalization, thinking aloud,* or *inner speech.* Rehearsal is a rote memory strategy that does not promote meaningful processing of information. In most academic situations, it is not the most effective strategy for remembering. As students learn other more sophisticated strategies, rehearsal as a study strategy is used less often (Rafoth, Leal, and DeFabo, 1993).

According to Hayes (1981,1989), there are two ways information can be lost in short-term memory:

- **Displacement**—Putting a new chunk of information in short-term memory displaces an old chunk because short-term memory capacity is limited.
- **Decay**—Information is lost in short-term memory because it's not rehearsed.

Rehearsing—repeating a message to ourselves—is one way to hold a message in short-term memory for a longer period of time. Consider the following situations where rehearsal is common:

1. remembering a name;
2. remembering a phone number;
3. remembering a locker combination;
4. remembering a short shopping list;
5. remembering directions to complete a task;
6. remembering directions to a location;
7. remembering a word while you look it up in the dictionary;
8. remembering a phone number;
9. remembering how to spell a word; and
10. remembering a page number.

Have students add to this list. Discuss other occasions for "talking yourself" through a process by rehearsing information. Without rehearsal, information stored in short-term memory will decay within 15–20 seconds.

●●●●●

LEARNING STRATEGY

The adolescent will use a variety of strategies for remembering information.

MEANINGFUL RELATIONSHIPS STRATEGY

(ADAPTED FROM BRAGSTAD AND STUMPF, 1982, 1987)

PURPOSE

To recognize the effect that meaning or recognizing relationships among items has on memory

Semantic organization is a strategy that gradually develops during grades two through five (Rafoth, Leal, and DeFabo, 1993). Although students group and categorize items in the early elementary grades, they rarely use this strategy spontaneously to study until adolescence.

Write the following list where everyone can see it:

way	on	their
this	my	school
to	?	did
friends	a	morning
tire	have	flat

Inform the students that they will have 15 seconds to memorize the list, and that then they will have to write all they can recall. (The order of the items in the list is not important.) Compare numbers of recalled items among students and compare strategies used by each of them to recall the above items. Were any strategies more efficient than others? Were any items easier to recall? Did the position of a word in the list affect recall?

Next, write the following sentence where everyone can see it. Again, after allowing students to study it for 15 seconds, ask them to record what they remember:

Did my friends have a flat tire on their way to school this morning?

Compare the first and second memory tasks. Discuss the following:

- Which of the two memory tasks was easier? Why might the words arranged as a question be easier to recall than the list?
- What did you notice about the items recalled? Did the position of the item in the list make the item easier to recall? (People tend to recall more from the beginning and end of a list or session, tend to remember unique items, and tend to remember items associated with one another.)
- How did the meaning or the relationship among items aid memorization of the words? How might this strategy help you to study for an exam? (E.g., information organized for memorization will have more meaning if you relate it to what you already know or relate it to what was previously studied.)

●●●●●

LEARNING STRATEGY

The adolescent will use a variety of strategies for remembering information.

CATEGORIZING STRATEGY

PURPOSE

To become aware of the efficiency in categorizing information to be memorized

Larger amounts of information can be reduced to smaller chunks of information by categorizing according to common characteristics. An organizational system for remembering, such as categorizing, promotes semantic processing of the material being memorized, and that in turn makes it easier to remember. The following activity, adapted from Bragstad and Stumpf (1982, 1987), emphasizes the efficiency of categorizing as a memory strategy.

Present students with 15 to 20 items on a tray. Examples of what might be gathered are the following:

paper clip	fork	quarter
comb	hairbrush	pin
penny	credit card	coffee cup
nail file	pencil	paper plate
eraser	spoon	tape
tack	photograph	pen
key	dime	

Allow students 45 seconds to study the tray before removing or covering it. Then, ask students to record all the items they can recall.

Compare and explore the various student responses and the numerous strategies they used to recall the items. Discuss possible ways to categorize the objects on the tray (such as items found in a wallet, in a kitchen, or in a desk).

Repeat this exercise with the same items, encouraging students to use categorization as a memory device. What changes in student performance are noticeable?

Have students generate occasions when categorization might be an appropriate strategy. Examples follow:

lists of people, places, or things;

dates or events;

steps in a sequence;

vocabulary words;

main points/supporting ideas; and

grocery lists.

●●●●●

LEARNING STRATEGY

The adolescent will use a variety of strategies for remembering information.

Refer to the lists created by students in the "Awareness of Memory Use" activity, page 258. Could a categorization strategy be applied to any of the items that are difficult for the students to remember?

Continue this exercise using content materials from students' classes. Discuss the categorical relationships that exist and how the relationships can be used to help memorize information:

Biology—classes and phyla of living things
classes and types of diseases
categories of parasites and predators

English—parts of speech
parts of a sentence
meanings of words in a novel read by the class

Social Studies—advantages/disadvantages of the Industrial Revolution
events leading to World War I

Categories are frequently hierarchical. Paying attention to the hierarchical arrangement of material is also a powerful memory tool (Hayes, 1981).

MNEMONIC DEVICES

PURPOSE

To create mnemonic devices and to discuss the occasions for using them

Mnemonic devices are formulas or aids used to improve the recall of information, particularly listed items, steps in a sequence, etc. (For example, music students recall the acronym FACE as a strategy for remembering the spaces of the treble staff.)

Mnemonic devices can be unique or catchy words or sentences. For instance, in memorizing the following list of rivers in Wisconsin, the sentence "Wise men stay near fire in blizzards" could be created using the initial letters of each river:

Wisconsin
Mississippi
St. Croix
Namekagon
Flambeau
Iron
Brule

Generate other examples of mnemonic devices. Together with students, develop a one-word (e.g., FACE) or sentence mnemonic device for remembering the following:

1. five cities in Ohio: Cleveland, Akron, Cincinnati, Dayton, Columbus;
2. six countries in Europe: Poland, Czechoslovakia, Hungary, Rumania, Bulgaria, Turkey;
3. the three kinds of neurons in mammals: sensory, motor, and associative;
4. the steps for self-correcting assignments: check for capitalization, organization, punctuation, spelling;
5. four southern states: Florida, Alabama, North Carolina, Georgia;
6. steps in starting a car: press clutch, start ignition, put in gear;
7. sources of vitamin C: strawberries, oranges, grapefruit;
8. metals used in the United States: copper, lead, zinc, aluminum, nickel, uranium;

●●●●●

LEARNING STRATEGY

The adolescent will use a variety of strategies for remembering information.

9. stages of succession after a forest fire: burned ground, annuals, meadow, aspen, firs; and

10. the last five presidents of the United States: Clinton, Bush, Reagan, Carter, Ford.

Discuss occasions in the students' current classes when use of a mnemonic memory strategy would be appropriate, such as making lists or putting steps in a sequence.

Provide students with lists of names, objects, events, or steps (or let students generate their own lists of content material from their current classes). Have students develop a mnemonic device to remember the material. Give students five minutes to develop the device. Check their retention of the lists. Check again at the end of class.

Refer to the lists created by students in the "Awareness of Memory Use" activity, page 258. Could a mnemonic strategy be applied to any of the items that are difficult for students to remember?

VISUAL IMAGERY STRATEGY

PURPOSE

To construct visual images as a strategy for remembering

Constructing visual images, referred to as *mental* or *visual imagery* or *visualization,* while studying or reading information is an elaboration strategy for remembering. *Mental imagery* is "seeing" an object in one's mind in the absence of the concrete visual object (Kaniel, 1995). The most effective visualizations focus on relevant visual attributes. Also, images or pictures that form connections are useful aids, while separated images are not (Hayes, 1989). Students begin to spontaneously use visual elaboration strategies by age 10 or 11 (Rafoth, Leal, and DeFabo, 1993). Adolescents who produce their own images (rather than using educator-provided images) perform better at remembering information.

Present students with the following fantasy:

> You are a contestant on your favorite television game show. You have the opportunity to win $10,000 if you can open the treasure chest in front of you. You are given the following directions to examine for 20 seconds, after which time they will be removed. You will have to remember the directions and follow them in the exact order given.
>
> 1. Turn the trunk upside down.
> 2. Remove the strap.
> 3. Insert the key.
> 4. Twist the key to the left.
> 5. Hold the button in.
> 6. Open the trunk.

What visual strategies could be used to remember the steps? (One possible strategy would be to visualize performing each action in the order given. The image could begin with an overturned trunk bound with a strap. Imagine the key in your left hand to remember to turn it to the left. Hold in the button with your right hand.)

●●●●●

LEARNING STRATEGY

The adolescent will use a variety of strategies for remembering information.

Visual images can be used to remember the meanings of unfamiliar vocabulary terms or names of persons you meet. The more outrageous these images are, the easier they are to remember. The following are some examples:

- bovine—to remember this vocabulary term, imagine a cow eating a vine with a large bow around its neck.
- John Gallup—to remember the name of this person just met, visualize him on a galloping horse with his name, John, inscribed on the saddle.

Require students to bring to class five new vocabulary items for memorization. As a group, discuss visual images that might be powerful memory aids.

Refer to the lists created by students in the "Awareness of Memory Use" activity, page 258. Could a visual imagery strategy be applied to any of the items that are difficult for students to remember?

DAILY "FORGETFULNESS": BREAKING THE NORMAL PATTERN

(ADAPTED FROM PROJECT STILE, 1979)

PURPOSE

To become aware of breaking a pattern as a strategy for remembering

This strategy is probably most appropriate for those students who continually "forget" to follow directions or complete tasks such as these:

- bringing materials to class;
- bringing lunch money;
- bringing athletic shoes for physical education;
- bringing permission slips;
- putting their names on their papers; or
- keeping appointments.

Breaking the normal pattern is like "tying a string around your finger." The "string" should be an outlandish circumstance that jars the memory. Give students the following example:

> To remember to take lunch money in the morning, tie your coat sleeve in a knot or tie your shoes together; when you see the knot, you will remember why you tied it and then will remember your lunch money.

Breaking the pattern should not be substituted for a more organized memory approach (e.g., making lists, taking notes, or making checklists), but when all other strategies fail, students can rely on this strategy.

Challenge students to come up with examples of their own patterns of "forgetfulness." What techniques will they use to break these patterns?

●●●●●

LEARNING STRATEGY

The adolescent will use a variety of strategies for remembering information.

TIME-SAVING FUNCTIONS

PURPOSE

To become aware of the time-saving function of text elements

Recall that *text*, in this chapter, refers to all forms of reading, including textbooks, magazines, teacher handouts, etc. Explain the general ways in which authors and publishers structure text (e.g., chapter titles, index, table of contents, headings and subheadings, glossary, etc.). Identify the various parts of a text the students are using in one of their courses. Discuss the functions of those parts and the time-saving aspects.

Modeling the proper use of these text elements and providing practice is the best way to ensure students use text structure to improve their studying (Gall, Gall, Jacobsen, and Bullock, 1990). Be sure to analyze a number of different texts (including textbooks, magazines, teacher handouts, and brochures or pamphlets).

Before engaging in the following activity, prepare a list of information you would like students to locate in a particular text. Two copies of the chosen text are required for this activity. To illustrate the time-saving features of elements in texts, stage a contest between two groups of students. Direct one group to locate information you request using text elements such as the index, table of contents, or glossary; direct the other group to locate the same information without using the text elements. Analyze the results by asking the following questions:

- Which group finished first?
- Which group was most efficient?

If a student's goal is to complete homework as quickly and efficiently as possible, would it be prudent to use the text elements for their intended purposes?

●●●●●●

LEARNING STRATEGY

The adolescent will use text efficiently.

MAIN IDEA CLUES

PURPOSE

To discuss and discover clues to an author's purpose

Require students to bring at least one of their textbooks to class for this activity. Using one of the students' current textbooks, examine chapter titles. Have students predict the overall content of the chapter. Direct students to locate examples of boldface letters, italicized words, underlined information, words in a different font or type size, or words printed in all capital letters. Relate reasons for the author's decision to emphasize the words or concepts.

Ask students to predict main ideas based on the bold-faced headings, italicized words, etc. How can this information be used to save time?

Review another textbook and chapter within it for other main idea clues. Some texts include main idea statements in the margin. Others include summaries and review questions at the end of the chapter that cue students to main ideas or the author's purpose. Look for differing examples. Assign each student to skim or scan a chapter in his or her textbook and to predict the main ideas. Have students share their predictions with the group.

Direct students' attention to the organizational techniques authors use in writing texts. For example, a world history textbook might present a major historical event by first describing the cause and then describing the effect or the consequence of the event. This pattern would most likely be used throughout the chapter.

Using their own textbooks, challenge students to describe the author's organizational patterns in a chosen chapter, section, or paragraph. The following describe commonly used patterns of organization (also refer to the speakers' organizational patterns discussed on page 92 in Chapter 5):

1. cause/effect;
2. sequence of events; and
3. comparisons: qualities, advantages, disadvantages.

LEARNING STRATEGY

The adolescent will use text efficiently.

AWARENESS ACTIVITY

PURPOSE

To develop an awareness of color coding as a perceptual system for segregating the components of a whole

LEARNING STRATEGY

The adolescent will use color coding as a strategy for efficient studying.

Color coding or highlighting of important information is an effective study strategy if students are challenged to do the coding. When authors or teachers highlight all the important information, students are deprived of separating the foreground from the background and thus lose the opportunity to develop an effective memory strategy (Sylwester, 1995).

Present students with examples of various perceptual systems used to differentiate parts of a whole. Include objects whose parts are numbered, alphabetized, or colored. Some of these examples might be included:

- maps with colored parts;
- a stack of library books with Dewey Decimal numbers visible;
- numbered pages from a book;
- a chart with colored bars or profiles;
- a collection of multicolored cups;
- a set of driver's licenses (different colors for probationary and regular);
- a picture of variously colored cars in a parking lot;
- a worksheet with red-ink corrections;
- advertisements with important messages in brilliant colors;
- a picture of a woman with cosmetically accented lips, eyes, and lashes; or
- a dictionary.

Encourage students to add other examples of parts differentiated from the whole by a perceptual system. Discuss the various perceptual systems that each item uses to attract attention (e.g., the alphabet, a numbering system, colors).

Parts of objects can be made to stand out from the whole object in various ways. The system used to emphasize the parts of a whole are dependent on our needs. If our need is to visually separate important information for quick review in studying, which system might be most efficient? Discuss the perceptual coding system of highlighting information using color. Ask questions such as the following:

- How do maps use color to differentiate parts? Are there consistent colors used in maps (blue to indicate water, green to indicate land, etc.)?

- How would color help you identify your cup within a group?
- Why does the department of transportation use different colors for different driver's licenses?
- In looking for your car in a crowded parking lot, how would color provide cues for locating it?
- Why do instructors often use different (red) colored pens to correct your work?
- What purpose do cosmetics serve in accenting a face?
- How do ads use contrasting colors to sell their ideas?
- Would advertisements have the same effect if colors were not complementary?
- What other systems rely on color to separate or identify parts quickly and efficiently? (E.g., transportation systems use road signs and traffic lights; family and consumer education classes often color-code kitchen utensils for each separate kitchen; hospitals color-code floor equipment; reading, spelling, and math programs often color-code the grade levels.)

WHAT TO COLOR?

PURPOSE

To determine specific information to color-code

Present an example of text in which main ideas within a paragraph are highlighted with a particular color and important details are highlighted with a different color. Also present a sample of a student's notes that have been color-coded. At the same time, present a comparison sample of overindulged coloring. Ask questions such as the following:

- What parts of the text appear to "catch your eye"?
- What kind of information is highlighted in color?
- Why would different colors be used for different types of information?
- Is it possible to highlight too much information? What happens when too much information is highlighted? Is there still the effect of differentiating the parts?

Discuss the advantages of using color coding as a strategy for studying (e.g., it helps the student recall information, provides for a quick review, encourages understanding of main ideas, calls attention to important information, and encourages use of another modality for studying).

The following ideas offered by Bragstad and Stumpf (1982) are suggestions for discerning what to mark. Direct students to consider highlighting the following:

1. the main idea of the article or paragraph—the author's purpose and subject;
2. major concepts;
3. significant details;
4. items in a series ("baseball, football, and basketball are popular...);
5. introduction to a series ("four ways to...");
6. transitional words and phrases ("however, in addition to..."); and
7. new vocabulary words and key terms.

To successfully code an article, passage, or notes requires reading the text, questioning what was read to determine the main idea, and then highlighting. Several paragraphs may have to be read to determine the central idea.

LEARNING STRATEGY

The adolescent will use color coding as a strategy for efficient studying.

COLOR-CODING MATERIAL

PURPOSE

To develop the skill of color coding

Provide or require students to have several light-colored markers, preferably yellow, pink, light green, or blue. (Pens made especially for highlighting are available at school supply stores or bookstores.) Create an overhead transparency of several paragraphs found in students' current texts. The following is an example:

> The energy an object has as it moves is called *energy of motion* or *kinetic energy*. The faster your bike moves, the more energy of motion it has. The energy of motion increases dramatically as weight and speed increase. Once you understand the natural law concerning energy of motion, you can adjust to traffic situations ahead of time.

Display the transparency paragraphs. As a class, decide which information should be highlighted.

Collect and print more examples of paragraphs found in students' current texts or class notes on three-by-five-inch index cards. The following are examples:

> In referring to clothing, keep these three terms in mind: fads, fashions, and styles. Fads come and fads go rapidly. Fashions are slower to be accepted but stay popular for a longer period of time. Styles are the fashion of the moment or refer to a particular fashion.

●●●●●●●

LEARNING STRATEGY

The adolescent will use color coding as a strategy for efficient studying.

> *Alternating current* (AC) is an electric current that reverses directions in a circuit at regular intervals. The circuits in your home have alternating current. When the electricity is on, free electrons in the wires vibrate with back and forth movement. For example, in a 60-cycle home circuit, the electrons vibrate 60 times per second.

> Java has become one of the most densely populated areas in the world. On average, between 1,500 and 2,000 people live on every square mile of this important Indonesian island. Djakarta, in Western Java, is the capital and largest city in Indonesia.

Require students to individually highlight information on the cards. Guide them by asking the following questions:

- What information is important enough to remember? What information will be important to review for an exam?
- What details might be important to highlight? Are there any new vocabulary words to remember?

Require each student to bring to class a textbook, reading assignment, or notes from a current course. Paper clip acetate sheets to students' materials as overlays for practice highlighting. Highlight information on the pages as a group at first, and encourage discussion when differences of opinion occur. When completed, compare the pages with and without color. Using relevant materials from the students' content area classes (e.g., social studies, English) ensures that this strategy is generalized to other study situations.

A caution regarding highlighting materials that are school property may not be necessary, but this most likely will be a common query of students. Most instructors/principals will be supportive of color coding school materials for the purpose of improving students' knowledge. Students, most likely, will be reluctant to color without permission. Obviously, students can color-code personal property and handouts or articles for assignments.

ANALYZING PAST EXAM ERRORS

PURPOSE

To identify causes of errors on previous exams written by students

If students have been concerned about past test performance, identification of errors is the first step toward improvement. Direct students to bring to class exams previously written (or these could be collected from classroom teachers). Guide students to analyze test errors by answering some of the following questions:

- Were there correct answers written in the wrong place?
- Were any errors due to illegible handwriting?
- Were any problems accidentally skipped?
- Were there vocabulary words on the test that were hard to understand (e.g., *compare, define,* etc.)?
- Were key words in the directions misinterpreted?
- How many items contained information not studied?
- How many errors were due to inadequate preparation?
- Were items marked wrong because time ran out?
- What type of test items were most problematic?

Determining causes of errors on exams can lead to any of the following activities, depending on the needs of students. Share the following test-taking strategies with students as general rules for success:

- Develop a positive attitude.
- Determine information that will be included on the exam.
- Prepare by studying.
- Know the vocabulary.
- Look for clues on an exam.
- Use time-management strategies during the exam.

●●●●●●●●

LEARNING STRATEGY

The adolescent will improve test performance.

TRADE SECRETS

PURPOSE

To assess students' knowledge of test preparation

Ask students to sit in a circle. Designate one student as the leader. Give him or her a pencil and a sheet of paper. Have the lead student begin by writing down one "trade secret" he or she uses to prepare for an exam and then passing the paper to the next student. Encourage each student, in turn, to share a different test-taking preparatory task and to write it down. Continue this activity until no one can contribute a task not previously mentioned.

Cut the individual tasks into strips and, as a group, sequence the tasks according to which should be completed first, second, third, etc. Are there any tasks that could be carried out simultaneously? (This may require a group estimate of time required to complete activities.)

- Have any tasks been omitted?
- Are any tasks unnecessary?
- How much time commitment is required for each task?

Discuss the benefits of preparing for test taking. How is test performance affected by inadequate preparation? What risks are taken by "cramming" for tests? What other factors can affect test performance?

LEARNING STRATEGY

The adolescent will improve test performance.

INTERVIEW SURVEY

PURPOSE

To recognize "expert" test takers' strategies for exam preparation

Since "experts" can provide firsthand accounts of the "how to" of their successes, an interview or survey of successful students may provide insight regarding effective test preparation.

Require students to interview five of their peers who they believe are "experts" at taking exams. As a group, decide which questions would be appropriate to ask. Create a survey form containing the questions. The following questions are examples:

- How soon before the test do you begin to study?
- How do you know what to study?
- What do you study?
- How often do you study?

Compare expert strategies with those currently in use. What steps could be taken to change current strategies?

The interview/survey technique may be helpful in determining the "what to study" question for a class exam. Remind students to question their instructors when unsure of exam contents. (Refer to Chapter 7, "Question-Asking Strategies.")

LEARNING STRATEGY

The adolescent will improve test performance.

PREPARATION THROUGH MANAGED STUDY

PURPOSE

To differentiate study techniques for various exam types

The type of exam determines how one studies. For instance, given the following comparisons, discuss as a group how different or similar the study strategies would be:

ESSAY/ SHORT ANSWER	versus	MULTIPLE-CHOICE QUESTIONS
List five events leading to the start of the Civil War.		Which of the following are events leading to the Civil War? a. The surrender of Fort Sumter b. The forming of the Confederate states c. The election of John Breckinridge as president

DEFINITIONS	versus	MATCHING	
Define *symmetrical.*		1. Symmetrical	a. upright
Define *vertical.*		2. Diagonal	b. a line in a slanting position
Define *diagonal.*		3. Vertical	c. a well-balanced arrangement of parts

LEARNING STRATEGY

The adolescent will improve test performance.

TRUE-FALSE	versus	SENTENCE COMPLETION
T or F George Washington was our first president.		______________ was our first president.

Essay/short answer exams require a student to have a complete or "whole" understanding of the subject materials. Objective tests, on the other hand, require a better understanding of details. Objective tests include true-false statements, multiple-choice items, sentence completion, and matching. Essays may require more application of the knowledge learned, while objective tests generally have one correct answer.

Discuss with students how to determine the type of test they will be taking. How can they get information about an upcoming exam?

DETERMINING WHAT TO STUDY

PURPOSE

To determine what subject matter should be studied

The benefits of study strategies discussed previously, including memory strategies, time management, and color coding, will become apparent to the student as he or she prepares for an exam. Understanding how class notes and highlighted textual information relate to test taking is imperative. If students recognize the continuity between strategies and assignments, they will determine important information to review for the exam more easily. Discuss clues to determining the kind of information that might be included on a test:

- What clues do instructors use to guide students to testable information?
- Do individual instructors have a certain style for giving clues?
- What are key words used by instructors to cue students?

Have students share cues used by instructors in their content area courses. Examples follow:

- "The test will cover…";
- "You might want to know…";
- "An important concept you are responsible for knowing…";
- "…will be on Wednesday's exam"; and
- "When you read p. 21, notice the…."

Guide students in determining how they will note the "cues" given by their instructors.

LEARNING STRATEGY

The adolescent will improve test performance.

TEST TAKING: RECOGNIZE CLUES

PURPOSE

To recognize syntactical clues on exams

Using the following list of examples, discuss possible syntactical clues to answers present in each example:

1	Check the errors you find below.	Clue: plural marker *s* implies more than one error
2	Mark the picture that is correct.	Clue: singular *picture* implies one answer
3	A bear is an __________.	Clue: *an* implies answer will begin with a vowel
4	The __________ are coming.	Clue: *are* implies plural answer
5	Choose all answers	Clue: *all answers* implies more than one apply
6	A __________.	Clue: *a* implies an answer beginning with a consonant
7	Advantages / Disadvantages ________ ________ ________ ________ ________ ________	Clue: the three lines in each column might imply three answers
8	A __________ engine was invented by Rudolf Diesel.	Clue: a descriptor or adjective is implied
9	The main function of calcium is to __________.	Clue: *to* is part of an infinitive clause; it implies the answer will be a verb form
10	What dietary recommendations would you give to maintain good health?	Clue: plural *recommendations* implies at least two

Review past exams with students. Identify syntactical clues on the exams.

LEARNING STRATEGY

The adolescent will improve test performance.

TEST TAKING: VOCABULARY CLUES

(ADAPTED FROM PROJECT STILE, 1979, AND ALLEN, MASON, AND MCKEAN, 1982)

PURPOSE

To recognize the effect of absolute terminology on a statement's meaning

LEARNING STRATEGY

The adolescent will improve test performance.

Frequently contained in true-false statements and multiple-choice items are vocabulary terms whose presence may appear insignificant but which serve to control the meaning of the statement.

Discuss the importance of *and/or* in multiple-choice items. Given a response choice *A and B* implies that both answers must be correct, while the response choice *A or B* is correct if only one of the choices is appropriate. Additionally, statements containing the following terms indicate an absolute condition; that is, there are not any exceptions to the statements:

all	none	invariably
never	always	best
every	exactly	worst

The following words modify the condition of "absoluteness" in a statement:

some	usually	sometimes
seldom	many	often
most		

Present students with statements containing these terms and have them identify those that are absolute. Considering the absolute nature of some of these terms, would the statement be true or false? What word could be substituted to make a true statement false? A false statement true?

1. Sometimes February has 28 days.
2. All fires are dangerous.
3. First period never begins at 3:15.
4. The train is always late.
5. Thanksgiving is never in July.
6. Sometimes the temperature drops below zero.
7. The president usually resides at the White House.
8. Many birds can fly.
9. None of the above are true.

10 All birds fly south for the winter.

11 Most astronauts are men.

12 The bus usually runs daily.

13 All Japanese persons are short.

14 Pepper invariably causes a sneeze.

15 We seldom have a winter without snow.

16 The worst pain one can experience is a toothache.

17 One hundred pennies are exactly equal to $1.

18 Every month has 31 days.

19 McDonald's makes the best hamburgers.

20 Winter invariably includes snow and cold weather.

Examine students' past exams and identify absolutes and modified absolutes. What effect does a small piece of false information have on a statement that is otherwise true? To be true, all parts of a statement must be true, including the absolute and modified absolute terms.

TEST TAKING: TEST VOCABULARY

PURPOSE

To comprehend test vocabulary and perform according to directions

Additional barriers often faced in a test situation are vocabulary terms whose meanings are unclear to students. A misinterpreted key or clue word in a test item could (1) lead the student to provide only part of the information (e.g., when asked to "compare and contrast" the bicycle and the motorcycle as forms of transportation, the student might discuss similarities only); and (2) lead the student to provide information, but not within the constraint of a key word definition (when asked to "define" the word *perpendicular*, the student might give examples of perpendicular items instead of writing the definition).

The following list contains words commonly found on essay exams. Duplicate this list (see Appendix S) and distribute it to students. Students might also identify and add vocabulary terms most often used by their instructors. Have a dictionary handy and be prepared to modify the definitions given.

analyze	examine the parts of an item and discuss how they are related
compare	look at two or more items and show how they are the same or different
contrast	compare two or more items to show differences between them
criticize	give your opinion or judgment about the positive and negative points
define	give the meaning of
describe	write about it, "paint a picture" with words; do so in a logical sequence
diagram	make a drawing, graph, or chart and label its parts
discuss	talk something over, looking at positive and negative points
enumerate	list facts using numbers
evaluate	give your opinion of the importance of something; give advantages and disadvantages

LEARNING STRATEGY

The adolescent will improve test performance.

explain	make something clear that is not understood; tell how something happened or how to do something
hypothesize	think about what would happen if...
illustrate	explain your answer in writing and make it clear using examples, stories, pictures, charts, diagrams
interpret	explain the meaning of something, using examples to make it clear
justify	give a reason for or defend something; give evidence
list	produce answers in words or sentences and number them
outline	list a plan that gives only the main ideas; summarize showing how the ideas are organized
prove	give evidence or argue that something is true
relate	show how one thing is connected to or similar to another
review	examine and talk about the important parts of something; perhaps discuss positive and negative points
state	tell; express precisely; sentences should be brief and should omit details
summarize	give only the main points of a thing or event, not details or examples
trace	follow the development of (the history of) something from beginning to end

COMPARE AND CONTRAST TEST-TAKING TERMS

PURPOSE

To recognize similarities and differences of test terminology

LEARNING STRATEGY

The adolescent will improve test performance.

Using the vocabulary terms from the "Test Taking: Test Vocabulary" activity, page 287, have students group the words into categories with similar meanings. For example:

- list/enumerate;
- discuss/describe/explain;
- prove/justify; and
- compare/contrast.

Require students to explain why they grouped the terms together and to discuss the similarities and differences of the words in each group. Students' answers will vary.

VOCABULARY TEST

PURPOSE

To demonstrate comprehension of test vocabulary terms by performing the action

Using ideas familiar to the students, require them to perform the action given in the following statements:

1. Discuss going to the basketball game Friday night.
2. Hypothesize what an evening with the president of the United States would be like.
3. Describe your brother's new car.
4. Compare your blue jeans to another student's jeans.
5. Summarize yesterday's lesson.
6. Define the word *test.*
7. Describe the accident you saw on Fifth Street and Main.
8. Evaluate your progress in this class.
9. Review the school play.
10. List the names of persons attending this class.
11. Diagram the walk from the office to this class.
12. Analyze the mistakes you made on your last exam.
13. Contrast your hairstyle with mine.
14. Enumerate the reasons for wearing a bike helmet.
15. Explain your being out past curfew last night.
16. Justify leaving the school building at noon.
17. Interpret this signal (motion hello or good-bye).
18. How does the bell ringing relate to this class?
19. Illustrate how $1,000 would make you feel right now.
20. Outline your plans for cleaning your bedroom.

LEARNING STRATEGY

The adolescent will improve test performance.

21. Prove you are the age you tell me you are.
22. State your name and address.
23. Trace your walk from home to school.
24. Criticize the Dallas Cowboys football team.
25. Compare and contrast junior high school with elementary school.

VOCABULARY TASK

PURPOSE

To demonstrate comprehension of test vocabulary terms by performing the action

●●●●●●●●●

LEARNING STRATEGY

The adolescent will improve test performance.

Generate a list of topics to use for this activity or use topics listed on the next page. Write test-taking terms on three-by-five-inch index cards. (The terms are reprinted in Appendix T.) Name a topic, and then instruct students to each pick a card. Direct them to perform the action required in relation to the topic given. Review the following example:

TOPIC

Columbus discovered America.

Analyze how he came to be a famous explorer.

Discuss when his journey was made and how a similar voyage would be different today.

Explain why Columbus was chosen to make his now-famous voyage.

Prove that he landed in America and not Asia.

Trace his adventure from beginning to end.

State the names of his ships.

Pretend you are Columbus and **justify** your trip to the Queen of Spain.

Diagram the trip he made.

Hypothesize the outcome if Columbus had landed in Canada.

Compare Columbus discovering America with the first man landing on the moon.

Define *discovery*.

Outline a trip like Columbus made.

Pretend you are a Native American Indian and **criticize** the statement, "Columbus discovered America."

Example topics include these:

1. A butterfly is an insect.
2. The eagle is our national bird.
3. You want to attend the Friday night basketball game.
4. Television is the best invention ever created.
5. Acid rain pollutes the environment.
6. Immunizations prevent the spread of disease.
7. The earth is round.
8. Health care should be nationalized.
9. The drinking age for citizens should be uniform in all states.
10. The football season should be all year long.

WHAT KINDS OF LISTS CAN YOU MAKE?

PURPOSE

To generate examples related to test vocabulary terms

For this activity, pair students. Then write one of the test vocabulary terms (see Appendix T) where everyone can see it. Direct each pair to generate examples of things or events to which the vocabulary term could be applied. For example, given the term *evaluate*, challenge each pair to list items that could be evaluated.

Give students a time limit of two to three minutes. At the expiration of the time limit, have groups compare responses. Direct them to give their rationale for including an item if challenged by another pair of students.

LEARNING STRATEGY

The adolescent will improve test performance.

10 SURVIVAL LANGUAGE STRATEGIES

This chapter approaches survival language in three ways:

1. It suggests activities in survival-language environments. These activities facilitate the adolescent's independent functioning as a family member, student, consumer, citizen, participant of leisure, and employee. Educators are reminded to examine the "functional reality" underlying objectives for teaching survival language (Valletutti and Bender, 1982). Inspired by Larson and McKinley (1987, 1995) and Valletutti and Bender (1982), activities call for examination of the student's perspective and consideration of the context in which the learning task will be performed, thereby preserving the "functional essence" of the activities.

2. The chapter provides basic word lists containing word elements, including word roots, prefixes, and suffixes, as a survival strategy for helping students ascertain meaning from words that are unfamiliar to

them. Using methods described by Crais (1990), Devine (1981), Hamersky (1993) and Nelson (1993), the chapter describes a meta-approach to increasing student's lexical skills.

3. The chapter provides basic "interest" lists for the survival of the professional providing intervention. The lists are provided as examples of the kinds of topics in which adolescents may be interested. Adolescents' motivation to participate in activities can be heightened by developing strategies using topics of interest to them.

VOCABULARY FOR COMMON DAILY LIVING SITUATIONS

Independent functioning in daily living situations at home, at work, or in the community require numerous survival language skills. We need only to reflect on our own daily experiences to realize the vast amount of language required for survival in today's society. Adolescents whose thinking, speaking, and listening are impaired tend to have deficits in survival language (Larson and McKinley, 1995). These adolescents may need help in developing the daily living skills needed to make the transition to adulthood (Paul, 1995).

In considering survival language skills, the concern is focused on the understanding and use of underlying vocabulary or concepts necessary to successfully and independently complete particular daily living tasks. Chronological age expectations are set for these skills even for adolescents with much younger age-level, cognitive abilities. This is because survival language is so basic to independent living that adolescents without these skills stand out as "odd" or "different" to their peers and to adults (Larson and McKinley, 1995). Larson and McKinley summarize the survival language skills that must be intact for adequate functioning in academic, vocational, and social settings:

1. comprehending language for specific situations (e.g., school classroom, restaurant, grocery store);
2. comprehending language for multisituational settings (e.g., money, signs);
3. producing language for specific situations; and
4. producing language for multisituational settings.

In addition, Valletutti and Bender (1982) present six environments and roles to consider when addressing survival language:

1. at home, as a family member;
2. at school, as a student;
3. in the marketplace, as a consumer of goods and services;
4. in the community, as a citizen;
5. in society, as a participant of leisure; and
6. in the workplace, as a producer of goods or services.

The basic word lists included in this chapter's activities are intended as examples of the types of survival language appropriate for adolescents. The sizes of the lists are purposely restricted; professionals are encouraged to extend these lists to include the survival language terminology appropriate to the needs of the adolescents in the region in which they reside.

The activities for the survival word groups were adapted from or inspired by Valletutti and Bender (1982), in whose resource manual, *Teaching Functional Academics,* educators are reminded to examine the "functional reality" underlying objectives for teaching and to consider the context in which the learning task will eventually be used. The older the adolescent, the more imperative it is that the adolescent's program emphasize the survival language skills that are not intact.

SURVIVAL IN UNDERSTANDING NEW VOCABULARY WORDS

Direct teaching of vocabulary words through drills, exercises, word lists, and memorization is the way many of us learned new words when we were students. However, when considering the needs of students who have language and learning problems and whose memory systems for nonmeaningful information are already taxed, this approach seems nonproductive. In fact, it would be a monumental task, if not impossible, especially when considering that there are more than 600,000 words in the English language (Devine, 1981).

Vocabulary acquisition is a lifelong process. Professionals can teach students strategies for dealing with new words and new meanings. "Word power" can be improved in students using approaches such as the following described by Devine (1981):

1. Teach students key root words from which many other words have developed.
2. Teach common prefixes and suffixes that assist students in getting at the meanings of unfamiliar words.
3. Give regular practice in using context clues. (p. 128)

A *word root,* as defined by *The American Heritage Dictionary* (1993), is the element that carries the main component of meaning in a word; *prefixes* and *suffixes* are affixed before or after root words to produce derivatives that change the root word meaning. As early as first grade, students are introduced to word combinations that form new words, such as the compounds *doghouse* and *pancake.* The English language grows mainly by the process of compounding; whole words may be combined, or word roots, prefix, or suffix parts may be joined into compound forms (*World Book Encyclopedia,* 1981). And so it is that meaningful word elements are combined to form new words such as *telegraphic, megabusiness,* and *user-friendly.*

Students confront unfamiliar words on a daily basis and in a variety of communicative settings, including those of listening and reading. Crais (1990) discusses research that indicates by 6 years of age, children are adding approximately five word roots per day to their lexicons. Knowledge of word elements in the forms of word roots, prefixes, and suffixes provides external clues to word meanings and expands another facet of daily survival: understanding new vocabulary terms confronted. Crais (1990) describes teaching a root word strategy as a "meta" approach to increasing student's lexical skills.

In the study of word elements, direct teaching of all elements of words (i.e., word roots, prefixes, and suffixes) is impractical and nonmeaningful. The majority of word elements must be acquired by abstracting meaning in the context in which the word is used. A meaningful approach might be to dissect a new word and its elements, recognize elements in other familiar words, and then observe how certain words containing the same element are related in meaning. For example, in exploring the word root *tele,* meaning distance, students might generate words formed from the "tele word family" such as *telegraph, telephone, telescope, television, telegraphic,* and *telepathy.* Students could then define the words and consider the relationships of their meanings. Words taught in sets tend to be learned better in association and in contrast to each other (Nelson, 1993).

Nelson (1993) also suggests establishing meaningful contexts to encourage individuals of all ages to add new words to their lexicons. Hamersky (1993) presents visual strategies to assist in establishing meaningful contexts; students integrate new words with words that are already familiar to them using a visual format. For instance, in using the above example, the professional could employ the visual strategy known as a word map to illustrate the similarities and differences among the words *telegraph, telephone, telescope, television, telegraphic,* and *telepathy* (see Figure 10.1.)

Stauffer (1942) identified 15 prefixes that account for 82 percent of the most frequently used words in

FIGURE 10.1

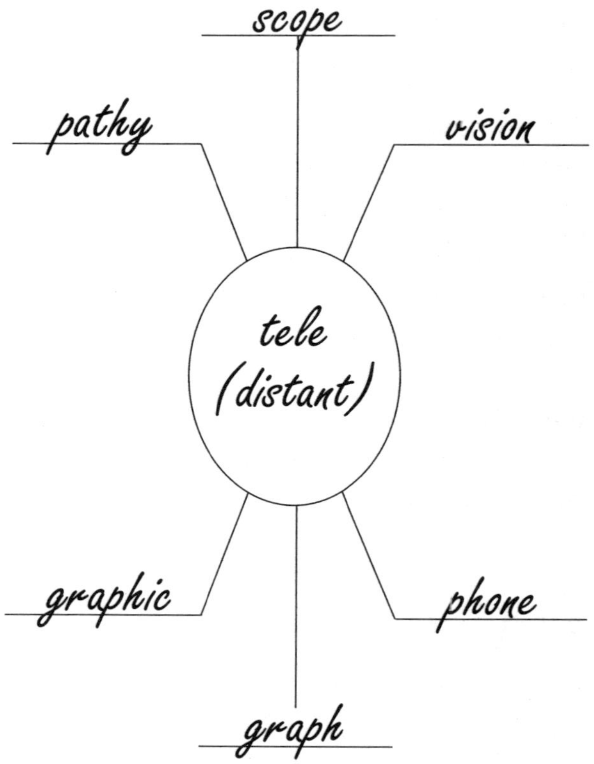

general reading for children. They are *ab, ad, be, com, de, dis, en, ex, in (into), in (not), pre, pro, re, sub,* and *un.* Additionally, Brown (1952) claims the 14 words in Table 10.1 may be used to decipher the meanings of more than 14,000 English words. These prefixes and word roots, as well as others, are included in this chapter's activities.

The lists in Tables 10.2, 10.3, and 10.4 are included as references to the study of word parts. They are adapted from World Book Encyclopedia (1981). While the list of word roots is organized alphabetically, the prefixes and suffixes are grouped in categories most representative of their meaning. They are organized in this way to communicate the relationships existing in the ways they are used.

TABLE 10.1
BROWN'S 14 WORDS

WORD	PREFIX 1		PREFIX 2		ROOT WORD
precept			pre (before)	+	capere (take, seize)
detain			de (away from)	+	tenere (hold, have)
intermittent			inter (between)	+	mittere (send)
offer			ob (against)	+	ferre (bear, carry)
insist			in (into)	+	stare (stand)
monograph			mono (one, alone)	+	graphein (write)
epilogue			epi (upon)	+	legein (say, study)
aspect			ad (towards, to)	+	specere (see)
uncomplicated	un (not)	+	com (with)	+	plicare (fold)
nonextended	non (not)	+	ex (out of)	+	tendere (stretch)
reproduce	re (back, again)	+	pro (forward)	+	ducere (lead)
indisposed	in (not)	+	dis (apart from)	+	ponere (put, place)
oversufficient	over (above)	+	sub (under)	+	facere (make, do)
mistranscribe	mis (wrong)	+	trans	+	scribere (write)

TABLE 10.2
ROOT WORDS

ROOT	MEANING	EXAMPLE
alt	tall, high	altitude
angle, angul	corner	rectangle
annus	year	annual
aqua	water	aquarium
arch	chief	hierarchy
arm	weapon	armor
aster, astro	star	astronaut
athl, athlon	prize, contest	athlete

(continued)

TABLE 10.2—*Continued*

ROOT	MEANING	EXAMPLE
aud	hear	audience
belli	war	belligerent
bio	life	biopsy
cap	head	capital
cardi	heart	cardiac
ced, ceed	go, yield	precede
cens	judge	censorship
cept	take, receive, catch	conception
cide	kill	suicide
circ	ring, around	circus
clud	shut	exclude
cogn	know	recognize
cracy, crat	rule	bureaucrat
cred	believe	credibility
crim	judge, accuse	discriminate
crit	separate, judge	critic
deb	owe	debit
demos	people	democracy
dent	tooth	dental
derm	skin	dermatitis
dia, die	day	per diem
dic, dict	say	contradict
do	give	donate
doc	teach	documentary
dorm	sleep	dormant
dyn	power	dynamite
ego	I	egocentric
em, empt	buy, obtain	redemption
emia, hemia	blood	leukemia
enni	year	perennial
equ	equal, even, just	equator
err	wander	erratic
esth	feeling	anesthetic
fac	make, do	manufacture
fer	carry, bear	infer
fid	faith	bona fide

(continued)

TABLE 10.2—*Continued*

ROOT	MEANING	EXAMPLE
fin	end	finale
firm	steady	confirmation
fix	fasten	prefix
flam	blaze	inflammable
flex	bend	flexible
fract, frag	break	fracture
fug	flee	refuge
funct	perform	malfunction
gam	marriage	monogamy
gen	race, birth	generation
geo	earth	geology
gnos	know	diagnose
gon	angle	polygon
grad	step	graduation
gram	letter, written	telegram
graph	write	graphics
grat	please, thank	gratitude
hom	man	homicide
homo	same	homonym
ident	same	identification
ign	fire	ignition
junct	join	conjunction
jus	law, right	justification
lat	side	lateral
lect	gather, choose	collect
lect, leg	read	lector
lev	raise, lift	leverage
litera	letter	literal
magni	great	magnificent
mal	bad	malignant
man	hand	manipulate
mand	order	mandatory
memoria	memory	commemorate
meter	measure	perimeter
metr	measure	symmetrical
miss	send, let go	missile

(continued)

TABLE 10.2—*Continued*

ROOT	MEANING	EXAMPLE
mor	custom	morale
mort	death	mortality
mot	move	promote
nat	born	innate
nom	law, arrangement	astronomy
nov	new	novelty
numer	number	numerator
ocul	eye	binoculars
onym	name	antonym
path	feel, suffer	sympathy
ped	foot	pedestrian
pen, pun	punishment	penitentiary
phon	sound	phonograph
photo	light	photography
pod, pus	foot	tripod
quer, quest	seek, ask	query
rect	straight, right	erect
referre	carry back	referent
rupt	break	interrupt
scope	watch	microscope
scrib, script	write	inscription
sec, sect	cut	intersect
sen	old	senile
tele	distant	telescope
temp	time, season	contemporary
terrere	to frighten	terrorize
thermo	heat	thermometer
tom	cut	appendectomy
topos	place, spot	topical
tox	poison	intoxication
tract	pull, draw, drag	extract
vaca, vacu	empty, hollow	vacate
vapor	steam	evaporate
vari	different, various, spotted	variant
vit	live	vitamin
viv	live	survive
zo	animal	zoologist

TABLE 10.3 PREFIXES
DIRECTIONAL

PREFIX	MEANING	EXAMPLE
a-	on	aboard
ab-	from	absent
ad-	to	adjunct, adhere
ante-	before	antecedent
circu-/circum-	around, about	circumvent
co-/col-	with	coincident
com-	together, with	compact
con-	together	connect
de-	down	dejected
de-	away	deflect
dia-	through, between	diagnosis
dis-	apart from	disarm
e-	out	eject
en-	in	encircle
endo-	inside, within	endocrine
epi-	upon, in addition	epitaph
ex-	out	exit
extra-	outside, beyond	extraordinary
im-	into	implant
in-	into	inhale
infra-	below	infrastructure
inter-	between, among	interracial
intra-/intro-	within	introspective
meta-	beyond	metaphysics
mid-	middle point	midweek, midway
para-	beside	paraprofessional
per-	thoroughly, throughout	permanent
peri-	around, near, about	perimeter
pro-	forward	progress
pro-	in front	prologue
re-	back	rebate
retro-	back	retroactive
sub-	under	subsoil
super-	over	supernatural
sym-	together, with	symmetry
syn-	together, with	synthesis
trans-	across, over	transatlantic
ultra-	beyond	ultraviolet

(continued)

TABLE 10.3—*Continued*

NEGATIVE

PREFIX	MEANING	EXAMPLE
a-	not, without	amoral
anti-	against	antidote
contra-	against	contrary
counter-	against	counterbalance
de-	away	dehydrate
dis-	not	disobey
dis-	opposite	disarrange
dys-	bad	dystrophy
il-	not	illegible
im-	not	immovable
in-	not	inactive
ir-	not	irregular
mis-	wrong	misbehave
non-	not	nonstop
ob-	against, opposite	obstruct
pseudo-	false	pseudonym
un-	not	unsure

DESCRIPTORS

PREFIX	MEANING	EXAMPLE
eu-	well, good	eulogy
hetero-	different	heterosexual
homo-	same	homogeneous
hyper-	over, beyond	hyperactive
hypo-	under, too little	hypochondriac
macro-	large, long	macrometer
mega-	large	megaphone
micro-	small	microscope
neo-	new	neonate
pen-	almost	peninsula
pro-	in place of	pronoun
pro-	in favor of	pro-American
quasi-	partly	quasi-humorous
re-	again	repeat
vice-	in place of	vice-principal

(continued)

TABLE 10.3—*Continued*

TIME

PREFIX	MEANING	EXAMPLE
ante-	before	antecedent
post-	after	postpone
pre-	before	precede
pro-	before	prophecy

NUMBER

PREFIX	MEANING	EXAMPLE
bi-	two, twice	biceps
cent-	hundred	centennial
dec-	ten	decimal
demi-	half	demigod
di-	two	diphthong
du-	two	dual
hemi-	half	hemisphere
hept-/sept-	seven	heptagon
iso-	equal	isosceles
kilo-	1,000	kilogram
milli-	1/1,000	millisecond
mono-	one	monotone
multi-	many	multicolored
non-/novem-	nine	novena
octa-/octo-	eight	octagon
omni-	all	omnipotent
pan-	all	panorama
penta-	five	pentagon
poly-	many	polygamy
proto-	first	prototype
quad-/quart-/quartr-	four	quadrangle
quin-	five	quintet
semi-	half	semicircle
sex-/hex-	six	sextet, hexagon
tetra-	four	tetrachloride
tri-	three	trimester
uni-	one	universe

(continued)

TABLE 10.4 SUFFIXES

STATE OF BEING

SUFFIX	MEANING	EXAMPLE
-acy/-cy	office, rank of, state of	infancy
-ance	state of	importance
-ancy	state of	vacancy
-ant	state of, condition of	radiant
-ation	state of, quality of, result of	occupation
-dom	state of	wisdom
-ence	state, quality, condition of	confidence
-ency	quality of, state of	frequency
-hood	state of, quality of, condition of	womanhood
-ion	state of	ambition
-ism	state of, condition of	racism
-ism	doctrine, system	realism
-ity	state of	necessity
-ment	state of	amazement
-ness	state of, quality of, condition of	greatness
-osis	abnormal condition, state of	hypnosis
-ship	state of, profession, art, skill	ownership
-wise	way, manner, respect	clockwise
-y	condition or quality of being	jealousy

SMALL

SUFFIX	MEANING	EXAMPLE
-cule/-ule	small	capsule
-et/-ette	small	dinette
-icle	little	particle
-ie	little	cutie
-kin	little	lambkin
-let	small	bracelet
-ling	small	duckling
-y	small	dolly

(continued)

TABLE 10.4—*Continued*

CHARACTERISTIC OF

SUFFIX	MEANING	EXAMPLE
-al	relating to	royal
-an	relating to	American
-ary	characterized by, relating to	military
-ese	of or having to do with	Japanese
-esque	in the manner, style of, like	picturesque
-ial	in the manner, related to	industrial
-ian	in the manner, related to	physician
-ic	of the nature of, characterized by	angelic
-ical	of the nature of, characterized by	critical
-ine	like, characterized by, pertaining to	feminine
-ious	characterized by	gracious
-ish	like, pertaining to	clownish
-like	like	homelike
-ly	characteristic of, in the manner of	fatherly
-oid	like, resembling	asteroid
-ous	possessing the qualities of	poisonous
-ster	one belonging to, characterized by	mobster, youngster
-y	full of	cloudy

FEMININE GENDER

SUFFIX	MEANING	EXAMPLE
-ess	feminine ending	actress
-ette	feminine ending	usherette
-ine	feminine ending	heroine

(continued)

TABLE 10.4—*Continued*

PERSON/PLACES

SUFFIX	MEANING	EXAMPLE
-age	place of	orphanage
-arian	person who, place where, object which	librarian
-ary	person who, place where, object which	secretary
-er/-or*	person connected with	carpenter
-eur	agent	chauffeur
-ery/-ry	place where	bakery
-ier/-yer*	person who, place where	cashier
-ist	person who	bicyclist
-or*	person who	auditor
-orium	place for, object used for	natatorium
-ory	place where	laboratory

*makes word into a noun

WORDS MADE INTO NOUNS

SUFFIX	MEANING	EXAMPLE
-ade	process, action	blockade
-and/-end	to be done	dividend
-ant/-ent	person who	resident
-ation	process, action	continuation
-atory	process, action, place where	reformatory
-ic	to form nouns	public
-ings	noun associated with the verb form	earnings
-ion	action, process	construction
-ism	action, process	baptism
-ment	action, process	government

NOUNS MADE INTO ADJECTIVES

SUFFIX	MEANING	EXAMPLE
-able/-ible/-ble	can be done	lovable
-able/-ible/-ble	inclined to	perishable
-en	to make or made of	golden
-ful	enough to fill	beautiful
-less	without	fruitless

(continued)

TABLE 10.4 SUFFIXES—*Continued*
MISCELLANEOUS

SUFFIX	MEANING	EXAMPLE
-ate	to make, cause to be	radiate
-ectomy	surgical removal	tonsillectomy
-er	comparative degree	faster
-est	comparative degree	largest
-fy	make of, form into	amplify
-ing	present participle	walking
-ing	material	roofing
-ise/-ize	subject to, make, carry on	sterilize
-itis	inflammatory disease	bronchitis
-logy	science of	biology
-ry	collection of	jewelry

SURVIVAL LANGUAGE FOR THE ADULT MEDIATOR

Adult mediators who reside with adolescents in their homes have the advantage of recognizing the ever-changing interests of this age group. For those, however, who find themselves experiencing a generation gap, basic "interest" lists for the "survival" of the adult mediator are included. The lists were generated by Midwestern adolescents, but regional differences in adolescents exist and rapid changes in their interests occur. The lists, intended as examples of topics of which educators may want to be cognizant, are captured on pages 341–345.

ACTIVITIES TO ENHANCE SURVIVAL LANGUAGE STRATEGIES

SURVIVAL LANGUAGE SKILLS

● Understanding and use of vocabulary pertaining to food, food preparation, grocery shopping, and restaurants

●● Understanding and use of vocabulary pertaining to personal independence, hygiene, and health

●●● Understanding and use of vocabulary pertaining to transportation

●●●● Understanding and use of vocabulary pertaining to math, money, and banking

●●●●● Understanding and use of vocabulary pertaining to entertainment, crafts, hobbies, and sports

●●●●●● Understanding and use of vocabulary pertaining to comprehension of word elements

●●●●●●● Knowledge of each adolescent's culture

FUNCTIONAL VOCABULARY

PURPOSE

To present vocabulary that commonly occurs in daily living situations

LEARNING STRATEGY

The adolescent will understand and use vocabulary related to food, food preparation, grocery shopping, and restaurants encountered independently in daily living situations.

The following vocabulary list, as well as lists in subsequent activities for survival language strategies, are adapted from numerous sources (Adams, Flowers, and Woods, 1978; Brigance, 1981; Greatsinger, 1976a, 1976b; Richey, 1978, 1980).

The following words are representative of vocabulary items that adolescents should have within their repertoire pertaining to food. While these words may be defined and discussed in an isolated activity, it would be more functional to have students learn them in the context of the suggested activities that follow the lists.

Food	Food Preparation	Grocery Shopping	Restaurants
appetizer	blanch	canned goods	à la carte
bars	broil	cashier	brunch
batter	brown	condiments	buffet
beverages	chop	convenience store	cafeteria
caffeine free	coffeemaker	coupons	check
calories	colander	customer	cocktails
carbohydrates	Dutch oven	dairy case	coffeehouse
casserole	frying pan	deli	cuisine
cholesterol	grate	drive-up	deli
citrus	griddle	expiration date	drive-through
dips	grill	express lane	diner
dressing	knead	freeze-dried	entrée
fat free	liquefy	fresh	family size
grains	marinate	frozen foods	fast food
greens	microwave	generic	gratuity
junk food	mince	meat counter	in a basket
low fat	pare	natural foods	jumbo
low sodium	pinch	organic	kiddie menu
lite	preserve	packaged	maitre d'
pasta	pureé	produce	on tap
pastry	sauté	proof of purchase	reservation
reduced fat	season	spices	short stack
saturated fat	simmer	sodium free	snack bar
sauces	steam	sugar free	soft drinks
seafood	stir fry	sweetless lane	super size
sodium	strain	UPC symbol	tip
starch	substitute	USDA Grade-A	vending machine
	wok		wine list

FOOD/FOOD PREPARATION/ GROCERY SHOPPING/ RESTAURANTS ACTIVITIES

PURPOSE

To learn survival vocabulary by participating in functional activities

LEARNING STRATEGY

The adolescent will understand and use vocabulary related to food, food preparation, grocery shopping, and restaurants encountered independently in daily living situations.

The following 10 activities are suggested ways to learn the language of food, food preparation, grocery shopping, and restaurants in a meaningful context.

1. Challenge students to plan a balanced lunch menu for a 3-year-old, including the beverage and a food item from each of the levels in the food pyramid. What considerations were made based on the age of the child?

2. Guide students in preparing a shopping list for the menu planned in task 1. In what grocery store department will each ingredient be found (e.g., produce, frozen foods, canned goods, baking needs)? What size packages will be appropriate?

3. Using the size terminology found on a menu, have students organize terms such as the following from small to large servings: *medium, small, large, jumbo, family size, super size.*

4. Instruct students to predict the size and price of meals, the menu, and the atmosphere of various kinds of restaurants—fast-food, hamburger joint, cafeteria, dining room, deli, etc. How does a consumer determine these characteristics in an eating establishment? How will the time of day affect the choice of a restaurant? How does the purpose of the meal determine where one will eat?

5. Have adolescents name foods that might be available in a vending machine and then describe probable locations of vending machines.

6. Help adolescents determine the amount of tip appropriate for a particular meal. What considerations should be made when tipping?

7. Tell students to name foods they would expect to be entrées, desserts, foods served à la carte, appetizers, etc.

8. With students, list foods that might be found in the produce section of a grocery store. Where might the produce section be found? (E.g., most refrigerated units are located on the outside walls of the store.) How or where will these products be stored at home?

9. Gather recipes, then give them to the adolescents. Discuss how the recipes might be organized in a recipe box (e.g., lasagna in a main meal section, cauliflower dip with appetizers). Give the adolescents additional meal ideas, then discuss how to find the recipe in a file or in a cookbook.

10. Given food preparation action words (e.g., pureé, chop, liquefy, microwave, broil), have students describe the appliances that would perform these actions (e.g., blender, food processor, microwave oven, broiler in oven).

FUNCTIONAL VOCABULARY

PURPOSE

To present vocabulary that commonly occurs in daily living situations

LEARNING STRATEGY

The adolescent will understand and use vocabulary related to personal independence, hygiene, and health needed in daily living situations.

The following words are representative of vocabulary items that adolescents should have within their repertoire pertaining to personal independence, hygiene, and health. While these words may be defined and discussed in an isolated activity, it would be more functional to have students learn them in the context of the suggested activities that follow the lists.

Body Awareness

abdomen/abdominal
AIDS
alcoholism
allergy/allergic
bacteria/bacterial infection
benign
bladder
blood test
blood pressure
bowels
cancer
cardiac/coronary
drug addiction
exercise
heart rate
ideal weight
indigestion
inflammation
malignant
nausea
pores
pulse
sensitivity
sinus
stress
stroke
tumor
urine specimen
vaccination
venereal disease
virus/viral infection

Clothing Care

100% wool
100% cotton
chlorine bleach
degreaser
delicate
Do not bleach
Do not dry in direct sunlight
Drip dry
Dry clean only
fabric softener
Flame-retardant
Hand wash
Lay flat to dry
Lycra
Machine wash, cold
Machine wash, warm
No iron, if decorated
permanent press
polyester/Dacron
prewash
shrink
Sponge spots with damp cloth
steam iron
Tumble dry low
Turn inside out to wash
Use only nonchlorine bleach
Wash before wearing
Wash with like colors
Wash separately

Shopping/Nonfoods

appliances
as advertised
automotive
cashier
clerk
consumer
cosmetics
credit card
credit check
deposit
discount store
dressing room
electronics
exchange
ladies' fashions
layaway
mail order
mall/plaza
notions
novelties
outlet store
pharmacy
raincheck
rebate
receipt
refund
register
return
service department
sporting goods
sundries
warranty

Pharmacy

antibiotic
antifungal
antihistamine
antioxidant
antiperspirant
antiseptic
caplet
capsule
chewable
compress
contraceptive
daily dosage
decongestant
dental floss
disinfectant
dispensing
generic
hydrogen peroxide
hypoallergenic
insect repellent
laxative
maximum strength
pain reliever
over-the-counter drugs
prescription
refill prescription
safety cap
salve/ointment
sterilize
symptoms
sunscreen/sunblock
temporary relief
vitamin/mineral

Warning Labels

Active Ingredients
Avoid Contact with Eyes
Caution: Contents Under Pressure
Caution/Eye Irritant
Caution: Not for Personal Use
Combustible Mixture
Danger High Voltage
Do Not Breathe Fumes
Do Not Exceed Recommended Daily Dosage
Do Not Incinerate Container
Do Not Induce Vomiting
Do Not Use Internally
Do Not Use if Seal Is Broken
Do Not Use Near Cooking Appliances
Fatal or Harmful if Swallowed
Fire Extinguisher
Flammable Substance
For External Use Only
If Rash Occurs, Discontinue Use
In Case of Contact, Flush with Water
Keep Out of Reach of Children
Not Recommended for Use with...
Prohibited
Refrigerate After Opening
Shake Well Before Using
Store Away from Heat
This Is Not a Toy! Keep Away From Children!
Use with Adequate Ventilation
Vapor Harmful

PERSONAL INDEPENDENCE/ HYGIENE/HEALTH ACTIVITIES

PURPOSE

To learn survival vocabulary by participating in functional activities

LEARNING STRATEGY

The adolescent will understand and use vocabulary related to personal independence, hygiene, and health needed in daily living situations.

The following 10 activities are suggested ways to learn the language of personal independence, hygiene, and health.

1. Given ailments/diseases such as the following, challenge adolescents to describe the body parts that might be affected: nausea, a cold, a coronary, a stroke, alcoholism.

2. Together with students, name diseases or ailments and then group them in the categories of "communicable" and "noncommunicable." Discuss the incubation period for the communicable diseases. What can students do to prevent contracting a communicable disease?

3. Help students identify the fabric types of the clothes they are wearing, then describe the appropriate washer and dryer (and iron) settings for laundering them. What kind of detergent and water temperature would be appropriate? What other types/colors of clothes could be safely washed together? Discuss how to determine the type of care required for particular clothes.

4. Provide students with a collection of warning labels from household items. What do each of the warnings mean? Where else might students encounter the given warning label? What are the consequences of disregarding various warning labels? What steps could be taken to remedy a problem created by disregarding a warning label?

5. Discuss safe storage locations for a list of items with various labels. How might the storage area change if a 2-year-old lived in the home?

6. Have students imagine they are shopping in a large discount store. In what department would they find an electric iron? An oil filter? A box of Band-Aids? A camera? A spool of thread? A garden hose? Have students name other items they might find in the notions department, the automotive department, ladies' fashions, the garden center, etc.

7. Discuss under what conditions an exchange of merchandise might be made. What about a refund? How are these transactions different from a return of merchandise? Where would the transactions be made? Are there any limiting conditions (time limit, return with receipt, tags on unused merchandise) that usually exist?

8. Gather and provide adolescents with direction labels from over-the-counter medications and prescription drugs. Guide them in formulating a plan for taking the proper dosages, including a description of the dosage (e.g., number of tablets necessary), the appropriate time of day to take the medicine, and the means of drug administration (e.g., taken orally, applied to skin, etc.). If students became ill after taking medication, what would they do? What do the various instructions ("apply liberally," "do not use internally") for administering the drugs mean?

9. List symptoms of ailments where everyone can see them. Help students name an over-the-counter drug that might relieve the symptoms. What cautions should students follow? What are the age restrictions for the drug? Should the medication be administered to a child? Who might be a good resource for answers to these questions? What are "generic" drugs? Are they safe to use?

10. Discuss symptoms that would require a doctor's visit. Present symptoms (e.g., blurred vision, intestinal pain, irritating rash) to the adolescents and ask them to determine the physician or specialist most appropriate to see. How is a family practice physician different from a specialist? How would they go about finding a physician or specialist?

FUNCTIONAL VOCABULARY

PURPOSE

To present vocabulary that commonly occurs in daily living situations

The following words are representative of vocabulary items that adolescents should have within their repertoire pertaining to transportation. While these words may be defined and discussed in an isolated activity, it would be more functional to have students learn them in the context of the suggested activities that follow the lists.

Driver's License	Car	Mass Transit
accelerate/decelerate	accelerator	accommodations
car length	air filter	Amtrak
clearance	alignment	arrival
collision	automatic choke	baggage claim
detour	carbon monoxide	boarding ramp/ boarding/on-board
DWI	carburetor	cancellation
Give 'em a Brake	clutch	concourse
hazard	coolant	connection
identification	cruise control	departure
implied consent	dimmer switch	depot
insurance	exhaust system	electronic devices
intoxicated	filter	fare
lane	flooded engine	fares subject to change
merge	fuel injection system	ferry
minor	fuel pump	gate
obstruct	high beam indicator	location/destination
oncoming	ignition	lodging
parallel	inflate	passport
pedestrian	insurability	rail pass
probationary	liability	schedule
prohibited	oil filter/oil change	shuttle
residential	owner's manual	subway
restriction	power steering	taxi
revocation/revoke	spark plugs	terminal
shoulder	title	token
suspended	tread	toll
tailgate	tune-up	transcontinental
traveler's advisory	unleaded/regular/ premium/diesel	transfer ticket
visibility	vehicle registration	traveler's check
zone		

LEARNING STRATEGY

The adolescent will understand and use vocabulary related to transportation used independently in daily living situations.

TRANSPORTATION ACTIVITIES

PURPOSE

To learn survival vocabulary by participating in functional activities

The following 10 activities suggest ways to learn the language of transportation.

1. Discuss what all forms of transportation have in common and what differentiates the many forms of transportation. What are the forms of transportation available in your area?

2. Present transportation terms and guide students in grouping the words according to the form of transportation to which they relate:

   Example:

Train	Airplane	All Forms of Transportation
Amtrak	pilot	baggage
conductor	flight attendant	departure gate
rail pass	electronic devices	concourse
		fare

3. Help students rank forms of transportation from least expensive to most expensive, and least convenient to most convenient.

4. Given travel brochures with vacation offerings, challenge students to plan a vacation and determine the total cost of the trip. Discuss vocabulary terms such as *round trip, one-way fare, per person, double occupancy, airfare additional, optional day, complimentary,* etc. Discuss what might not be included in the vacation offering. Then have adolescents determine the costs of lodging and meals for the trip. Compare the costs to the vacation offered through the travel brochure.

5. Given car parts, direct students to categorize them according to the location in which they might be found (e.g., engine, interior, exterior). Categorize parts or items according to convenience features (e.g., cruise control, air conditioning) versus necessary vehicle parts (e.g., exhaust system, fuel line).

6. Given situations such as the following, guide students in determining the options for resolving each problem and discuss how quickly they would need to deal with each situation:

●●●

LEARNING STRATEGY

The adolescent will understand and use vocabulary related to transportation used independently in daily living situations.

- You have a flat tire as you are driving down an interstate highway.
- You hear a knocking sound inside your car's engine.
- The CD player in your car is not working right.
- The oil light came on in your car and you are two blocks from home.
- Your battery is dead. You're parked in the grocery store parking lot.
- The air conditioning in your car doesn't seem to be cooling.
- You've locked your keys in the car.

7 Role-play a conversation between an auto owner and a mechanic. Instruct the owner to describe a malfunction of the automobile and the mechanic to ask appropriate questions to gain information about the malfunction.

8 Generate a list of highway terms such as the following: *interstate, expressway, four-lane, two-lane, county highway, town road.* Have students rank the terms from heavy traffic to light traffic, greatest number of lanes to least number of lanes, most rapid mode of highway travel to least rapid mode.

9 Role-play pedestrians who observed a traffic accident. Encourage adolescents to use appropriate terminology to describe the sequence of events, including *visibility, oncoming, head-on, merge, car length.*

10 Help students calculate the mileage from one destination to another. Given the parameters and schedule constraints of the different forms of transportation, direct them to determine the transportation that would get them to their destination the fastest. When would traveling by car be faster than traveling by plane? When would traveling by foot be faster than traveling by car?

FUNCTIONAL VOCABULARY

PURPOSE

To present vocabulary that commonly occurs in daily living situations

●●●●

LEARNING STRATEGY

The adolescent will understand and use vocabulary related to math, money, and banking used independently in daily living situations.

The following words are representative of vocabulary items that adolescents should have within their repertoire pertaining to math, money, and banking. While these words may be defined and discussed in an isolated activity, it would be more functional to have students learn them in the context of the suggested activities that follow the lists.

Math

180°
360°
angle
area
average
bisect
calculator
circumference
clockwise
counterclockwise
decimal
diagonal
diameter
dissect
divide
horizontal
mean
metric system
multiply
one-half
one-quarter
one-third
parallel
percent/percentage
perimeter
perpendicular
ratio
right angle
vertical
volume

Money/Banking

account
asset
balance due
bankrupt
certificate of deposit (CD)
charge account
check
collateral
compounded daily
credit card
credit rating
currency
debit
deduction
deposit
earning
endorse
installment
interest rate
liability
money market fund
money order
mortgage
mutual fund
penalty
principal
repossess
savings bond
statement
withdrawal

MATH/MONEY/ BANKING ACTIVITIES

PURPOSE

To learn survival vocabulary by participating in functional activities

LEARNING STRATEGY

The adolescent will understand and use vocabulary related to math, money, and banking used independently in daily living situations.

The following 10 activities are suggested ways to learn the vocabulary of math, money, and banking.

1. Compare and contrast the terms *circumference* and *diameter.* Discuss the purpose for knowing how to determine the circumference of an object (e.g., head circumference—hat size; neck circumference—shirt size; table circumference—to add trim to a tablecloth) and the diameter of an object (e.g., table diameter—tablecloth size; wheel rim diameter—tire size). What instrument would be used to measure circumference or diameter in the examples given? Have students generate more examples.

2. Have students demonstrate the rotations *clockwise* and *counterclockwise,* then describe situations where the terms might be used (e.g., rotation when playing cards, turning nuts and bolts, opening combination locks).

3. Compare and contrast the terms *perimeter* and *area.* Instruct students to name situations that would require knowing the area of an object (e.g., measuring carpeting or linoleum, determining if a carpet remnant will fit a particular room) and the perimeter of an object (e.g., measuring weatherstripping or a wallpaper border). What is the formula for determining area? What is the formula for determining perimeter? What resource could be used to find these formulas if they are forgotten?

4. Using a city map, challenge students to describe the streets in relation to one another using vocabulary such as *parallel, perpendicular, angle, right angle.* Where else have they heard these terms used? When would these terms be used in daily living situations (e.g., giving directions, driving a car, parallel parking)?

5. Guide students in classifying—positive (addition) and negative (subtraction)—the following money or banking-related terms: *withdrawal, deposit, asset, liability, deduction, interest, debit, credit.*

6. Direct students to compare and contrast various forms of money: currency, personal check, money order, traveler's check, cash, cashier's check, credit card, charge account. Give examples of when each form of money might be used.

7. Using the forms of money listed in the previous activity, what are the intended purposes of the various forms of money? Discuss advantages and disadvantages of each type in various settings. Rank the forms of money from least costly to the user to most costly to the user.

8. Directions for operation of a lawn mower require mixing gas and oil in a ratio of 2 to 1. Challenge students to calculate the amount of gasoline needed to combine with one quart of oil. What other situations might require a ratio mixture?

9. Present the students with various bills, monthly statements, transaction receipts, checks, accounts, summaries, etc. Have them identify the elements of each, such as signature, balance due, due date, withdrawal amount, deposits, payments made, account balance, subtotals, tax, account numbers.

10. Obtain a loan application from a bank. Tell students to pretend they make $20,000 a year performing janitorial services, they have no outstanding debts, and they are married with two children. Their spouse does not work outside of the home. Have them complete the application form using this information. What other information do they need?

FUNCTIONAL VOCABULARY

PURPOSE

To present vocabulary that commonly occurs in daily living situations

●●●●●

LEARNING STRATEGY

The adolescent will understand and use vocabulary related to entertainment, crafts, hobbies, and sports encountered independently in daily living situations.

The following words are representative of vocabulary items that adolescents should have within their repertoire pertaining to entertainment, crafts, hobbies, and sports. While these words may be defined and discussed in an isolated activity, it would be more functional to have students learn them in the context of the suggested activities following the lists.

Entertainment	**Crafts/Hobbies/Sports**
admission	aerobics
aisle	antiques
balcony	athletic club
Broadway play	backgammon
carnival	billiards
concert	bicycle trail
concession	bike lane
convention center	board game
documentary	collectibles
drama	counted cross-stitch
festival	etiquette
gallery	figure skating
intermission	Frisbee
marquee	in-line skating
motel/hotel	jogging
program	karate
recital	league
resort	macramé
sightseeing	Olympics
sports arena	racquetball
stadium	recreation
standing ovation	regulation
theatre	snorkeling
ticket center	spectator sport
usher	sports event
VCR	sportsmanship
video arcade	stenciling
video games	tour
video rentals	workout
will call	yoga

ENTERTAINMENT/CRAFTS/ HOBBIES/SPORTS ACTIVITIES

PURPOSE

To learn survival vocabulary by participating in functional activities

●●●●●

LEARNING STRATEGY

The adolescent will understand and use vocabulary related to entertainment, crafts, hobbies, and sports encountered independently in daily living situations.

The following 10 activities are suggested ways to learn the vocabulary of entertainment, crafts, hobbies, and sports.

1. Discuss resources available for learning about local entertainment (e.g., information centers, posters in grocery stores, newspapers, neighborhood flyers). How can entertainment information about cities or communities outside of the local area be obtained (e.g., travel bureaus, chambers of commerce, tourist information centers)?

2. Have students determine the kind of entertainment information given in their local newspaper. What information can be found in the yellow pages of the phone book? Review vocabulary terms found in the entertainment ads.

3. Direct students to choose one of the forms of entertainment found in task 2 and then plan an evening involving this entertainment. Challenge them to calculate the costs involved, the mileage, transportation to and from the activity, and an estimated time line.

4. Classify sports and sporting activities according to whether they are team or individual sports. Where would you call to find out if you could play on a city volleyball team? A local softball team? What is a spectator sport? How can tickets be purchased for a chosen spectator sport?

5. Name sports or hobbies. Have students list equipment that might be required for each and determine the places for purchasing the equipment (e.g., sporting goods stores, departments within a store, catalogs, newspaper for used sports equipment, thrift sales) or for renting the needed the equipment. Have students name equipment they might be able to rent (e.g., canoes, bikes, in-line skates, rafts). What are the advantages (e.g., allows you to try the sport before you buy equipment, less expensive to rent if you don't use the equipment very often) and disadvantages (e.g., costly if you do it often, deposit required) of renting equipment?

6. List types of festivals (e.g., folk, music, film, church). Allow students to share experiences they have had at festivals in the area. This will help others to know what festivals are available locally. What kinds of entertainment would be found at the various festivals?

7. Challenge students to think of a multitude of resources for learning about new crafts, hobbies, or sports (e.g., the yellow pages of the phone book, hobby shops, craft stores, technical colleges, evening classes, parks and recreation departments).

8. Poll students to determine their favorite forms of entertainment. Guide them in listing and defining terminology related to their favorite activities (e.g., bowling—*pins, strike, alley, gutter ball, spare, bowling ball, reset).*

9. Discuss with students the commonalities of all forms of entertainment. What characteristics differentiate various forms of entertainment?

10. Discuss reasons for participating in leisure activities (e.g., for enjoyment, to stay in shape, for relaxation, to reduce stress). Encourage each adolescent to report on his or her favorite leisure activity and, if possible, to demonstrate it to the group.

SYNTHESIZING WORD PARTS

PURPOSE

To develop an awareness of word parts in whole words and to become aware of words with similar parts

In English, words are "coined" by combining old words with new prefixes or suffixes (Devine, 1981) (e.g., *cyberspace* and *megabucks*). Most students are not aware that they can analyze the elements within a word to glean partial meaning of the word. In this section of *Daily Communication*, students are taught to analyze the parts of words as a strategy to deciphering their meaning. This strategy cannot alone determine the meaning of a word, as the context in which the word is used is also a powerful tool for determining meaning.

Refer to Tables 10.2 through 10.4 (pages 299–309) for this activity. First guide students to generalize the meanings of word elements for words with which they are familiar. Follow this step by analyzing unfamiliar words with similar word elements. If students have difficulty deciphering the meaning of an unfamiliar word, putting the word in the context of a sentence can help them ascertain the word meaning. Finally, guide students in generating words with similar meanings based on a word element (i.e., a prefix, suffix, or word root).

The following activities reinforce the analysis and synthesis of word elements to determine the meaning of vocabulary words.

Present words containing several word elements. Analyze the elements of each word. Provide students with the meaning of each element. Challenge them to synthesize the word elements and define the resulting word, and then to generate additional words that use the same word part.

1. If *poly* means *many* and *gon* means *angle*, what does *polygon* mean? Name other *poly* words (e.g., *polygamy, polyester, polymer)*. Name other *gon* words (e.g., *octagon, pentagon, hexagonal, trigonometry)*. What does each word mean?

2. If *ident* means *same* and *fy* means *make*, what does *identify* mean? Name other *ident* words (e.g., *identical, identity, identification)*. Name other *fy* words (e.g., *crucify, rectify)*. What does each word mean?

3. If *micro* means *small* and *scope* means *to watch*, what does *microscope* mean? Name other *micro* words (e.g., *micrometer, microphone)*. Name other *scope* words (e.g., *telescope, periscope)*. What does each word mean?

LEARNING STRATEGY

The adolescent will comprehend word elements as a strategy for understanding unfamiliar vocabulary and for expanding functional vocabulary use.

4. If *bi* means *two* and *enni* means *year*, what does *biennial* mean? Name other *bi* words (e.g., *bisect, biweekly*). Name other *enni* words (e.g., *perennial, centennial*). What does each word mean?

5. If *pre* means *before* and *ced* means *go*, what does *precede* mean? Name other *pre* words (e.g., *prehistoric, predict, premeditate*). Name other *ced* words (e.g., *recede, antecedent, concede*). What does each word mean?

Continue using the following words and elements, generating and defining similar words:

6	immortal	im		mort		al		
		not	+	death	+	relating to		
7	intoxication	in		tox		ic		ation
		into	+	poison	+	characterized by	+	state of
8	interruption	inter		rupt		ion		
		between	+	break	+	state of		
9	promote	pro		mote				
		forward	+	move				
10	perimeter	peri		meter				
		around	+	measure				
11	biology	bio		logy				
		life	+	science of				
12	homicide	hom		cide				
		man	+	kill				
13	audible	aud		ible				
		hear	+	can be done				
14	discriminate	dis		crim		in		ate
		apart from	+	judge	+	into	+	make or cause to be

15	contradict	contra		dict		
		against	+	say		
16	infer	in		fer		
		into	+	carry, bear		
17	inflammable	in		flam		able
		not	+	blaze	+	state of
18	geography	geo		graph		y
		earth	+	write	+	pertaining to
19	counterclockwise	counter		clock		wise
		against	+	clock	+	way, manner
20	pseudonym	pseudo		onym		
		false	+	name		

ANALYZING WORD PARTS

PURPOSE

To develop an awareness of word parts in whole words and to recognize how word parts change word meaning

Refer to Tables 10.2 through 10.4 (pages 299–309) for this activity. Introduce a word element to the students. If introducing a word root, present prefixes or suffixes that could be added to it. Analyze the change in meaning when each new element is added.

If introducing a prefix or suffix, present word roots. Analyze the prefix or suffix meaning and how its addition changes the meaning of the root words.

The following are examples:

1. Word root: *do* (give) — donate, donor, antidote
2. Word root: *acro* (high) — acrobat, acronym, acrophobia
3. Word root: *mers* (sink, dip) — submerse, immerse, submersion
4. Word root: *legal* (legal) — illegal, legalize, legitimate
5. Word root: *bio* (life) — biology, biologist, biopsy
6. Prefix: *hyper* (over, beyond) — hyperactive, hypercorrect, hypercritical
7. Word root: *crit* (judge) — criticize, critique, critic
8. Prefix: *hypo* (under, too little) — hypochondriac, hypocorrect, hyponasal

LEARNING STRATEGY

The adolescent will comprehend word elements as a strategy for understanding unfamiliar vocabulary and for expanding functional vocabulary use.

9	Suffix: *y* (small)	ducky dolly Timmy
10	Prefix: *ex* (out)	exhume exit ex-husband
11	Suffix: *like* (like)	childlike homelike fatherlike
12	Prefix: *bi* (two, twice)	biceps biennial bicycle
13	Word root: *vit* (life)	vital vitality vitamin
14	Word root: *photo* (light)	photograph photography photosynthesis
15	Word root: *tom* (cut)	tonsillectomy hysterectomy appendectomy
16	Prefix: *pro* (for, in favor of)	protest pro-American pro-choice
17	Prefix: *post* (after)	postprom postpone post-test
18	Suffix: *wise* (way, manner, respect)	clockwise counterclockwise likewise

19	Prefix: *sub* (under)	submarine submerse substandard
20	Suffix: *ment* (state of)	amusement amazement containment

SIMILAR MEANINGS

PURPOSE

To explore the similar meanings of prefixes and suffixes and the effect of adding them to root words

Using the information provided in Tables 10.2 through 10.4 (pages 299–309), group prefixes and/or suffixes of similar meaning. For example, the following prefixes form antonyms when added to a root word:

in, a, im, il, non, under, over

The following prefixes make the root word "bigger":

mega, hyper, poly, ultra, multi, extra, super

Present the following meanings and have students identify prefixes or suffixes that have similar meanings. Then have them generate words that contain each suffix or prefix.

1. before
2. in
3. against
4. not
5. after
6. state of
7. numbers
8. related to
9. make little
10. make feminine
11. back
12. over
13. out
14. in place of
15. large
16. away
17. like
18. make the opposite of
19. can be done
20. person who

●●●●●●

LEARNING STRATEGY

The adolescent will comprehend word elements as a strategy for understanding unfamiliar vocabulary and for expanding functional vocabulary use.

"WORD OF THE WEEK" CONTEST

PURPOSE

To generate words with similar roots, prefixes, and suffixes

Introduce one new word root, prefix, or suffix to the class weekly. To start, introduce one of the following most frequently used prefixes identified by Stauffer (1942) or those found in Brown's (1952) 14 words. These word elements may give students the "most mileage" for their efforts:

ab	ex	over
ad	in (into)	pre
be	in (not)	pro
de	inter	re
dis	mis	sub
en	mono	trans
epi	non	un

Word roots (based on Brown's [1952] 14 words) with Latin derivatives will be more challenging for students, since the connection to the Latin derivative is not always obvious. However, the challenge will be helpful to students. The word roots are:

capere (take, seize)	legein (say, study)	specere (see)
ducere (lead)	mittere (send)	stare (stand)
facere (make, do)	plicare (fold)	tendere (stretch)
ferre (bear, carry)	ponere (put, place)	tenere (hold, have)
graphein (write)	scribere (write)	

1. Keep a new root word, prefix, or suffix posted throughout the week and hold a contest to see who can gather the most words containing the word root, prefix, or suffix. Encourage students to search for words in their textbooks, at their jobs, or at home in newspapers or magazines.

2. Construct a "Word of the Week" box where students can submit their entries during the week. Require adolescents to define the words for the group as they place them in the box. Allow students to also create "new" words using the prefix, suffix, or word root of focus, provided they can define the new word and use it appropriately in context.

3. With the group, determine prizes of worth (computer time, time to play an educational board game, etc.) for the weekly winner.

LEARNING STRATEGY

The adolescent will comprehend word elements as a strategy for understanding unfamiliar vocabulary and for expanding functional vocabulary use.

4. On the final contest day, count the words entered per student, post the words where everyone can see them, and announce the winner.

5. Challenge students to create a word-element dictionary. Each week, have them record the new word element, its meaning, and examples in their dictionaries.

WORD CONNECTIONS

PURPOSE

To organize new words learned with other familiar words using a visual strategy

LEARNING STRATEGY

The adolescent will comprehend word elements as a strategy for understanding unfamiliar vocabulary and for expanding functional vocabulary use.

To vary the "Word of the Week" contest, post the words gathered by students using a word map. Encourage students to assist in the organization of the words. Integrating new words with familiar words helps students to see the relationship between the new words and the familiar words, thereby aiding word retrieval at a later time. An example word map follows for the word element *mis*.

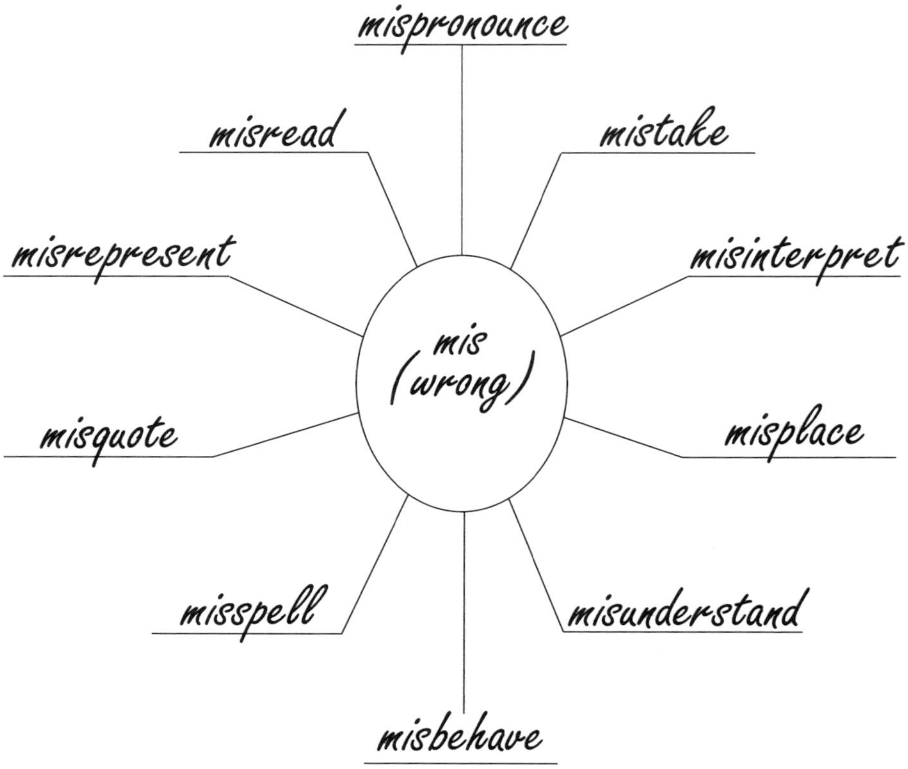

WORD CATEGORIES

PURPOSE

To define words with common roots, prefixes, and suffixes

Duplicate Appendix U onto heavy stock paper; cut into cards (or create cards relevant to students' needs). Prepare one set per pair of students.

Pair students. Have one student (the speaker) within the pair read the suffixes, prefixes, or word root and the category listed at the top of the card. Then direct the speakers to give definitions of the words given on the cards to their listening partners. Instruct the listeners to determine the words in that category based on the definitions given and the prefixes, suffixes, or word root given.

Announce a time limit. Assigning points or distributing play money for words guessed adds interest to this activity. Have the speakers and listeners reverse roles and pick new cards.

Simplify this activity by having the speaker write the category and prefixes, suffixes, or word roots where the listener can see them.

Vary this activity by having one speaker give the clues to the large group. To add interest, give a point or token to the first listener to guess each word.

SUFFIXES

1. **(-ule, -et [-ette], -icle)**
   little
   ringlet
   statuette
   capsule
   minuscule
   particle

2. **(-or, -er, -ier)**
   persons
   donor
   cashier
   auditor
   lawyer
   instructor
   director

3. **(-arian, -ian, -ist)**
   persons
   socialist
   chemist
   physician
   bicyclist
   librarian
   comedian

4. **(-orium, -ory, -ary, -atory)**
   places
   auditorium
   laboratory
   sanctuary
   observatory
   planetarium

5. **(-ish, -ster, -ly)**
   characteristic of
   childish
   timely
   Jewish
   motherly
   youngster
   gangster

6. **(-ship, -hood, -ism)**
   state of
   manhood
   censorship
   racism
   ownership
   hardship
   hypnotism

●●●●●●

LEARNING STRATEGY

The adolescent will comprehend word elements as a strategy for understanding unfamiliar vocabulary and for expanding functional vocabulary use.

7 (-itis, -ance, -ancy)
state of
bronchitis
resistance
truancy
arthritis
avoidance
vacancy

8 (-logy)
science of
biology
geology
theology
psychology
zoology
archaeology

9 (-ful)
enough to fill
mouthful
meaningful
handful
joyful
wonderful
spoonful

PREFIXES

10 (in-, non-, un-)
negative
nonstop
inactive
unsure
informal
nonsense
unsafe

11 (bi-, di-)
two
dissect
biennial
bisect
diphthong
bicycle
dilemma

12 (en-, in-, im-)
in, into
include
encircle
inhale
immerse
encase
implant

13 (contra-, counter-)
against
contradict
counterbalance
contraband
contrast
counterclockwise
counteract

14 (re-)
again
repeat
reorganize
rename
renew
remodel
repossess

15 (micro-)
small
microphone
microscope
microfilm
microsecond
microwave
microorganism

16 (mid-)
middle
midriff
Midwestern
midnight
midterm
midair
midpoint

17 (pro-)
directional
promote
provide
proceed
produce
progress
project

WORD ROOTS

18 **(graph)**
write
telegraph
paragraph
graphite
biography
autograph
geography

19 **(onym)**
name
antonym
homonym
acronym
synonym
pseudonym
anonymous

20 **(cide)**
kill
germicide
pesticide
suicide
homicide
herbicide
insecticide

DICTIONARY GAME

PURPOSE

To apply knowledge of word parts to unfamiliar words

Direct one student to look in the dictionary for a word composed of at least two word elements. The word should be one he or she thinks no other student will know. Direct the student to announce this word to the group. Have each person write possible definitions for this word, based on his or her knowledge of word parts, on a piece of paper. Instruct the student with the dictionary to write the actual meaning of the word on a piece of paper.

Tell the student with the dictionary to collect all definitions and read each to the group, including the actual definition, numbering them as he or she is reading. Have each student decide which definition he or she thinks is correct and write the number of the definition on a piece of paper.

Announce the number of the actual definition. Use a scoring system, such as the one following, to keep track of correct choices.

> Score 1 point if someone selects your definition.
>
> Score 1 point if you select the appropriate definition.
>
> Score 1 point if you wrote an acceptable definition.

Use the dictionary to verify the exact definition(s) for the selected word.

To reduce the competition, have each student try to better his or her own score from the last time the activity was used.

LEARNING STRATEGY

The adolescent will comprehend word elements as a strategy for understanding unfamiliar vocabulary and for expanding functional vocabulary use.

THE WORLD OF SPORTS

PURPOSE

To present the current baseball, basketball, football, and hockey teams

LEARNING STRATEGY

As a means toward better communication, the adult mediator will develop some knowledge of the cultural objects that bind together the adolescent's community.

A frequent topic of conversation among adolescents is sports. The following lists summarize the current professional sports teams. Adult mediators are urged to keep the lists up-to-date as changes occur.

MAJOR LEAGUE BASEBALL

National League	American League
Atlanta Braves	Baltimore Orioles
Chicago Cubs	Boston Red Sox
Cincinnati Reds	California Angels
Colorado Rockies	Chicago White Sox
Florida Marlins	Cleveland Indians
Houston Astros	Detroit Tigers
Los Angeles Dodgers	Kansas City Royals
Montreal Expos	Milwaukee Brewers
New York Mets	Minnesota Twins
Philadelphia Phillies	New York Yankees
Pittsburgh Pirates	Oakland Athletics
San Diego Padres	Seattle Mariners
San Francisco Giants	Texas Rangers
	Toronto Blue Jays

NATIONAL BASKETBALL ASSOCIATION

Eastern Conference	Western Conference
Atlanta Hawks	Dallas Mavericks
Boston Celtics	Denver Nuggets
Charlotte Hornets	Golden State Warriors
Chicago Bulls	Houston Rockets
Cleveland Cavaliers	Los Angeles Clippers
Detroit Pistons	Los Angeles Lakers
Indiana Pacers	Minnesota Timberwolves
Miami Heat	Phoenix Suns
Milwaukee Bucks	Portland Trail Blazers
New Jersey Nets	Sacramento Kings
New York Knicks	San Antonio Spurs
Orlando Magic	Seattle SuperSonics
Philadelphia Seventy-Sixers	Utah Jazz
Toronto Raptors	Vancouver Grizzlies
Washington Bullets	

NATIONAL FOOTBALL LEAGUE

American Football Conference

Buffalo Bills
Cincinnati Bengals
Cleveland Browns
Denver Broncos
Houston Oilers
Indianapolis Colts
Jacksonville Jaguars
Kansas City Chiefs
Los Angeles Raiders
Miami Dolphins
New England Patriots
New York Jets
Pittsburgh Steelers
San Diego Chargers
Seattle Seahawks

National Football Conference

Atlanta Falcons
Carolina Panthers
Chicago Bears
Dallas Cowboys
Detroit Lions
Green Bay Packers
Los Angeles Rams
Minnesota Vikings
New Orleans Saints
New York Giants
Philadelphia Eagles
Phoenix Cardinals
San Francisco Forty-Niners
Tampa Bay Buccaneers
Washington Redskins

NATIONAL HOCKEY LEAGUE

Wales Conference

Boston Bruins
Buffalo Sabres
Hartford Whalers
Montreal Canadiens
New Jersey Devils
New York Islanders
New York Rangers
Philadelphia Flyers
Pittsburgh Penguins
Quebec Nordiques
Washington Capitals

Campbell Conference

Calgary Flames
Chicago Black Hawks
Detroit Red Wings
Edmonton Oilers
Los Angeles Kings
Dallas Lone Stars
St. Louis Blues
San Jose Sharks
Toronto Maple Leafs
Vancouver Canucks
Winnipeg Jets

THE WORLD OF TELEVISION, SPORTS, AND MUSIC

PURPOSE

To present television stars, movie stars, music groups, and sports figures known to adolescents

LEARNING STRATEGY

As a means toward better communication, the adult mediator will develop some knowledge of the cultural objects that bind together the adolescent's community.

The following lists were developed by Midwestern adolescents between the ages of 12–20 years. They are not intended to be exhaustive, but rather to reflect current preferences by a select group of youth. They are representative of the types of lists helpful for adult mediators to compile within their own locale, since stars, music groups, and sports figures will vary greatly with geographical location.

TV AND MOVIE STARS

Tim Allen
Roseanne Arnold
Drew Barrymore
Warren Beatty
Beavis & Butthead
Candice Bergen
Mayim Bialik
Jonathan Brandis
Matthew Broderick
Candice Cameron
Kirk Cameron
John Candy
Dean Cane
Jim Carrey
Dana Carvey
Sean Connery
Kevin Costner
Cindy Crawford
Tom Cruise
Billy Crystal
Macaulay Culkin
Jamie Lee Curtis
Ted Danson
Johnny Depp
Danny DeVito
Phil Donahue
Mike Douglas
Clint Eastwood
Emilio Estevez
Erik Estrada
Chris Farley
Harrison Ford
Jodi Foster
Michael J. Fox
Mel Gibson
Sarah Gilbert
Whoopi Goldberg
Brian Austin Green
Tom Hanks
Woody Harrelson
Neil Patrick Harris
Ethan Hawke
Dustin Hoffman
Cathy Ireland
Jenni Jones
Shay Jordan
Michael Keaton
Nicole Kidman
Val Kilmer
Ricki Lake
Martin Lawrence
Jay Leno
David Letterman
Demi Moore
Kate Moss
Eddie Murphy
Bill Murray
Chris O'Donnell
Al Pacino
Stone Phillips
Brad Pitt
Maury Povich
Jason Priestley
Dan Rather
Robert Redford
Keanu Reeves
Michael Richards
Julia Roberts
Winona Ryder
Adam Sandler
Arnold Schwarzenegger
Steven Segal
Jerry Seinfeld
Charlie Sheen
Grant Show
Richard Simmons
Christian Slater
Will Smith
Jerry Springer
Sharon Stone
Keifer Sutherland
Patrick Swayze
Jean-Claude Van Damme
Vanna White
Robin Williams
Bruce Willis
Oprah Winfrey

MUSIC GROUPS

Aaliyah
AC/DC
Ace of Base
Aerosmith
Air Supply
All-4-One
Anthrax
Amy Grant
Belly
Bette Midler
Billy Joel
Blackstreet
Blind Melon
Bon Jovi
Bonnie Raitt
Boyz II Men
Brandy
Bruce Springsteen
The Cars
Changing Faces
Collective Soul
The Cranberries
Dave Matthews Band
Def Leppard
The Doors
Eagles
Elton John
En Vogue
Enigma
Eric Clapton
Garth Brooks
Genesis
George Strait
Gillette
Grateful Dead
Great White
Green Day
Green Jelly
Guns N' Roses
Hammer
Hi-Five
Hole
Hootie & the Blowfish
Ice Cube
Immature
Jade
Jamie Walters
Janet Jackson
Jeff Foxworthy
Jimi Hendrix
John Mellencamp
Kansas
Kiss
Lyle Lovett
Madonna
Mariah Carey
Marky Mark
Mary J. Blige
Melissa Etheridge
Men at Large
Metallica
Michael Bolton
Michael Jackson
Mick Jagger
Montel Jordan
Motley Crue
Mr. Big
Nine Inch Nails
Nirvana
Pantera
Paul Simon
Paula Abdul
Pearl Jam
Prince
Queen Latifah
R. Kelly
Red Hot Chili Peppers
R.E.M.
Rolling Stones
Rush
Salt-N-Pepa
Seal
Sheryl Crow
Slaughter
Slayer
Smashing Pumpkins
Snow
Soundgarden
Stevie Nicks
Sting
Stone Temple Pilots
Styx
Subway
TLC
Tevin Campbell
Tom Petty
Tone-Loc
U2
Usher
Ugly Kid Joe
Vanessa Williams
Vanilla Ice
Weird Al Yankovich
White Lion
Whitney Houston
Wings
Weezer
ZZ Top
Zhane'

SPORTS FIGURES

Andre Agassi
Troy Aikman
Roberto Alomar
Kenny Anderson
Mario Andretti
Michael Andretti
Vin Baker
Charles Barkley
Bonnie Blair
Larry Bird
Riddick Bowe
Muggsy Bogues
Jennifer Capriati
Joe Carter
Ki-Jana Carter
Sam Cassell
Michael Chang
Derrick Coleman
Kerry Collins
Randall Cunningham
Todd Day
Clyde Drexler
Tyus Edney
Julius Erving
Chris Evert
Patrick Ewing
Brett Favre
Michael Finley
George Foreman
Scott Goodyear
Steffi Graf
Wayne Gretzky
Ken Griffey, Jr.
Rashard Griffith
Anfernee Hardaway
Grant Hill
Robert Horry
Michael Irvin
Kareem Abdul-Jabbar
Bo Jackson
Dan Jansen
Kevin Johnson
Larry Johnson
Magic Johnson
Michael Jordan
Shawn Kemp
Nancy Kerrigan
Jackie Joyner Kersee
Jason Kidd
Toni Kukoc
Christian Laettner
Karl Malone
Danny Manning
Dan Majerle
Jamal Mashburn
Reggie Miller
Steve McNair
Harold Miner
Paul Molitor
Joe Montana
Alonzo Mourning
Joe Namath
Martina Navratilova
Ed O'Bannon
Hakeem Olajuwon
Shaquille O'Neal
Robert Parish
Scottie Pippen
Terry Porter
Bobby Rahal
Glen Rice
Jerry Rice
Isaiah Rider
Cal Ripken, Jr.
David Robinson
Glenn Robinson
Jeremy Roenick
Nolan Ryan
Pete Sampras
Barry Sanders
Deion Sanders
Sterling Sharpe
Emmitt Smith
Joe Smith
Jerry Stackhouse
John Stockton
Frank Thomas
Isiah Thomas
Thurman Thomas
Wayman Tisdale
Al Unser, Jr.
Nick Van Exel
Rasheed Wallace
Spud Webb
Chris Webber
Reggie White
Dominique Wilkins
Katarina Witt
Kristi Yamaguchi
Steve Young

APPENDICES

ADDITIONAL RESOURCES FOR OLDER STUDENTS

RESOURCE	AREA OF MODIFICATION	SUGGESTED AGE OR GRADE
ALP: Active Listening Program (1986) van der Laan, C. Thinking Publications Eau Claire, WI	Listening	Grade 6–Adult
Cartoon Cut-Ups: Teaching Figurative Language and Humor (1995) Hamersky, J. Thinking Publications Eau Claire, WI	Social Communication Thinking Metalinguistics	Grades 4–8
Communicate (1986) Mayo, P., and Waldo, P. Thinking Publications Eau Claire, WI	Listening Speaking	Grades 5–12
Conversations: A Framework for Language Intervention (1995) Hoskins, B. Thinking Publications Eau Claire, WI	Speaking Listening Social Communication	Grades 5–Adult
CORT Thinking Lessons (1981) deBono, E. Pergamon Press New York, NY	Thinking	Grades 5–12
Daily Problem Solving Activities: Transitioning to Independence (1993) Gruen, A., and Gruen, L. Thinking Publications Eau Claire, WI	Thinking Listening Survival Language Writing	Grade 10–Adult
Face To Face: Facilitating Adolescent Communication Experiences (1993) Marquis, M.A. Communication Skill Builders Tucson, AZ	Speaking Listening Social Communication	Ages 12–19
Figurative Language: A Comprehensive Program (1992) Gorman-Gard, K. Thinking Publications Eau Claire, WI	Speaking Metalinguistics Thinking	Grades 4–12
Guidebook for Teaching Study Skills and Motivation (2nd ed.) (1987) Bragstad, B., and Stumpf, S. Allyn and Bacon Boston, MA	Study Skills	Grades 5–12

RESOURCE	AREA OF MODIFICATION	SUGGESTED AGE OR GRADE
Job-Related Social Skills: A Curriculum for Adolescents with Special Needs (1991) Montague, M., and Lund, K. Exceptional Innovations Ann Arbor, MI	Social Communication	Ages 15–22
Just for Laughs (1993) Spector, C. Communication Skill Builders Tucson, AZ	Thinking Metalinguistics Listening	Age 10–Adult
Let's Talk: Intermediate Level (1984) Wiig, E., and Bray, C. Psychological Corporation Austin, TX	Speaking	Grades 5–10
Life Skills Workshop: An Active Program for Real-Life Problem Solving (1992) Hannon, K., and Thompson, M. LinguiSystems East Moline, IL	Survival Language	Age 12–Adult
Life Works: A Transition Program for High School Students (1994) Dalke, C., and Howard, D. LinguiSystems East Moline, IL	Survival Language	High School
The Magic of Stories: Literature-Based Language Intervention (1995) Strong, C., and Hoggan North, K. Thinking Publications Eau Claire, WI	Thinking Listening Speaking Narrative Skills	Grades K–8
Make-It-Yourself Barrier Activities: Barrier Activities for Speakers and Listeners (1987) Schwartz, L., and McKinley, N. Thinking Publications Eau Claire, WI	Thinking Listening Speaking Writing	Grades K–Adult
Mind Benders (1978) Harnadek, A. Midwest Publications Pacific Grove, CA	Thinking	Grades 7–12
PALS: Pragmatic Activities in Language and Speech (1988) Davis, B. Pro-Ed Austin, TX	Speaking Listening Reading Writing	Secondary Level

RESOURCE	AREA OF MODIFICATION	SUGGESTED AGE OR GRADE
POW! Personal Power! (1992) Gajewski, N., and Mayo, P. Thinking Publications Eau Claire, WI	Thinking Speaking Listening Social Communication	Ages 11–18
Pragmatic Language Trivia for Thinking Skills (1990) Marquis, M.A. Communication Skill Builders Tucson, AZ	Thinking Speaking Listening Social Communication	Ages 11–18
Problem Solver (1986) Waldo, P. Thinking Publications Eau Claire, WI	Thinking Speaking	Grades 5–12
Referential Communication: Barrier Activities for Speakers and Listeners (Part One and *Part Two)* (1985) McKinley, N., and Schwartz, L. Thinking Publications Eau Claire, WI	Thinking Listening Speaking Writing	Grades K–5 (Part One) and Grade 6–Adult (Part Two)
Scripting: Social Communication for Adolescents (1994) Mayo, P., and Waldo, P. Thinking Publications Eau Claire, WI	Speaking Social Communication	Grades 5–12
Skillstreaming the Adolescent: A Structured Learning Approach to Teaching Prosocial Skills (1980) Goldstein, A., Sprafkin, R., Gershaw, N., and Klein, P. Research Press Champaign, IL	Thinking Social Communication	Ages 12–18
Social Language for Teens: Tackling Real-Life Situations (1993) Turnbow, G., and Proctor, D. LinguiSystems East Moline, IL	Listening Speaking Social Communication Nonverbal Communication	Grades 6–12
SSS: Social Skill Strategies (Book A and *Book B)* (1989) Gajewski, N., and Mayo, P. Thinking Publications Eau Claire, WI	Thinking Speaking Social Communication Nonverbal Communication	Grades 6–12
Social Communication: Activities for Improving Peer Interactions and Self-Esteem (1992) Marquis, M.A., and Addy-Trout, E. Thinking Publications Eau Claire, WI	Thinking Social Communication Listening	Grades 6–12

RESOURCE	AREA OF MODIFICATION	SUGGESTED AGE OR GRADE
A Sourcebook of Adolescent Pragmatic Activities (Revised) (1994) Weinrich, B., Glaser, A., and Johnston, E. Communication Skill Builders Tucson, AZ	Speaking Listening Nonverbal Communication	Grades 7–12
Study Smart: An Educational Activity to Reinforce Study Skills (1990) Mayo, P., Gajewski, N., and Rajek, A. Thinking Publications Eau Claire, WI	Study Skills	Grades 5–12
Teaching Functional Academics: A Curriculum Guide for Adolescents and Adults with Learning Problems (1982) Bender, M., and Valletutti, P. Pro-Ed Austin, TX	Survival Language	Grade 9–Adult
Teaching Study Skills: A Guide for Teachers (1981) Devine, T. Allyn and Bacon Boston, MA	Study Skills	Grades 5–12
Thinking with Language, Grades 4–6 (1992) Krassowski, E. Burke Communication Skill Builders Tucson, AZ	Thinking Speaking	11–16 years
Transfer Activities: Thinking Skill Vocabulary Development (1986) Mayo, P., and Gajewski, N. Thinking Publications Eau Claire, WI	Thinking Study Skills Writing	Grades 5–12
Vocabulary Maps (1993) Hamersky, J. Thinking Publications Eau Claire, WI	Thinking Listening Speaking	Grades 5–12
The Walker Social Skills Curriculum—The ACCESS Program: Adolescent Curriculum for Communication and Effective Social Skills (1988) Walker, H., Todis, B., Holmes, D., and Horton, G. Pro-Ed Austin, TX	Social Communication Study Skills	"Middle and High School"
Word Finding Intervention Program (1993) German, D. Communication Skill Builders Tucson, AZ	Word Finding	Children–Adults
Warm-Up Exercises: Calisthenics for the Brain (Books I, II, III) (1984, 1985, and 1992) Kisner, R., and Knowles, B. Thinking Publications Eau Claire, WI	Listening Speaking	Grades 5–12

CONTRACT

I, ____
Name

will do the following by ______________________________.
Date

1.

2.

3.

Level of Performance:

Evaluation Plan:

Consequences:

Signed: ______________________________

____

Date: ______________________________

© 1995 Thinking Publications

Duplication permitted for educational use only.

ENHANCING STUDENT SELF-EVALUATION

1. **Involve the student.**
   Develop positive relationships with adolescents that communicate "I care" and "I believe in you."

2. **Focus on present behavior.**
   When dealing with the present incident, do not bring up past mistakes.

3. **Encourage value judgments.**
   Have students evaluate their own behaviors. Is the behavior helping you get what you want? Is it helping others? Is it against the rules? Why do we need rules?

4. **Make a plan.**
   Help students develop strategies to deal with similar situations in the future. Put these plans on paper.

5. **Get a commitment.**
   If appropriate, use a written contract. Follow up, check back, reinforce.

6. **Don't accept excuses.**
   If things go wrong, replan strategies rather than accept excuses.

7. **Seek responsibility, not punishment.**
   Students need help in developing a sense of ownership of, and responsibility for, their behaviors. Punishment relieves students from responsibility.

8. **Never give up.**
   Persist with adolescents so they know you care. Giving up can reinforce negative self-concepts.

© 1995 Thinking Publications

Duplication permitted for educational use only.

LISTENING QUESTIONNAIRE

Name ____________________

Date ____________________

Mark each statement as true or false.

________ 1 Teachers or friends who don't listen to me aren't smart enough to appreciate my ideas.

________ 2 Teaching students to listen is like teaching them to breathe.

________ 3 I've already developed good listening skills because I have to listen all the time in school.

________ 4 It is more important to be good speakers than good listeners because we learn by talking.

________ 5 It is more important to be good readers than good listeners.

________ 6 I think I have been adequately trained to listen at school and home.

________ 7 Students should not have to work at listening to class lectures.

________ 8 I can't stand to listen to people who talk about ideas that sound crazy.

________ 9 It doesn't matter if I stop listening because I don't miss much.

________ 10 I'm a good listener when I want to be.

© 1995 Thinking Publications

Duplication permitted for educational use only.

LISTENING STRATEGIES—MAIN IDEA CARDS

MAIN IDEA

People in different locations see different patterns of stars.

© 1995 Thinking Publications Appendix E
Duplication permitted for educational use only.

MAIN IDEA

Music can be relaxing.

© 1995 Thinking Publications Appendix E
Duplication permitted for educational use only.

MAIN IDEA

House exteriors are usually built with the most available and least expensive materials (e.g., wood, brick, mud).

© 1995 Thinking Publications Appendix E
Duplication permitted for educational use only.

MAIN IDEA

Students cannot charge lunch tickets at school.

© 1995 Thinking Publications Appendix E
Duplication permitted for educational use only.

MAIN IDEA

Pets require consistent care and attention.

© 1995 Thinking Publications Appendix E
Duplication permitted for educational use only.

MAIN IDEA

Computers are commonplace in homes.

© 1995 Thinking Publications Appendix E
Duplication permitted for educational use only.

MAIN IDEA

My brother hates mathematics.

© 1995 Thinking Publications Appendix E
Duplication permitted for educational use only.

MAIN IDEA

We can learn from past mistakes.

© 1995 Thinking Publications Appendix E
Duplication permitted for educational use only.

MAIN IDEA

Hard work is usually, but not always, rewarded.

© 1995 Thinking Publications Appendix E
Duplication permitted for educational use only.

MAIN IDEA

We have no definite proof that life exists on other planets.

© 1995 Thinking Publications Appendix E
Duplication permitted for educational use only.

MAIN IDEA

People can learn to listen better (than their present skill level).

© 1995 Thinking Publications Appendix E
Duplication permitted for educational use only.

MAIN IDEA

Citizens have a responsibility to their country.

© 1995 Thinking Publications Appendix E
Duplication permitted for educational use only.

MAIN IDEA

All colors are tolerable, but my favorite one is red.

© 1995 Thinking Publications Appendix E
Duplication permitted for educational use only.

MAIN IDEA

Schools should be open 12 months a year.

© 1995 Thinking Publications Appendix E
Duplication permitted for educational use only.

MAIN IDEA

Athletes should be required to adhere to strict academic standards.

© 1995 Thinking Publications Appendix E
Duplication permitted for educational use only.

MAIN IDEA

Loud music can cause hearing loss.

© 1995 Thinking Publications Appendix E
Duplication permitted for educational use only.

MAIN IDEA

Seat belts save lives.

© 1995 Thinking Publications Appendix E
Duplication permitted for educational use only.

MAIN IDEA

Money doesn't buy as much as it used to.

© 1995 Thinking Publications Appendix E
Duplication permitted for educational use only.

MAIN IDEA

Football practice can be boring.

© 1995 Thinking Publications Appendix E
Duplication permitted for educational use only.

MAIN IDEA

Helmets protect motorcyclists from injury.

© 1995 Thinking Publications Appendix E
Duplication permitted for educational use only.

REFERENTIAL COMMUNICATION ACTIVITIES

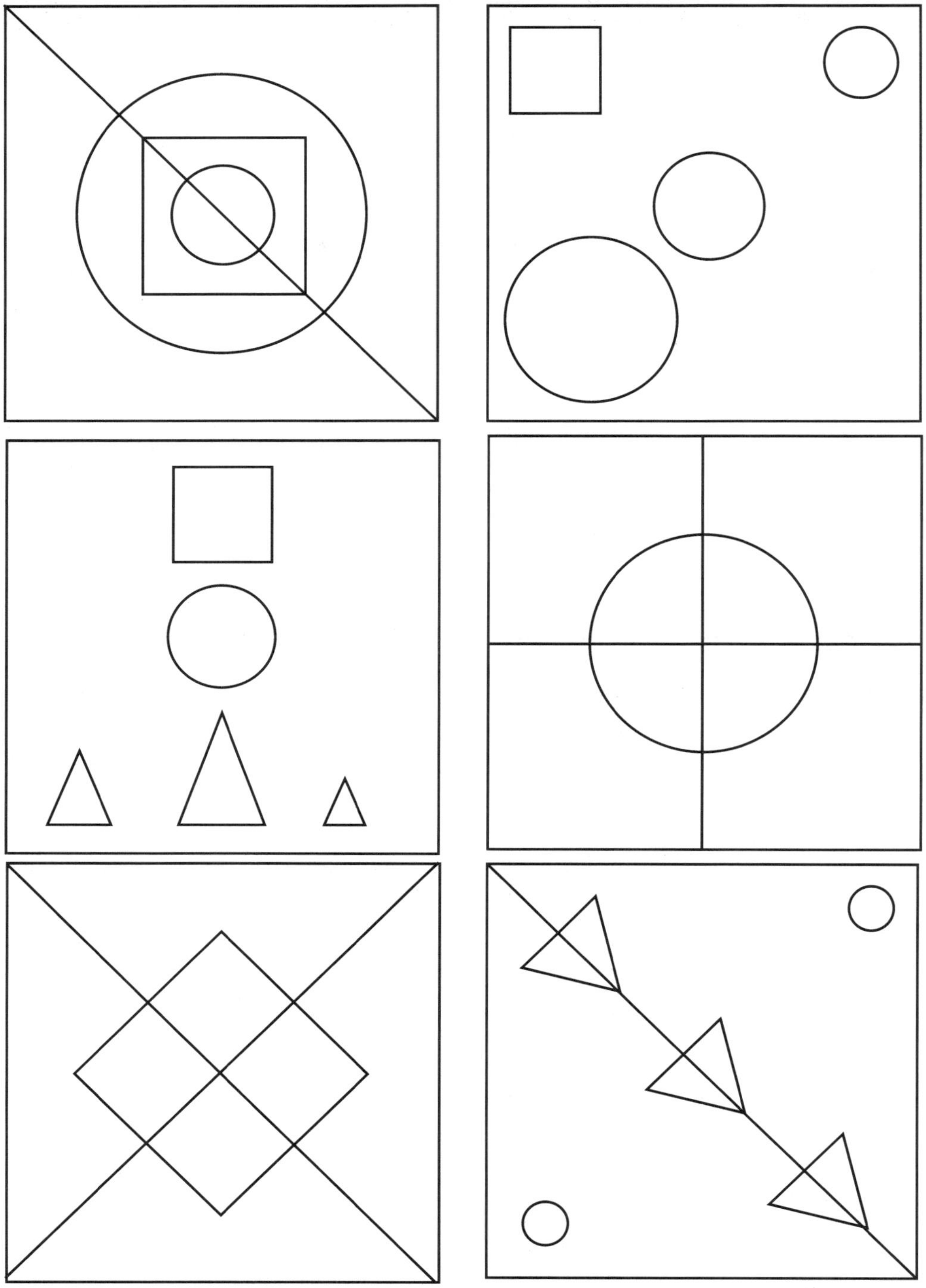

© 1995 Thinking Publications

Duplication permitted for educational use only.

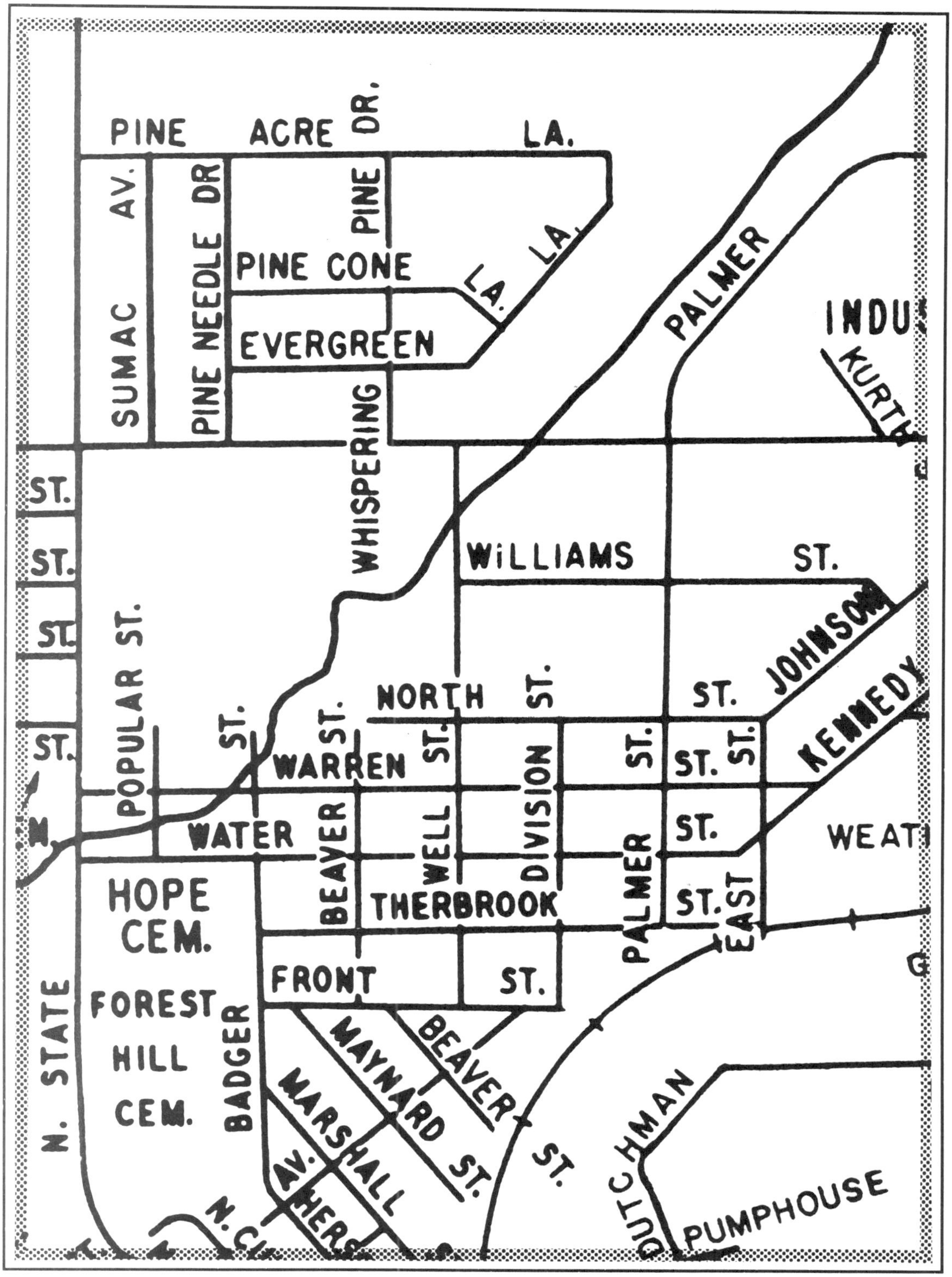

© 1995 Thinking Publications

Duplication permitted for educational use only.

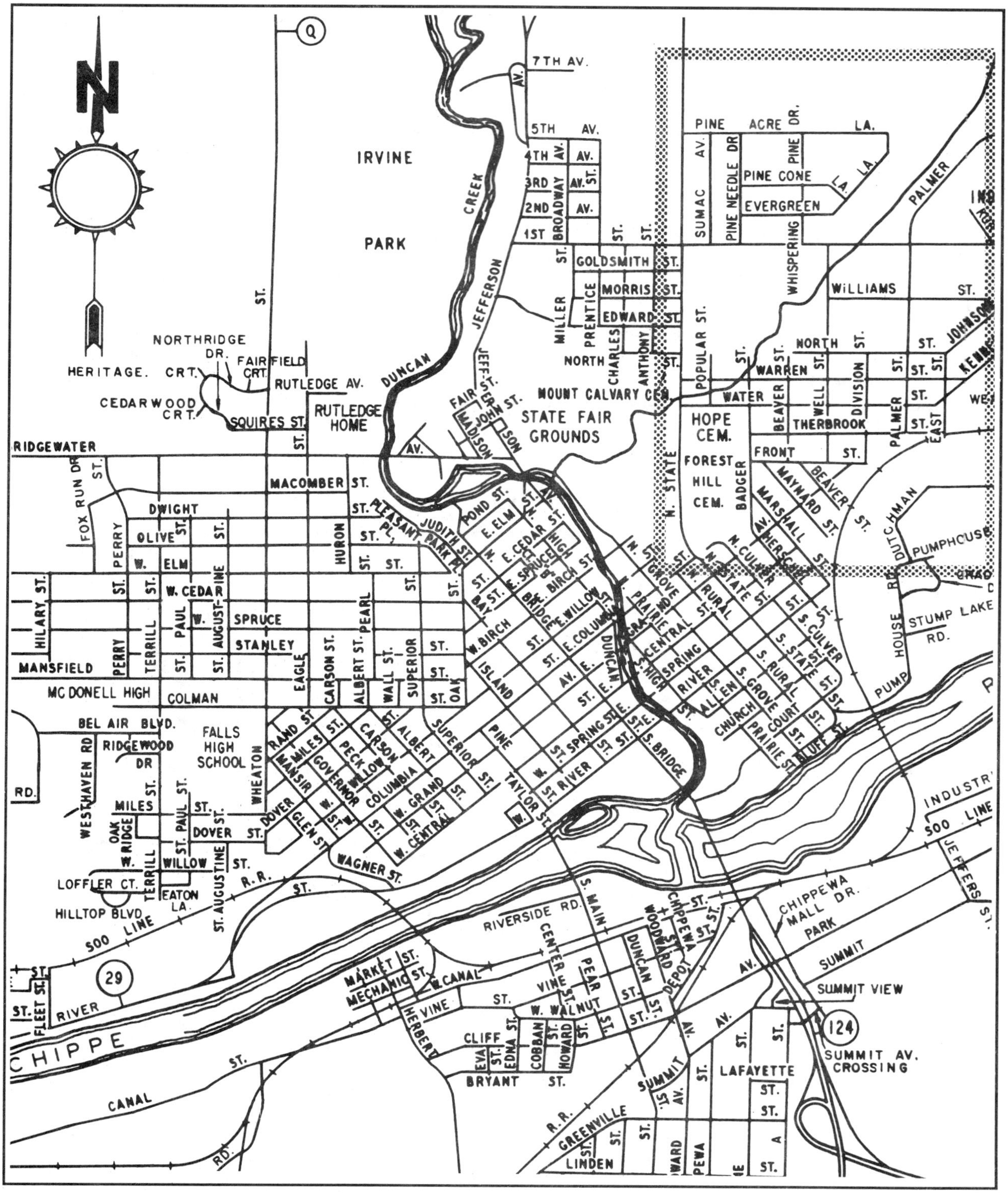

© 1995 Thinking Publications

Duplication permitted for educational use only.

CONVERSATIONAL STARTERS I

SPEAKER ROLE
STUDENT

LISTENER ROLE
STUDENT

What is the most interesting thing you've done this week?

© 1995 Thinking Publications Appendix G: Starters I
Duplication permitted for educational use only.

SPEAKER ROLE
STUDENT

LISTENER ROLE
STUDENT

What was the funniest thing that ever happened at your home?

© 1995 Thinking Publications Appendix G: Starters I
Duplication permitted for educational use only.

SPEAKER ROLE
STUDENT

LISTENER ROLE
STUDENT

How would I look up the name of this school in the telephone book?

© 1995 Thinking Publications Appendix G: Starters I
Duplication permitted for educational use only.

SPEAKER ROLE
STUDENT

LISTENER ROLE
STUDENT

Who was the best teacher you ever had? Why?

© 1995 Thinking Publications Appendix G: Starters I
Duplication permitted for educational use only.

SPEAKER ROLE
STUDENT

LISTENER ROLE
STUDENT

How do you buy hunting and fishing licenses in this state?

© 1995 Thinking Publications Appendix G: Starters 1
Duplication permitted for educational use only.

SPEAKER ROLE
STUDENT

LISTENER ROLE
STUDENT

What clothes do you wish you could buy right now?

© 1995 Thinking Publications Appendix G: Starters I
Duplication permitted for educational use only.

SPEAKER ROLE
STUDENT

LISTENER ROLE
STUDENT

How would I get to the best theater around here?

© 1995 Thinking Publications Appendix G: Starters I
Duplication permitted for educational use only.

SPEAKER ROLE
STUDENT

LISTENER ROLE
STUDENT

Where is a good place to eat around here? Why?

© 1995 Thinking Publications Appendix G: Starters I
Duplication permitted for educational use only.

SPEAKER ROLE
STUDENT

LISTENER ROLE
STUDENT

Who is your favorite singer or group? Why?

© 1995 Thinking Publications Appendix G: Starters I
Duplication permitted for educational use only.

SPEAKER ROLE
STUDENT

LISTENER ROLE
STUDENT

How do you get to your house from here?

© 1995 Thinking Publications Appendix G: Starters I
Duplication permitted for educational use only.

SPEAKER ROLE
STUDENT

LISTENER ROLE
STUDENT

What happened on your favorite TV show the last time you saw it?

© 1995 Thinking Publications Appendix G: Starters I
Duplication permitted for educational use only.

SPEAKER ROLE
STUDENT

LISTENER ROLE
STUDENT

What kind of job would you like to have some day?

© 1995 Thinking Publications Appendix G: Starters I
Duplication permitted for educational use only.

SPEAKER ROLE
STUDENT

LISTENER ROLE
STUDENT

What kinds of food do you like to eat?

© 1995 Thinking Publications Appendix G: Starters I
Duplication permitted for educational use only.

SPEAKER ROLE
STUDENT

LISTENER ROLE
STUDENT

What do your parents do (for work)?

© 1995 Thinking Publications Appendix G: Starters I
Duplication permitted for educational use only.

SPEAKER ROLE
STUDENT

LISTENER ROLE
STUDENT

If you could move to any place in the world, where would you go?

© 1995 Thinking Publications Appendix G: Starters I
Duplication permitted for educational use only.

SPEAKER ROLE
STUDENT

LISTENER ROLE
STUDENT

What are your brothers and sisters like?

© 1995 Thinking Publications Appendix G: Starters I
Duplication permitted for educational use only.

SPEAKER ROLE
STUDENT

LISTENER ROLE
STUDENT

What do you usually do during summer vacation?

© 1995 Thinking Publications Appendix G: Starters I
Duplication permitted for educational use only.

SPEAKER ROLE
STUDENT

LISTENER ROLE
STUDENT

If you could buy a car right now, what kind would you get?

© 1995 Thinking Publications Appendix G: Starters I
Duplication permitted for educational use only.

SPEAKER ROLE
STUDENT

LISTENER ROLE
STUDENT

What kind of jobs do you have to do at home?

© 1995 Thinking Publications Appendix G: Starters I
Duplication permitted for educational use only.

SPEAKER ROLE
STUDENT

LISTENER ROLE
STUDENT

What classes are you going to take next year? (Or for seniors, what are you going to be doing next year?)

© 1995 Thinking Publications Appendix G: Starters I
Duplication permitted for educational use only.

CONVERSATIONAL STARTERS II

SPEAKER ROLE
STUDENT

LISTENER-ASSUMED ROLE
A NEW STUDENT IN SCHOOL

LISTENER-POSED QUESTION
I'm a new student here. What rules are there about being in the hallway, missing school, and things like that?

© 1995 Thinking Publications Appendix G: Starters II
Duplication permitted for educational use only.

SPEAKER ROLE
STUDENT

LISTENER-ASSUMED ROLE:
THE GUIDANCE COUNSELOR

LISTENER-POSED QUESTION
What kind of job do you think you're interested in?

© 1995 Thinking Publications Appendix G: Starters II
Duplication permitted for educational use only.

SPEAKER ROLE
STUDENT

LISTENER-ASSUMED ROLE
THE SCHOOL PRINCIPAL

LISTENER-POSED QUESTION
How are your classes going?

© 1995 Thinking Publications Appendix G: Starters II
Duplication permitted for educational use only.

SPEAKER ROLE
STUDENT

LISTENER-ASSUMED ROLE
THE MATH TEACHER

LISTENER-POSED QUESTION
What do you think would make this class a better one for you?

© 1995 Thinking Publications Appendix G: Starters II
Duplication permitted for educational use only.

SPEAKER ROLE
STUDENT

LISTENER-ASSUMED ROLE
A PARENT

LISTENER-POSED QUESTION
Who are you hanging around with most these days?

© 1995 Thinking Publications Appendix G: Starters II
Duplication permitted for educational use only.

SPEAKER ROLE
STUDENT

LISTENER-ASSUMED ROLE
A YOUNGER STUDENT

LISTENER-POSED QUESTION
What teachers do you think I should avoid when I get to that school?

© 1995 Thinking Publications Appendix G: Starters II
Duplication permitted for educational use only.

SPEAKER ROLE
STUDENT

LISTENER-ASSUMED ROLE
A SCHOOL COACH

LISTENER-POSED QUESTION
Why aren't you going out for any sports this year?

© 1995 Thinking Publications Appendix G: Starters II
Duplication permitted for educational use only.

SPEAKER ROLE
STUDENT

LISTENER-ASSUMED ROLE
A SCHOOL NURSE

LISTENER-POSED QUESTION
What can you tell me about the last physical examination you had?

© 1995 Thinking Publications Appendix G: Starters II
Duplication permitted for educational use only.

SPEAKER ROLE
STUDENT

LISTENER-ASSUMED ROLE
A SCHOOL PSYCHOLOGIST

LISTENER-POSED QUESTION
What kind of achievement tests do you remember taking in the last few years?

© 1995 Thinking Publications
Duplication permitted for educational use only.
Appendix G: Starters II

SPEAKER ROLE
STUDENT

LISTENER-ASSUMED ROLE
A FRIEND OF YOUR PARENTS

LISTENER-POSED QUESTION
What kind of classes are you taking this year and how do you like them?

© 1995 Thinking Publications
Duplication permitted for educational use only.
Appendix G: Starters II

Appendix G: Starters II

Appendix G: Starters II

CONVERSATIONAL STARTERS III

SPEAKER-ASSUMED ROLE
A TEACHER

LISTENER-ASSUMED ROLE
A STUDENT

LISTENER-POSED QUESTION
How can I make up the test I will miss on Friday?

© 1995 Thinking Publications Appendix G: Starters III
Duplication permitted for educational use only.

SPEAKER-ASSUMED ROLE
A BABY SITTER

LISTENER-ASSUMED ROLE
A CONCERNED PARENT

LISTENER-POSED QUESTION
How will you go about contacting the fire department or police station if you need to?

© 1995 Thinking Publications Appendix G: Starters III
Duplication permitted for educational use only.

SPEAKER-ASSUMED ROLE
A PRINCIPAL OR HEADMASTER

LISTENER-ASSUMED ROLE
A STUDENT

LISTENER-POSED QUESTION
What do I have to do to get permission to be gone for a couple of days next week?

© 1995 Thinking Publications Appendix G: Starters III
Duplication permitted for educational use only.

SPEAKER-ASSUMED ROLE
A CUSTOMER IN A RESTAURANT

LISTENER-ASSUMED ROLE
A WAITER OR WAITRESS

LISTENER-POSED QUESTION
What would you like to order to eat today?

© 1995 Thinking Publications Appendix G: Starters III
Duplication permitted for educational use only.

SPEAKER-ASSUMED ROLE
A NURSE

LISTENER-ASSUMED ROLE
A SICK PERSON

LISTENER-POSED QUESTION
How can I get rid of this cold?

© 1995 Thinking Publications Appendix G: Starters III
Duplication permitted for educational use only.

SPEAKER-ASSUMED ROLE
A CUSTOMER

LISTENER-ASSUMED ROLE
A STORE CLERK

LISTENER-POSED QUESTION
What kind of clothes are you looking for today?

© 1995 Thinking Publications Appendix G: Starters III
Duplication permitted for educational use only.

SPEAKER-ASSUMED ROLE
A STORE OWNER

LISTENER-ASSUMED ROLE
A YOUNG SHOPPER

LISTENER-POSED QUESTION
What can I buy for my mother that is under 10 dollars?

© 1995 Thinking Publications Appendix G: Starters III
Duplication permitted for educational use only.

SPEAKER-ASSUMED ROLE
A POLICE OFFICER

LISTENER-ASSUMED ROLE
A MOTORIST IN THE SCHOOL PARKING LOT, ALMOST OUT OF GAS

LISTENER-POSED QUESTION
How do I get to the closest gas station from here?

© 1995 Thinking Publications Appendix G: Starters III
Duplication permitted for educational use only.

SPEAKER-ASSUMED ROLE
A PATIENT

LISTENER-ASSUMED ROLE
A DOCTOR

LISTENER-POSED QUESTION
How have you been feeling lately?

© 1995 Thinking Publications Appendix G: Starters III
Duplication permitted for educational use only.

SPEAKER-ASSUMED ROLE
A PARENT OF A SMALL CHILD

LISTENER-ASSUMED ROLE
A YOUNG PARENT

LISTENER-POSED QUESTION
What do you do when your child doesn't listen to you?

© 1995 Thinking Publications Appendix G: Starters III
Duplication permitted for educational use only.

SPEAKER-ASSUMED ROLE
A PARENT

LISTENER-ASSUMED ROLE
A PRINCIPAL

LISTENER-POSED QUESTION
What do you think we should do about your son skipping school?

© 1995 Thinking Publications Appendix G: Starters III
Duplication permitted for educational use only.

SPEAKER-ASSUMED ROLE
A DOG OWNER

LISTENER-ASSUMED ROLE
A POTENTIAL DOG OWNER

LISTENER-POSED QUESTION
How much does it cost to take care of a dog? I don't know anything about the shots they need or how much food they eat.

© 1995 Thinking Publications Appendix G: Starters III
Duplication permitted for educational use only.

SPEAKER-ASSUMED ROLE
A SEMI-TRUCK DRIVER WHO LOVES THE JOB

LISTENER-ASSUMED ROLE
A PERSON INTERESTED IN TRUCK DRIVING

LISTENER-POSED QUESTION
What is it you like about truck driving?

© 1995 Thinking Publications Appendix G: Starters III
Duplication permitted for educational use only.

SPEAKER-ASSUMED ROLE
A GRANDFATHER, GRANDMOTHER, OR OLDER PERSON

LISTENER-ASSUMED ROLE
A PERSON INTERESTED IN THE PAST

LISTENER-POSED QUESTION
What were things like when you were growing up?

© 1995 Thinking Publications Appendix G: Starters III
Duplication permitted for educational use only.

SPEAKER-ASSUMED ROLE
A PROBATION OFFICER

LISTENER-ASSUMED ROLE
A JUVENILE OFFENDER

LISTENER-POSED QUESTION
What happens if you catch me not going to school?

© 1995 Thinking Publications Appendix G: Starters III
Duplication permitted for educational use only.

SPEAKER-ASSUMED ROLE
A CAR OWNER

LISTENER-ASSUMED ROLE
A CURIOUS CHILD

LISTENER-POSED QUESTION
How do you know when your car has a flat tire? How do you fix it?

© 1995 Thinking Publications Appendix G: Starters III
Duplication permitted for educational use only.

SPEAKER-ASSUMED ROLE
A HOMEOWNER

SPEAKER-ASSUMED ROLE
A FELLOW HOMEOWNER

LISTENER-POSED QUESTION
How can I find a good electrician and a plumber to fix some things in my home?

© 1995 Thinking Publications Appendix G: Starters III
Duplication permitted for educational use only.

SPEAKER-ASSUMED ROLE
THE MANAGER OF A FAST-FOOD RESTAURANT

LISTENER-ASSUMED ROLE
A PERSON INTERVIEWING FOR A JOB

LISTENER-POSED QUESTION
What kind of job openings do you have right now?

© 1995 Thinking Publications Appendix G: Starters III
Duplication permitted for educational use only.

SPEAKER-ASSUMED ROLE
AN OLDER BROTHER

LISTENER-ASSUMED ROLE
A YOUNGER BROTHER

LISTENER-POSED QUESTION
How did you get your first date?

© 1995 Thinking Publications Appendix G: Starters III
Duplication permitted for educational use only.

SPEAKER-ASSUMED ROLE
AN EXPERIENCED WILDERNESS CAMPER

LISTENER-ASSUMED ROLE
A NOVICE CAMPER

LISTENER-POSED QUESTION
If you were going on a camping trip and couldn't get to a grocery store in the next two weeks, what would you buy?

© 1995 Thinking Publications Appendix G: Starters III
Duplication permitted for educational use only.

CONVERSATIONAL STARTERS—TOPIC MAINTENANCE

MAIN OBJECTIVE OF LISTENER

To talk about weekend plans

© 1995 Thinking Publications Appendix G: Topic Maintenance
Duplication permitted for educational use only.

MAIN OBJECTIVE OF LISTENER

To talk about the last time you were sick

© 1995 Thinking Publications Appendix G: Topic Maintenance
Duplication permitted for educational use only.

MAIN OBJECTIVE OF LISTENER

To talk about what fun you had going out to eat last night

© 1995 Thinking Publications Appendix G: Topic Maintenance
Duplication permitted for educational use only.

MAIN OBJECTIVE OF LISTENER

To talk about a car driving experience you have had, or would like to have

© 1995 Thinking Publications Appendix G: Topic Maintenance
Duplication permitted for educational use only.

MAIN OBJECTIVE OF LISTENER

To talk about the best TV show you have seen recently

© 1995 Thinking Publications Appendix G: Topic Maintenance
Duplication permitted for educational use only.

MAIN OBJECTIVE OF LISTENER

To talk about a car accident you have seen or heard about

© 1995 Thinking Publications Appendix G: Topic Maintenance
Duplication permitted for educational use only.

MAIN OBJECTIVE OF LISTENER

To talk about how it would feel to be an only child

© 1995 Thinking Publications Appendix G: Topic Maintenance
Duplication permitted for educational use only.

MAIN OBJECTIVE OF LISTENER

To talk about what you would have done if you had not come to school today

© 1995 Thinking Publications Appendix G: Topic Maintenance
Duplication permitted for educational use only.

MAIN OBJECTIVE OF LISTENER

To talk about the kind of entertainment you like

© 1995 Thinking Publications Appendix G: Topic Maintenance
Duplication permitted for educational use only.

MAIN OBJECTIVE OF LISTENER

To talk about pets your family has owned or that you would like to own

© 1995 Thinking Publications Appendix G: Topic Maintenance
Duplication permitted for educational use only.

MAIN OBJECTIVE OF LISTENER

To talk about what you typically do on your birthday

© 1995 Thinking Publications Appendix G: Topic Maintenance
Duplication permitted for educational use only.

MAIN OBJECTIVE OF LISTENER

To talk about how much money you wish you had right now

© 1995 Thinking Publications Appendix G: Topic Maintenance
Duplication permitted for educational use only.

MAIN OBJECTIVE OF LISTENER

To talk about your least favorite season of the year

© 1995 Thinking Publications Appendix G: Topic Maintenance
Duplication permitted for educational use only.

MAIN OBJECTIVE OF LISTENER

To talk about food that makes you gag

© 1995 Thinking Publications Appendix G: Topic Maintenance
Duplication permitted for educational use only.

MAIN OBJECTIVE OF LISTENER

To talk about how it would feel if parents still arranged marriage partners for their children

© 1995 Thinking Publications Appendix G: Topic Maintenance
Duplication permitted for educational use only.

MAIN OBJECTIVE OF LISTENER

To talk about what radio station you listen to most of the time and why

© 1995 Thinking Publications Appendix G: Topic Maintenance
Duplication permitted for educational use only.

MAIN OBJECTIVE OF LISTENER

To talk about what cartoon character(s) you like best

© 1995 Thinking Publications Appendix G: Topic Maintenance
Duplication permitted for educational use only.

MAIN OBJECTIVE OF LISTENER

To talk about what you would like to alter about your appearance

© 1995 Thinking Publications Appendix G: Topic Maintenance
Duplication permitted for educational use only.

MAIN OBJECTIVE OF LISTENER

To talk about what you hope gets changed/fixed soon in your house

© 1995 Thinking Publications Appendix G: Topic Maintenance
Duplication permitted for educational use only.

MAIN OBJECTIVE OF LISTENER

To talk about how far behind (or ahead) you are with your homework

© 1995 Thinking Publications Appendix G: Topic Maintenance
Duplication permitted for educational use only.

MAIN OBJECTIVE OF SPEAKER

To ask if you can copy a page of homework

© 1995 Thinking Publications Appendix G: Topic Maintenance
Duplication permitted for educational use only.

MAIN OBJECTIVE OF SPEAKER

To talk about what you would like to do this weekend if you could do anything in the world

© 1995 Thinking Publications Appendix G: Topic Maintenance
Duplication permitted for educational use only.

MAIN OBJECTIVE OF SPEAKER

To talk about how frustrated you are with your parents

© 1995 Thinking Publications Appendix G: Topic Maintenance
Duplication permitted for educational use only.

MAIN OBJECTIVE OF SPEAKER

To talk about what you're hungry for right now (or will be later today)

© 1995 Thinking Publications Appendix G: Topic Maintenance
Duplication permitted for educational use only.

MAIN OBJECTIVE OF SPEAKER

To talk about the worst movie you have ever seen

© 1995 Thinking Publications Appendix G: Topic Maintenance
Duplication permitted for educational use only.

MAIN OBJECTIVE OF SPEAKER

To talk about football—how well you like it or dislike it

© 1995 Thinking Publications Appendix G: Topic Maintenance
Duplication permitted for educational use only.

MAIN OBJECTIVE OF SPEAKER

To talk about how things have been going at school

© 1995 Thinking Publications Appendix G: Topic Maintenance
Duplication permitted for educational use only.

MAIN OBJECTIVE OF SPEAKER

To talk about the last new clothes that were bought for you

© 1995 Thinking Publications Appendix G: Topic Maintenance
Duplication permitted for educational use only.

MAIN OBJECTIVE OF SPEAKER

To talk about how much you like or dislike being outside in the weather you're having right now

© 1995 Thinking Publications Appendix G: Topic Maintenance
Duplication permitted for educational use only.

MAIN OBJECTIVE OF SPEAKER

To talk about the worst teacher you have ever had

© 1995 Thinking Publications Appendix G: Topic Maintenance
Duplication permitted for educational use only.

MAIN OBJECTIVE OF SPEAKER

To talk about what your family usually does on national holidays like July 4th or Thanksgiving

© 1995 Thinking Publications Appendix G: Topic Maintenance
Duplication permitted for educational use only.

MAIN OBJECTIVE OF SPEAKER

To talk about a trip to a zoo you have taken or wish you could take

© 1995 Thinking Publications Appendix G: Topic Maintenance
Duplication permitted for educational use only.

MAIN OBJECTIVE OF SPEAKER

To talk about your favorite holiday

© 1995 Thinking Publications Appendix G: Topic Maintenance
Duplication permitted for educational use only.

MAIN OBJECTIVE OF SPEAKER

To talk about the kind of house you would like to live in some day

© 1995 Thinking Publications Appendix G: Topic Maintenance
Duplication permitted for educational use only.

MAIN OBJECTIVE OF SPEAKER

To talk about motorcycles you have ridden or would like to ride

© 1995 Thinking Publications Appendix G: Topic Maintenance
Duplication permitted for educational use only.

MAIN OBJECTIVE OF SPEAKER

To talk about what TV or cable channel you watch most and why

© 1995 Thinking Publications Appendix G: Topic Maintenance
Duplication permitted for educational use only.

MAIN OBJECTIVE OF SPEAKER

To talk about the kinds of physical exercise you like to do best

© 1995 Thinking Publications Appendix G: Topic Maintenance
Duplication permitted for educational use only.

MAIN OBJECTIVE OF SPEAKER

To tell someone about the hardest work you think you have ever done

© 1995 Thinking Publications Appendix G: Topic Maintenance
Duplication permitted for educational use only.

MAIN OBJECTIVE OF SPEAKER

To talk about how you wish your mother or father would change

© 1995 Thinking Publications Appendix G: Topic Maintenance
Duplication permitted for educational use only.

MAIN OBJECTIVE OF SPEAKER

To talk about a favorite friend you had as a small child

© 1995 Thinking Publications Appendix G: Topic Maintenance
Duplication permitted for educational use only.

CONVERSATIONAL STARTERS—TOPIC CHANGES

MAIN OBJECTIVES OF SPEAKER

a. To ask for a ride home after tomorrow night's game

b. To tell about the book that caught on fire during a science experiment

© 1995 Thinking Publications Appendix G: Topic Changes
Duplication permitted for educational use only.

MAIN OBJECTIVES OF SPEAKER

a. To tell what you'd like to do during summer vacation

b. To tell about your favorite actor

© 1995 Thinking Publications Appendix G: Topic Changes
Duplication permitted for educational use only.

MAIN OBJECTIVES OF SPEAKER

a. To tell about your fight with your father this morning and how you felt

b. To suggest that the room would be more comfortable if windows could be opened to let in fresh air

© 1995 Thinking Publications Appendix G: Topic Changes
Duplication permitted for educational use only.

MAIN OBJECTIVES OF SPEAKER

a. To tell about the hardest subject you are taking right now

b. To talk about your favorite aunt, uncle, or cousin

© 1995 Thinking Publications Appendix G: Topic Changes
Duplication permitted for educational use only.

MAIN OBJECTIVES OF SPEAKER

a. To describe what your daily routine is before arriving at school

b. To ask what kind of music your friend would like to listen to right now

© 1995 Thinking Publications Appendix G: Topic Changes
Duplication permitted for educational use only.

MAIN OBJECTIVES OF SPEAKER

a. To explain how well you like the location of your locker at school

b. To talk about what annoys you most at home

© 1995 Thinking Publications Appendix G: Topic Changes
Duplication permitted for educational use only.

MAIN OBJECTIVES OF SPEAKER

a. To tell about the worst storm you ever lived through

b. To ask if your friend would like something to drink

© 1995 Thinking Publications Appendix G: Topic Changes
Duplication permitted for educational use only.

MAIN OBJECTIVES OF SPEAKER

a. To talk about what your favorite song is right now

b. To ask if your friend has ever had to have an eye exam

© 1995 Thinking Publications Appendix G: Topic Changes
Duplication permitted for educational use only.

MAIN OBJECTIVES OF SPEAKER

a. To ask what time it is

b. To ask what homework your friend has to do tonight

© 1995 Thinking Publications Appendix G: Topic Changes
Duplication permitted for educational use only.

MAIN OBJECTIVES OF SPEAKER

a. To ask if your friend has ever gone to a wedding and what it was like (or what he or she thinks it would be like)

b. To ask if your friend has ever gone camping and what it was like (or what he or she thinks it would be like)

© 1995 Thinking Publications Appendix G: Topic Changes
Duplication permitted for educational use only.

MAIN OBJECTIVES OF SPEAKER

a. To ask if there's anything exciting going on this weekend

b. To tell about the last party you went to

© 1995 Thinking Publications Appendix G: Topic Changes
Duplication permitted for educational use only.

MAIN OBJECTIVES OF SPEAKER

a. To talk about what you think your family would do if there was a nuclear attack

b. To ask if your friend has ever considered joining the military after high school

© 1995 Thinking Publications Appendix G: Topic Changes
Duplication permitted for educational use only.

MAIN OBJECTIVES OF SPEAKER

a. To tell about the funniest teacher you know, or the one who tells the best jokes

b. To tell about a hotel that you have stayed at, or think would be fun to stay at

© 1995 Thinking Publications Appendix G: Topic Changes
Duplication permitted for educational use only.

MAIN OBJECTIVES OF SPEAKER

a. To tell about the most expensive food you think you have ever eaten

b. To ask if your friend likes the weather today

© 1995 Thinking Publications Appendix G: Topic Changes
Duplication permitted for educational use only.

MAIN OBJECTIVES OF SPEAKER

a. To tell about your parents' computer knowledge

b. To ask if your friend has a favorite computer game and why it is so much fun to play

© 1995 Thinking Publications Appendix G: Topic Changes
Duplication permitted for educational use only.

MAIN OBJECTIVES OF SPEAKER

a. To ask where your friend buys clothing most of the time

b. To talk about how much makeup you like to see girls wearing at school

© 1995 Thinking Publications Appendix G: Topic Changes
Duplication permitted for educational use only.

MAIN OBJECTIVES OF SPEAKER

a. To ask what part of the day your friend likes best

b. To describe your favorite way to study (e.g., noisy/quiet, sitting up/lying down)

© 1995 Thinking Publications Appendix G: Topic Changes
Duplication permitted for educational use only.

MAIN OBJECTIVES OF SPEAKER

a. To explain whether or not you feel bored at school

b. To ask if your friend would like to get something to eat

© 1995 Thinking Publications Appendix G: Topic Changes
Duplication permitted for educational use only.

MAIN OBJECTIVES OF SPEAKER

a. To describe when you get yelled at most often at home

b. To describe something that you fear a great deal

© 1995 Thinking Publications Appendix G: Topic Changes
Duplication permitted for educational use only.

MAIN OBJECTIVES OF SPEAKER

a. To ask your friend how much time it takes to get from home to school

b. To tell something you like about your friend's clothing or appearance today

© 1995 Thinking Publications Appendix G: Topic Changes
Duplication permitted for educational use only.

CONVERSATIONAL STARTERS—TOPIC INTERRUPTIONS

INITIAL TOPIC:

Places you would like to visit

MAIN OBJECTIVE(S) OF SPEAKER:

To tell how mean your sister (or a friend) has been to you lately

© 1995 Thinking Publications Appendix G: Topic Interruptions
Duplication permitted for educational use only.

INITIAL TOPIC:

Clothes you would like to buy

MAIN OBJECTIVE(S) OF SPEAKER:

To ask if you can copy tomorrow's English assignment

© 1995 Thinking Publications Appendix G: Topic Interruptions
Duplication permitted for educational use only.

INITIAL TOPIC:

Famous people you would like to meet

MAIN OBJECTIVE(S) OF SPEAKER:

To express worry over passing math this year

© 1995 Thinking Publications Appendix G: Topic Interruptions
Duplication permitted for educational use only.

INITIAL TOPIC:

Who is dating whom at school

MAIN OBJECTIVE(S) OF SPEAKER:

To tell your friend he or she has to stop seeing someone and why

© 1995 Thinking Publications Appendix G: Topic Interruptions
Duplication permitted for educational use only.

INITIAL TOPIC:

The best pizza to eat

MAIN OBJECTIVE(S) OF SPEAKER:

To announce that your parents are out of town this weekend and talk about what to do while they're gone

© 1995 Thinking Publications Appendix G: Topic Interruptions
Duplication permitted for educational use only.

INITIAL TOPIC:

The best TV show you saw in the last week

MAIN OBJECTIVE(S) OF SPEAKER:

To complain that you have to do more chores than your brother does

© 1995 Thinking Publications Appendix G: Topic Interruptions
Duplication permitted for educational use only.

INITIAL TOPIC:

The car you wish your family owned

MAIN OBJECTIVE(S) OF SPEAKER:

To express disappointment in who won a recent game and to offer advice on what should have been changed

© 1995 Thinking Publications Appendix G: Topic Interruptions
Duplication permitted for educational use only.

INITIAL TOPIC:

The musical group you'd most like to hear in concert

MAIN OBJECTIVE(S) OF SPEAKER:

To ask if you can borrow some money to buy a candy bar

© 1995 Thinking Publications Appendix G: Topic Interruptions
Duplication permitted for educational use only.

INITIAL TOPIC:

The worst class in school

MAIN OBJECTIVE(S) OF SPEAKER:

To find out how much money your friend has to spend and where he or she gets it

© 1995 Thinking Publications Appendix G: Topic Interruptions
Duplication permitted for educational use only.

INITIAL TOPIC:

How parents should act when your friends come over

MAIN OBJECTIVE(S) OF SPEAKER:

To find out where one of your teachers lives

© 1995 Thinking Publications Appendix G: Topic Interruptions
Duplication permitted for educational use only.

INITIAL TOPIC:

The next party you hope to go to

MAIN OBJECTIVE(S) OF SPEAKER:

To talk about the last fight you had with your parent(s) or a friend

© 1995 Thinking Publications Appendix G: Topic Interruptions
Duplication permitted for educational use only.

INITIAL TOPIC:

Embarrassing things that have happened to you or to others

MAIN OBJECTIVE(S) OF SPEAKER:

To ask when summer vacation begins and what your friend is doing

© 1995 Thinking Publications Appendix G: Topic Interruptions
Duplication permitted for educational use only.

INITIAL TOPIC:

Grades you received that seemed unfair

MAIN OBJECTIVE(S) OF SPEAKER:

To complain that you lost a quarter in a vending machine

© 1995 Thinking Publications Appendix G: Topic Interruptions
Duplication permitted for educational use only.

INITIAL TOPIC:

Food you have eaten that tasted terrible

MAIN OBJECTIVE(S) OF SPEAKER:

To find out whether your friend has a curfew imposed by a parent(s)

© 1995 Thinking Publications Appendix G: Topic Interruptions
Duplication permitted for educational use only.

INITIAL TOPIC:

Your favorite relative(s)

MAIN OBJECTIVE(S) OF SPEAKER:

To find out who your friend thinks is the most popular boy or girl in school

© 1995 Thinking Publications Appendix G: Topic Interruptions
Duplication permitted for educational use only.

INITIAL TOPIC:

Things teachers do that you dislike

MAIN OBJECTIVE(S) OF SPEAKER:

To ask what tomorrow's math assignment is and to tell your friend there's a black smudge on his or her face

© 1995 Thinking Publications Appendix G: Topic Interruptions
Duplication permitted for educational use only.

INITIAL TOPIC:

How schools should be run

MAIN OBJECTIVE(S) OF SPEAKER:

To tell about the best gift you ever received and to find out what kinds of gifts your friend likes

© 1995 Thinking Publications Appendix G: Topic Interruptions
Duplication permitted for educational use only.

INITIAL TOPIC:

Part-time jobs you wish you could have while in high school

MAIN OBJECTIVE(S) OF SPEAKER:

To ask if you can borrow a comb and to complain that you have to be in by 10 p.m. this weekend

© 1995 Thinking Publications Appendix G: Topic Interruptions
Duplication permitted for educational use only.

INITIAL TOPIC:

The most fun times you have had with your family or friends

MAIN OBJECTIVE(S) OF SPEAKER:

To ask what time it is and to announce you are late and have to go

© 1995 Thinking Publications Appendix G: Topic Interruptions
Duplication permitted for educational use only.

INITIAL TOPIC:

Your favorite hairstyles and who has them

MAIN OBJECTIVE(S) OF SPEAKER:

To ask your friend what he or she is wearing to school tomorrow and to ask how much money he or she usually carries to school

© 1995 Thinking Publications Appendix G: Topic Interruptions
Duplication permitted for educational use only.

EVERYDAY QUESTIONS

Name ______________________________

Date ______________________________

DIRECTIONS: Write two examples of each question type in the spaces provided.

SITUATION	ASK INFORMATION	REQUEST ACTION	EMPHASIZE AN IDEA (RHETORICAL)
IN THE CLASSROOM			
AT HOME			
WITH PEERS			

© 1995 Thinking Publications

Duplication permitted for educational use only.

VARIABLES THAT INFLUENCE GAZING

MORE GAZING IS PREDICTED WHEN

- you are female.
- you are physically distant from your partner.
- you are discussing easy, impersonal topics.
- you have nothing else to look at.
- you are interested in your partner's reaction.
- you like/love your partner.
- you are of a lower status than your partner. (This may be reversed for interactants who are from Asian or Native American cultures, in which looking at an elder or an authority figure can be regarded as a sign of disrespect.)
- you are trying to dominate or influence your partner.
- you are listening rather than talking. (This may be reversed for interactants who are African-American. LaFrance and Mayo [1976] found that African-Americans gazed more while speaking, while Caucasians gazed more while listening.)

LESS GAZING IS PREDICTED WHEN

- you are male.
- you are physically close.
- you are discussing difficult, intimate topics.
- you have other relevant objects, people, or backgrounds to look at.
- you are not interested in your partner's reaction.
- you perceive yourself as a higher-status person than your partner. (Note the caveat mentioned previously.)
- you have a mental disorder like schizophrenia.
- you are embarrassed, ashamed, sad, submissive, or trying to hide something.
- you are talking rather than listening. (Note the caveat mentioned previously.)

© 1995 Thinking Publications

Duplication permitted for educational use only.

FACIAL EXPRESSIONS

SURPRISE

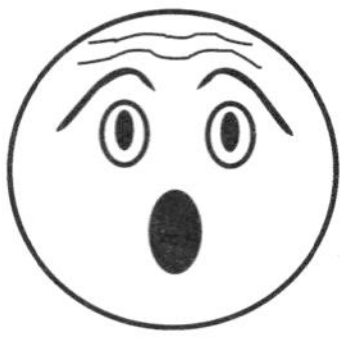

- Eyebrows are raised, curved and high.
- Skin below brow is stretched.
- Forehead has horizontal wrinkles all the way across.
- Eyelids are wide open; the sclera (white of the eye) shows above and below the iris.
- Jaw drops; lips and teeth are parted, but with no tension or stretching of the mouth.

FEAR

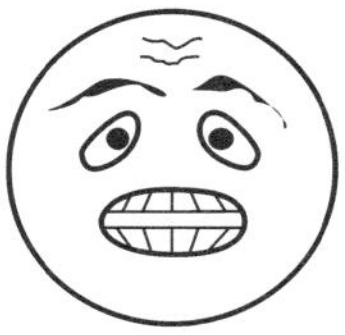

- Brows are raised and drawn together.
- Forehead has wrinkles in center area only.
- Upper eyelids are raised; lower eyelids are tensed and drawn up.
- Mouth opens; lips are tense or stretched and drawn back.

DISGUST

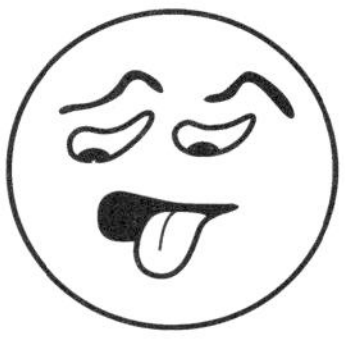

- Upper lip is raised; lower lip is raised and pushed up to the upper lip, or lowered and protruded slightly.
- Nose is wrinkled.
- Cheeks are raised.
- Brow is lowered; upper eyelids are lowered.

ANGER

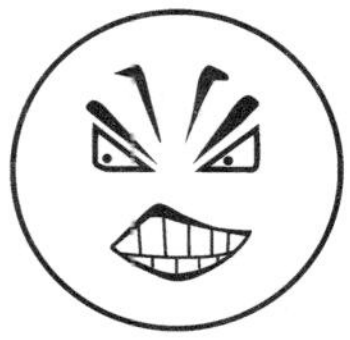

- Brows are lowered and drawn together; vertical lines appear between the brows.
- Eyes have a hard stare and may appear to bulge.
- Lips either pressed together firmly or open, as if shouting.

HAPPINESS

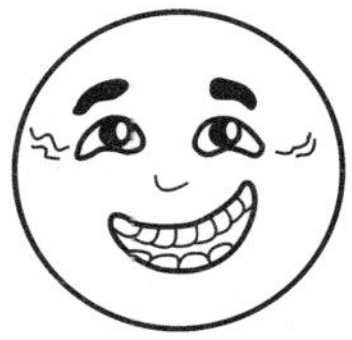

- Corners of lips drawn back and up (i.e., forming a smile).
- Cheeks are raised.
- Wrinkles extend down the nose to the outer edges beyond the lip corners.
- "Crow's foot" wrinkles go outward from the corners of the eyes.

SADNESS

- Inner corners of eyebrows are drawn up.
- Inner corners of the upper eyelids are raised.
- Corners of the lips are down; the lips may be trembling.

© 1995 Thinking Publications

Duplication permitted for educational use only.

ENCODING AND DECODING EMBLEMS

COMMANDS

Sit down beside me

© 1995 Thinking Publications Appendix K
Duplication permitted for educational use only.

COMMANDS

Be silent/Hush

© 1995 Thinking Publications Appendix K
Duplication permitted for educational use only.

COMMANDS

Come here

© 1995 Thinking Publications Appendix K
Duplication permitted for educational use only.

COMMANDS

I can't hear you

© 1995 Thinking Publications Appendix K
Duplication permitted for educational use only.

COMMANDS

Wait/Hold it

© 1995 Thinking Publications Appendix K
Duplication permitted for educational use only.

COMMANDS

I warn you

© 1995 Thinking Publications Appendix K
Duplication permitted for educational use only.

COMMANDS

Get lost

© 1995 Thinking Publications Appendix K
Duplication permitted for educational use only.

COMMANDS

Follow me

© 1995 Thinking Publications Appendix K
Duplication permitted for educational use only.

COMMANDS

Time to go

© 1995 Thinking Publications Appendix K
Duplication permitted for educational use only.

COMMANDS

Stop

© 1995 Thinking Publications Appendix K
Duplication permitted for educational use only.

COMMANDS

Go the other way

© 1995 Thinking Publications Appendix K
Duplication permitted for educational use only.

COMMANDS

Got a cigarette?

© 1995 Thinking Publications Appendix K
Duplication permitted for educational use only.

COMMANDS

Look!

© 1995 Thinking Publications Appendix K
Duplication permitted for educational use only.

COMMANDS

Take it away

© 1995 Thinking Publications Appendix K
Duplication permitted for educational use only.

COMMANDS

Stay here

© 1995 Thinking Publications Appendix K
Duplication permitted for educational use only.

PHYSICAL STATE

I'm hot/It's hot

© 1995 Thinking Publications Appendix K
Duplication permitted for educational use only.

PHYSICAL STATE

Hard work

© 1995 Thinking Publications Appendix K
Duplication permitted for educational use only.

PHYSICAL STATE

Close shave

© 1995 Thinking Publications Appendix K
Duplication permitted for educational use only.

PHYSICAL STATE

I'm cold/It's cold

© 1995 Thinking Publications Appendix K
Duplication permitted for educational use only.

PHYSICAL STATE

I'm full

© 1995 Thinking Publications Appendix K
Duplication permitted for educational use only.

PHYSICAL STATE

I've got a headache

© 1995 Thinking Publications Appendix K
Duplication permitted for educational use only.

PHYSICAL STATE

I've got a toothache

© 1995 Thinking Publications Appendix K
Duplication permitted for educational use only.

PHYSICAL STATE

I've got an earache

© 1995 Thinking Publications Appendix K
Duplication permitted for educational use only.

PHYSICAL STATE

Tastes good

© 1995 Thinking Publications Appendix K
Duplication permitted for educational use only.

PHYSICAL STATE

I am smart

© 1995 Thinking Publications Appendix K
Duplication permitted for educational use only.

PHYSICAL STATE

How could I be so dumb?

© 1995 Thinking Publications Appendix K
Duplication permitted for educational use only.

INSULTS

The hell with you/Rejection

© 1995 Thinking Publications Appendix K
Duplication permitted for educational use only.

INSULTS

He's crazy/He's stupid

© 1995 Thinking Publications Appendix K
Duplication permitted for educational use only.

INSULTS

Shame on you

© 1995 Thinking Publications Appendix K
Duplication permitted for educational use only.

REPLIES

OK

© 1995 Thinking Publications Appendix K
Duplication permitted for educational use only.

REPLIES

No/I disagree

© 1995 Thinking Publications Appendix K
Duplication permitted for educational use only.

REPLIES

I don't know

© 1995 Thinking Publications Appendix K
Duplication permitted for educational use only.

REPLIES

Yes/I agree

© 1995 Thinking Publications Appendix K
Duplication permitted for educational use only.

REPLIES

Absolutely no!

© 1995 Thinking Publications Appendix K
Duplication permitted for educational use only.

REPLIES

I dislike it

© 1995 Thinking Publications Appendix K
Duplication permitted for educational use only.

REPLIES

I promise

© 1995 Thinking Publications Appendix K
Duplication permitted for educational use only.

REPLIES

Absolutely yes!

© 1995 Thinking Publications Appendix K
Duplication permitted for educational use only.

REPLIES

Hard to think about this/Thinking

© 1995 Thinking Publications Appendix K
Duplication permitted for educational use only.

REPLIES

I doubt it

© 1995 Thinking Publications Appendix K
Duplication permitted for educational use only.

AFFECT

I'm angry

© 1995 Thinking Publications Appendix K
Duplication permitted for educational use only.

AFFECT

I'm disgusted

© 1995 Thinking Publications Appendix K
Duplication permitted for educational use only.

AFFECT

I'm surprised

© 1995 Thinking Publications Appendix K
Duplication permitted for educational use only.

AFFECT

Whoopee/Hooray!

© 1995 Thinking Publications Appendix K
Duplication permitted for educational use only.

GREETINGS

Hello/Good-bye

© 1995 Thinking Publications Appendix K
Duplication permitted for educational use only.

UNCLASSIFIED

Me

© 1995 Thinking Publications Appendix K
Duplication permitted for educational use only.

UNCLASSIFIED

You

© 1995 Thinking Publications Appendix K
Duplication permitted for educational use only.

UNCLASSIFIED

Hitchhiking

© 1995 Thinking Publications Appendix K
Duplication permitted for educational use only.

UNCLASSIFIED

Counting

© 1995 Thinking Publications Appendix K
Duplication permitted for educational use only.

UNCLASSIFIED

Gossip

© 1995 Thinking Publications Appendix K
Duplication permitted for educational use only.

UNCLASSIFIED

Fighting

© 1995 Thinking Publications Appendix K
Duplication permitted for educational use only.

UNCLASSIFIED

Peace/Victory

© 1995 Thinking Publications Appendix K
Duplication permitted for educational use only.

UNCLASSIFIED

Good luck

© 1995 Thinking Publications Appendix K
Duplication permitted for educational use only.

UNCLASSIFIED

Money

© 1995 Thinking Publications Appendix K
Duplication permitted for educational use only.

UNCLASSIFIED

It's far away

© 1995 Thinking Publications Appendix K
Duplication permitted for educational use only.

UNCLASSIFIED

Suicide by gun

© 1995 Thinking Publications Appendix K
Duplication permitted for educational use only.

UNCLASSIFIED

Finished

© 1995 Thinking Publications Appendix K
Duplication permitted for educational use only.

ILLUSTRATORS—LINKING WITH SPEECH

SPOKEN MESSAGE

I really like the new English teacher. She's nice to me and lets me get assignments in late.

NONVERBAL MESSAGE

Matched

© 1995 Thinking Publications Appendix L
Duplication permitted for educational use only.

SPOKEN MESSAGE

I'm really not very comfortable. I ate a whole pizza by myself an hour ago.

NONVERBAL MESSAGE

Matched

© 1995 Thinking Publications Appendix L
Duplication permitted for educational use only.

SPOKEN MESSAGE

I would like everyone to remain seated. It should be just a few more minutes to wait. I'm as impatient as you are.

NONVERBAL MESSAGE

Mismatched

© 1995 Thinking Publications Appendix L
Duplication permitted for educational use only.

SPOKEN MESSAGE

The new math teacher is OK. You'd do all right in her class next year.

NONVERBAL MESSAGE

Mismatched

© 1995 Thinking Publications Appendix L
Duplication permitted for educational use only.

SPOKEN MESSAGE

My aunt is so disgusting. She comes to our house and eats all our food and never brings any. She's already so fat she wouldn't have to eat for a month.

NONVERBAL MESSAGE

Mismatched

© 1995 Thinking Publications Appendix L
Duplication permitted for educational use only.

SPOKEN MESSAGE

I wish we didn't have a test tomorrow. I'm really scared I'm going to flunk it.

NONVERBAL MESSAGE

Matched

© 1995 Thinking Publications Appendix L
Duplication permitted for educational use only.

SPOKEN MESSAGE

I have a friend who never comes to see me anymore. I really miss seeing her and wonder if I've done something to make her mad.

NONVERBAL MESSAGE

Mismatched

© 1995 Thinking Publications Appendix L
Duplication permitted for educational use only.

SPOKEN MESSAGE

I'm so angry at my dad. He promised to buy me new shoes, and now he says he won't because I got home late last night.

NONVERBAL MESSAGE

Mismatched

© 1995 Thinking Publications Appendix L
Duplication permitted for educational use only.

SPOKEN MESSAGE

I really like her new haircut. I wish I could get mine to look that way.

NONVERBAL MESSAGE

Matched

© 1995 Thinking Publications Appendix L
Duplication permitted for educational use only.

SPOKEN MESSAGE

The class is so boring. I recommend you don't take it next year. You'd be sorry.

NONVERBAL MESSAGE

Mismatched

© 1995 Thinking Publications Appendix L
Duplication permitted for educational use only.

SPOKEN MESSAGE

He said to take the second right turn to get to his house, but that took me down to the edge of the river. I was so lost and confused.

NONVERBAL MESSAGE

Matched

© 1995 Thinking Publications Appendix L
Duplication permitted for educational use only.

SPOKEN MESSAGE

My brother always beats me at computer games, but I'll show him. I've really been practicing, and I'm going to beat him.

NONVERBAL MESSAGE

Mismatched

© 1995 Thinking Publications Appendix L
Duplication permitted for educational use only.

SPOKEN MESSAGE

Mr. Roberts, the math teacher, always winks at Sue because he knows she has the answer. She's such a teacher's pet it's disgusting.

NONVERBAL MESSAGE

Matched

© 1995 Thinking Publications Appendix L
Duplication permitted for educational use only.

SPOKEN MESSAGE

Mr. Smith's dog just had puppies. He's going to be gone this weekend and asked me to look in on them every day. I'm really interested in seeing the little puppies.

NONVERBAL MESSAGE

Mismatched

© 1995 Thinking Publications Appendix L
Duplication permitted for educational use only.

SPOKEN MESSAGE

The grocery store window was broken yesterday, and they called my mom to see if I did it. I was with my friends near the store the night before, and they thought we did it. I can't believe they accused us.

NONVERBAL MESSAGE

Matched

© 1995 Thinking Publications Appendix L
Duplication permitted for educational use only.

SPOKEN MESSAGE

My grandmother just went into the hospital. She has terminal cancer, and they don't think she's going to live much longer. She's the only adult who cares about me.

NONVERBAL MESSAGE

Mismatched

© 1995 Thinking Publications Appendix L
Duplication permitted for educational use only.

SPOKEN MESSAGE

Mr. Jones said he'd give us two weeks to write our reports, and now he says he wants them Friday. I can't stand it when he does that.

NONVERBAL MESSAGE

Mismatched

© 1995 Thinking Publications Appendix L
Duplication permitted for educational use only.

SPOKEN MESSAGE

I hate it when teachers tell us what to do and how to act even when we're not in their classes. They're so mean to us.

NONVERBAL MESSAGE

Mismatched

© 1995 Thinking Publications Appendix L
Duplication permitted for educational use only.

SPOKEN MESSAGE

My mom just got a letter from her sister. She's coming to visit us for the whole month of December. Were we surprised! We don't even like her that much.

NONVERBAL MESSAGE

Matched

© 1995 Thinking Publications Appendix L
Duplication permitted for educational use only.

SPOKEN MESSAGE

I keep getting strange phone calls. As soon as I answer the phone, the person hangs up. It happens all the time, especially late at night. I'm getting scared.

NONVERBAL MESSAGE

Matched

© 1995 Thinking Publications Appendix L
Duplication permitted for educational use only.

LEARNING STYLE QUESTIONNAIRE

IDENTIFICATION INFORMATION

Name: ______________________________ Date: ______________

Grade: ______________________________ Class: ______________

Adult assisting you to complete this questionnaire: ______________________________

DIRECTIONS:

This is NOT a test. There are no right or wrong answers. The following items are simply a way to find out how you learn best. If an item is unclear, feel free to ask questions of the person administering this questionnaire.

The purpose of this questionnaire is to determine how you learn best, not how you like to learn a subject. For example, you might like to have the TV on while you are studying, but you study best when it is quiet. Also, you might like to study at night, but you are more productive if you study in the morning. *Learn best* means how you remember information the longest, attend to a task the best, or recall details and main ideas most easily. Knowing how you learn best will help us to help you to be more successful in school.

Before you begin to answer the questions, please write your name, the date, and other identification information requested in the space provided above.

Answer the following statements honestly about when, how, where, why, and with whom you learn best.

A subject important to me to learn is: ______________________________

I learn my most important subject best:

When?

1. Time (Check only one.)

   ______ Morning
   ______ Afternoon
   ______ Night
   ______ Other (explain): ______________________________
   ____

2. Timing (Check only one.)

   _____ Before meals
   _____ After meals

© 1995 Thinking Publications

Duplication permitted for educational use only.

I learn my most important subject best:

How?

1. Sound (Check only one.)

_____ Quiet
_____ Radio
_____ Conversation
_____ TV
_____ Music
_____ Noisy
_____ Other (explain): ____
____

2. Light (Check only one.)

_____ Dim
_____ Moderate
_____ Bright
_____ Other (explain): ____
____

3. Temperature (Check only one.)

_____ Cold
_____ Cool
_____ Warm
_____ Very warm
_____ Other (explain): ____
____

4. Intake (Check only one.)

_____ Eat foods
_____ Drink liquids
_____ Chew on something
_____ No eating, drinking, or chewing on anything while learning
_____ Other (explain): ____
____

© 1995 Thinking Publications Duplication permitted for educational use only.

I learn my most important subject best:

Where?

1. Place (Indicate your first choice.)

   _____ Home

   _____ School

2. Conditions (Within each place, rank the locations. 1 = The location where you learn best.)

   a. Home

   _____ Desk/Table
   _____ Bed
   _____ Floor
   _____ Straight chair
   _____ Soft chair
   _____ Couch
   _____ Other (explain): ____
   ____

   b. School

   _____ Desk/Table
   _____ Floor
   _____ Straight chair
   _____ Soft chair
   _____ Other (explain): ____
   ____

I learn my most important subject best:

Why? (Rank these items as to why you learn best. 1 = Your strongest reason for learning.)

_____ I want to.
_____ My teacher expects me to/demands it.
_____ My parent(s) expects me to/demands it.
_____ I'll get a reward such as:
    _____ money
    _____ better grades
    _____ privileges
_____ Other (explain): ____
____

© 1995 Thinking Publications *Duplication permitted for educational use only.*

I learn my most important subject best:

With whom? (Rank the top four. 1 = The best way to study the subject.)

_____ Alone
_____ A partner
_____ Small group (3–7)
_____ Large group (8 and above)
_____ Teacher(s)
_____ Parent(s)
_____ Sibling(s)
_____ Varied (explain): ____

____

Rank or check how you learn best in the following situations.

Inside the Classroom

1. Participating in the class (Rank the ways you learn best in the classroom. 1 = The way you learn important material the best.)

_____ Listening
_____ Reading
_____ Writing
_____ Speaking
_____ Doing
_____ Combination of the above
Please specify: ____

____

2. Participating in assignments within the classroom (Rank the top four assignments that help you learn the information best. 1 = The best way to learn via an assignment.)

_____ Worksheet questions
_____ Experiments
_____ Demonstrations
_____ Group projects
_____ Individual projects
_____ Written reports
_____ Oral reports
_____ Other (explain): ____

____

© 1995 Thinking Publications

Duplication permitted for educational use only.

3. Remembering main points from what the teacher says (Rank the top four. 1 = The best way to remember main points from what the teacher says.)

_____ Repeat the material to myself
_____ Think of a picture in my mind
_____ Make up words to remember main points in order
_____ Break ideas into smaller chunks
_____ Outline what the teacher says in writing
_____ Follow an outline that the teacher has provided
_____ Use rhyming words to recall main points
_____ Put main points into categories
_____ Audiotape what the teacher is saying and replay it later
_____ Other (explain): ____

____

____

4. Taking notes (Check only one.)

While listening to a lecture, I take notes when learning my most difficult subject as follows:

_____ Notes are key words
_____ Notes are attempts at complete sentences
_____ Notes are "doodles"
_____ Other (explain): ____

____

____

5. Asking questions of the teacher (Check only one.)

I learn my most important subject best if I ask questions:

_____ During class
_____ After class
_____ Before class
_____ Other (explain): ____

____

____

© 1995 Thinking Publications *Duplication permitted for educational use only.*

6. Remembering main points from a textbook (Rank the top four ways that you learn best from a textbook. 1 = The best way to remember main points from a textbook.)

_____ Look at headings and subheadings within the chapters
_____ Outline important ideas from the textbook
_____ Underline/highlight main points
_____ Write down questions to anticipate what a teacher will ask on a test
_____ Answer questions at the end of each chapter (if available)
_____ Follow along in the textbook while listening to an audiotape of the textbook
_____ Other (explain): ____

____

Outside the Classroom

1. Participating in outside classroom assignments (Rank the top two assignments that help you to learn an important subject best. 1 = The best way to learn via an assignment.)

_____ Preparing a written report
_____ Preparing for an oral report
_____ Answering questions from the textbook or worksheet
_____ Reading assigned information
_____ Other (explain): ____

____

2. Studying for a test (Rank the top four. 1 = The way you study best for a test.)

I learn best studying for a test in my most important subject when I:

_____ Read or reread the textbook the day before
_____ Read or reread the textbook 2–3 days before
_____ Listen or re-listen to audiotapes of what the teacher said
_____ Review the outline of my notes
_____ Review the outline provided by the teacher
_____ Predict questions to be on the test and answer them
_____ Rework problems assigned by the teacher
_____ Other (explain): ____

____

3. I learn my most important subject best when I study for __________ minutes each hour before taking a break.

Adapted from *Language Disorders in Older Students: Preadolescents and Adolescents* (pp. 278–284) by V. Lord Larson and N. McKinley, 1995, Eau Claire, WI: Thinking Publications. © 1995 by Thinking Publications. Adapted with permission.

© 1995 Thinking Publications *Duplication permitted for educational use only.*

IDEAL STUDYING AT HOME

Name ______________________

Date ______________________

	IDEAL	CURRENT	MAKE A CHANGE
WHEN			
Time			
Timing			
HOW			
Sound			
Light			
Temperature			
Intake			
WHERE			
Conditions			
WITH WHOM			
Alone			
With a partner (adult, peer, or sibling)			
In a small group			
In a team			
Varied			
I am going to make these changes in how I study at home:			

© 1995 Thinking Publications

Duplication permitted for educational use only.

TIME SCHEDULE

Name ______________________

Date ______________________

Day of Week ______________________

TIME	ACTIVITY	MINUTES

© 1995 Thinking Publications

Duplication permitted for educational use only.

Name ____________________

Date ____________________

Day of Week ____________________

ACTIVITY CATEGORY	MINUTES PER DAY	TOTAL MINUTES PER DAY

Total minutes in a day 1,440

Minus total minutes accounted for ____________

Total minutes free time ____________

© 1995 Thinking Publications

Duplication permitted for educational use only.

MONTHLY CALENDAR

Name ____________________

Date ____________________

Month ____________________

SUNDAY	MONDAY	TUESDAY	WEDNESDAY	THURSDAY	FRIDAY	SATURDAY

© 1995 Thinking Publications

Duplication permitted for educational use only.

WEEKLY ASSIGNMENT SCHEDULE

Name ______________________ Week of ______________________

Subject ______________________

Teacher ______________________

MONDAY	TUESDAY	WEDNESDAY	THURSDAY	FRIDAY

© 1995 Thinking Publications

Duplication permitted for educational use only.

"TO DO" LISTS

Name ______________________

Date ______________________

"TO DO" LIST		
A (MOST IMPORTANT)	B	C (LEAST IMPORTANT)

"TO DO" LIST					
	MONDAY	TUESDAY	WEDNESDAY	THURSDAY	FRIDAY
A					
B					
C					

© 1995 Thinking Publications

Duplication permitted for educational use only.

TEST TAKING—TEST VOCABULARY

analyze	examine the parts of an item and discuss how they are related
compare	look at two or more items and show how they are the same or different
contrast	compare two or more items to show differences between them
criticize	give your opinion or judgment about the positive and negative points
define	give the meaning of
describe	write about it, "paint a picture" with words; do so in a logical sequence
diagram	make a drawing, graph, or chart and label its parts
discuss	talk something over, looking at positive and negative points
enumerate	list facts using numbers
evaluate	give your opinion of the importance of something; give advantages and disadvantages
explain	make something clear that is not understood; tell how something happened or how to do something
hypothesize	think about what would happen if...
illustrate	explain your answer in writing and make it clear using examples, stories, pictures, charts, diagrams
interpret	explain the meaning of something, using examples to make it clear
justify	give a reason for or defend something; give evidence
list	produce answers in words or sentences and number them
outline	list a plan that gives only the main ideas; summarize showing how the ideas are organized
prove	give evidence or argue that something is true
relate	show how one thing is connected to or similar to another
review	examine and talk about the important parts of something; perhaps discuss positive and negative points
state	tell; express precisely; sentences should be brief and should omit details
summarize	give only the main points of a thing or event, not details or examples
trace	follow the development of (the history of) something from beginning to end

© 1995 Thinking Publications

Duplication permitted for educational use only.

TEST-TAKING VOCABULARY CARDS

ANALYZE

© 1995 Thinking Publications Appendix T
Duplication permitted for educational use only.

COMPARE

© 1995 Thinking Publications Appendix T
Duplication permitted for educational use only.

CONTRAST

© 1995 Thinking Publications Appendix T
Duplication permitted for educational use only.

CRITICIZE

© 1995 Thinking Publications Appendix T
Duplication permitted for educational use only.

DEFINE

© 1995 Thinking Publications Appendix T
Duplication permitted for educational use only.

DESCRIBE

© 1995 Thinking Publications Appendix T
Duplication permitted for educational use only.

DIAGRAM

© 1995 Thinking Publications Appendix T
Duplication permitted for educational use only.

DISCUSS

© 1995 Thinking Publications Appendix T
Duplication permitted for educational use only.

ENUMERATE

© 1995 Thinking Publications Appendix T
Duplication permitted for educational use only.

EVALUATE

© 1995 Thinking Publications Appendix T
Duplication permitted for educational use only.

EXPLAIN

© 1995 Thinking Publications Appendix T
Duplication permitted for educational use only.

HYPOTHESIZE

© 1995 Thinking Publications Appendix T
Duplication permitted for educational use only.

ILLUSTRATE

© 1995 Thinking Publications Appendix T
Duplication permitted for educational use only.

INTERPRET

© 1995 Thinking Publications Appendix T
Duplication permitted for educational use only.

JUSTIFY

© 1995 Thinking Publications Appendix T
Duplication permitted for educational use only.

LIST

© 1995 Thinking Publications Appendix T
Duplication permitted for educational use only.

OUTLINE

© 1995 Thinking Publications Appendix T
Duplication permitted for educational use only.

PROVE

© 1995 Thinking Publications Appendix T
Duplication permitted for educational use only.

RELATE

© 1995 Thinking Publications Appendix T
Duplication permitted for educational use only.

REVIEW

© 1995 Thinking Publications Appendix T
Duplication permitted for educational use only.

STATE

© 1995 Thinking Publications
Duplication permitted for educational use only.

Appendix T

SUMMARIZE

© 1995 Thinking Publications
Duplication permitted for educational use only.

Appendix T

TRACE

© 1995 Thinking Publications
Duplication permitted for educational use only.

Appendix T

Appendix T

WORD CATEGORY CARDS

SUFFIX

(-ule, -et [-ette], -icle)

little

ringlet

statuette

capsule

minuscule

particle

streamlet

© 1995 Thinking Publications Appendix U
Duplication permitted for educational use only.

SUFFIX

(-or, -er, -ier)

persons

donor

cashier

auditor

lawyer

instructor

director

© 1995 Thinking Publications Appendix U
Duplication permitted for educational use only.

SUFFIX

(-arian, -ian, -ist)

persons

socialist

chemist

physician

bicyclist

librarian

comedian

© 1995 Thinking Publications Appendix U
Duplication permitted for educational use only.

SUFFIX

(-orium, -ory, -ary, -atory)

places

auditorium

laboratory

sanctuary

observatory

planetarium

© 1995 Thinking Publications Appendix U
Duplication permitted for educational use only.

SUFFIX

(-ish, -ster, -ly)

characteristic of

childish
timely
Jewish
motherly
youngster
gangster

© 1995 Thinking Publications Appendix U
Duplication permitted for educational use only.

SUFFIX

(-ship, -hood, -ism)

state of

manhood
censorship
racism
ownership
hardship
hypnotism

© 1995 Thinking Publications Appendix U
Duplication permitted for educational use only.

SUFFIX

(-itis, -ance, -ancy)

state of

bronchitis
resistance
truancy
arthritis
avoidance
vacancy

© 1995 Thinking Publications Appendix U
Duplication permitted for educational use only.

SUFFIX

(-logy)

science of

biology
geology
theology
psychology
zoology
archaeology

© 1995 Thinking Publications Appendix U
Duplication permitted for educational use only.

SUFFIX

(-ful)

enough to fill

mouthful

meaningful

handful

joyful

wonderful

spoonful

© 1995 Thinking Publications Appendix U
Duplication permitted for educational use only.

PREFIX

(in-, non-, un-)

negative

nonstop

inactive

unsure

informal

nonsense

unsafe

© 1995 Thinking Publications Appendix U
Duplication permitted for educational use only.

PREFIX

(bi-, di-)

two

dissect

biennial

bisect

diphthong

bicycle

dilemma

© 1995 Thinking Publications Appendix U
Duplication permitted for educational use only.

PREFIX

(en-, in-, im-)

in, into

include

encircle

inhale

immerse

encase

implant

© 1995 Thinking Publications Appendix U
Duplication permitted for educational use only.

PREFIX

(contra-, counter-)

against

contradict

counterbalance

contraband

contrast

counterclockwise

counteract

© 1995 Thinking Publications Appendix U
Duplication permitted for educational use only.

PREFIX

(re-)

again

repeat

reorganize

rename

renew

remodel

repossess

© 1995 Thinking Publications Appendix U
Duplication permitted for educational use only.

PREFIX

(micro-)

small

microphone

microscope

microfilm

microsecond

microwave

microorganism

© 1995 Thinking Publications Appendix U
Duplication permitted for educational use only.

PREFIX

(mid-)

middle

midriff

Midwestern

midnight

midterm

midair

midpoint

© 1995 Thinking Publications Appendix U
Duplication permitted for educational use only.

PREFIX

(pro-)

directional

promote

provide

proceed

produce

progress

project

© 1995 Thinking Publications Appendix U
Duplication permitted for educational use only.

WORD ROOT

(graph)

write

telegraph

paragraph

graphite

biography

autograph

geography

© 1995 Thinking Publications Appendix U
Duplication permitted for educational use only.

WORD ROOT

(onym)

name

antonym

homonym

acronym

synonym

pseudonym

anonymous

© 1995 Thinking Publications Appendix U
Duplication permitted for educational use only.

WORD ROOT

(cide)

kill

germicide

pesticide

suicide

homicide

herbicide

insecticide

© 1995 Thinking Publications Appendix U
Duplication permitted for educational use only.

R

REFERENCES

Adams, A., Flowers, A., and Woods, E. (1978). *Reading for survival in today's society.* Santa Monica, CA: Goodyear Publishing.

Adler, M. (1983). *How to speak. How to listen.* New York: Macmillan.

Agency for Instructional TV. (1979). *"Think about" teacher's guide.* Bloomington, IN: Author.

Allen, B., Mason, J., and McKean, K. (1982). *Exceptions: A handbook for teachers of mainstreamed students.* Cushing, OK: Project Mainstream.

Alley, G., and Deshler, D. (1979). *Teaching the learning disabled adolescent: Strategies and methods.* Denver, CO: Love Publishing.

The American heritage dictionary (3rd ed.). (1992). Boston: Houghton Mifflin.

Arbuckle, D. (1970). *Counseling: Philosophy, theory, and practice* (2nd ed.). Boston: Allyn and Bacon.

Argyle, M., and Ingham, R. (1972). Gaze, mutual gaze, and proximity. *Semiotica, 6,* 32–49.

Armstrong, T. (1987). *In their own way: Discovering and encouraging your child's personal learning style.* New York: Tarcher/Putnam.

Armstrong, T. (1993a). *Multiple intelligences in the classroom.* Alexandria, VA: Association for Supervision and Curriculum Development.

Armstrong, T. (1993b). *7 kinds of smart.* New York: Tarcher/Putnam.

Ashear, V., and Snortum, J. (1971). Eye contact in children as a function of age, sex, social and intellective variables. *Developmental Psychology, 3,* 479.

Atwood, B. (1974). *Building independent learning skills.* Palo Alto, CA: Learning Handbooks.

Baggett, L. (1969, March). *Behavior that communicates understanding as evaluated by teenagers.* Paper presented at the American Personnel and Guidance Association Convention, Las Vegas, NV.

Baum, S.M., Renzulli, J.S., and Hebert, T.P. (1994a). *Reversing underachievement: Creative productivity as a systematic intervention.* Manuscript submitted for publication.

Baum, S.M., Renzulli, J.S., and Hebert, T.P. (1994b). *Reversing underachievement:*

Stories of success. Educational Leadership, 52(3), 48–52.

Benjamin, A. (1969). *The helping interview.* Boston: Houghton Mifflin.

Berensen, B., Mitchell, K., and Laney R. (1968). Level of therapist functioning: Types of confrontation and type of patient. *Journal of Clinical Psychology, 24,* 111–113.

Bergman, M. (1987). Social grace or disgrace: Adolescent social skills and learning disability subtypes. *Reading, Writing, and Learning Disabilities, 3,* 161–166.

Birdwhistell, R. (1970). *Kinesics and context.* Philadelphia, PA: University of Pennsylvania Press.

Boyce, N., and Larson, V. Lord. (1983). *Adolescents' communication: Development and disorders.* Eau Claire, WI: Thinking Publications.

Bragstad, B., and Stumpf, S. (1982). *A guidebook for teaching study skills and motivation.* Boston: Allyn and Bacon.

Bragstad, B., and Stumpf, S. (1987). *A guidebook for teaching study skills and motivation* (2nd ed.). Boston: Allyn and Bacon.

Bransford, J., Sherwood, R., Rieser, J., and Vye, N. (1986). Teaching thinking and problem solving: Research foundations. *American Psychologist, 41,* 1078–1089.

Bransford, J.D., and Vye, N.J. (1989). A perspective on cognitive research and its implications for instruction. In L. Resnick and L. Klopfer (Eds.), *Toward the thinking curriculum: Current cognitive research* (pp. 173–205). Alexandria, VA: Association for Supervision and Curriculum Development.

Brigance, A. (1981). *Inventory of essential skills.* North Billerica, MA: Curriculum Associates.

Brown, A.L., Campione, J.C., and Day, J. (1981). Learning to learn: On training students to learn from texts. *Educational Researcher, 10,* 14–24.

Brown, J.I. (1952). *Efficient reading.* Boston: Houghton Mifflin.

Cavior, N., and Donecki, P. (1973). Physical attractiveness, perceived attitude similarity and academic achievement as contributors to interpersonal attraction among adolescents. *Development Psychology, 9,* 44–54.

Cavior, N., and Howard, L. (1973). Facial attractiveness and juvenile delinquency among black and white offenders. *Journal of Abnormal Child Psychology, 1,* 202–213.

Cavior, N., and Lombardi, D. (1973). Developmental aspects of judgments of physical attractiveness in children. *Developmental Psychology, 8,* 67–71.

Chi, M.T. (1978). Knowledge structures and memory development. In R.S. Siegler (Ed.), *Children's thinking: What develops?* (pp. 73–96). Hillsdale, NJ: Erlbaum.

Chi, M.T., Bassok, M., Lewis, M.W., Reimann, P., and Glaser, R. (1988). *Self-explanations: How students study and use examples in learning to solve problems.* Pittsburgh, PA: Learning Research and Development Center.

Condon, W., and Ogston, W. (1966). Soundfilm analysis of normal and pathological behavior patterns. *Journal of Nervous and Mental Disease, 143,* 338–347.

Crais, E. (1990). World knowledge to word knowledge. World knowledge and language development: Development and disorders. *Topics in Language Disorders, 10*(3), 45–62.

Cromwell, R. (1963). A social learning approach to mental retardation. In N.R. Ellis (Ed.), *Handbook of mental deficiency* (pp. 41–91). New York: McGraw-Hill.

Cromwell, R. (1967). Personality evaluation. In A. A. Baumeister (Ed.), *Mental retardation: Appraisal, education and rehabilitation* (pp. 66–85). Chicago: Alden Publishing.

de Shazer, S. (1985). *Keys to solution in brief therapy.* New York: Norton.

de Shazer, S. (1988). *Clues: Investigating solutions in brief therapy.* New York: Norton.

de Shazer, S. (1991). *Putting difference to work.* New York: Norton.

Deshler, D.D., and Schumaker, J.B. (1986). Learning strategies: An instructional alternative for low-achieving adolescents. *Exceptional Children, 52,* 583–590.

Devine, T.G. (1981). *Teaching study skills.* Boston: Allyn and Bacon.

Dimitrovsky, L. (1964). The ability to identify the emotional meaning of vocal expressions at successive age levels. In J.R. Davitz (Ed.), *The communication of emotional meaning.* (pp. 69–86). New York: McGraw-Hill.

Dittman, A. (1972). Developmental factors in conversational behavior. *Journal of Communication, 22,* 404–423.

Drake, J. (1976). *Teaching critical thinking.* Danville, IL: Interstate Printers and Publishers.

Dunn, R. (1983, April). *Teaching students through their individual learning styles: A practical approach.* Presentation at the University of Wisconsin, Eau Claire.

Dunn, R., Beaudry, J., and Klavas, A. (1989). Survey of research on learning styles. *Educational Leadership, 46,* 50–58.

Dunn, R., Dunn, K., and Price, G. (1989). *Learning style inventory. LSI manual.* Lawrence, KS: Price Systems.

Dweck, C. (1986). Motivational processes affecting learning. *American Psychologist, 41,* 1040–1048.

Edmondson, W. (1981). *Spoken discourse: A model for analysis.* New York: Longman.

Ekman, P. (1965). Communication through nonverbal behavior: A source of information about an interpersonal relationship. In S. Tomkins and C. Izard (Eds.), *Affect, cognition and personality* (pp. 390–442). New York: Springer.

Ekman, P., and Friesen, W. (1972). Hand movements. *Journal of Communication, 22,* 353–374.

Ekman, P., Friesen, W., and Ellsworth, P. (1972). *Emotion in the human face: Guidelines for research and an integration of the findings.* New York: Pergamon Press.

Ekman, P., Friesen, W., and Tomkins, S. (1971). Facial affect scoring technique: A first validity study. *Semiotica, 3,* 37–58.

Ellis, E., and Friend, P. (1991). Adolescents with learning disabilities. In B. Wong (Ed.), *Learning about learning disabilities* (pp. 506–563). San Diego, CA: Academic Press.

Feuerstein, R. (1980). *Instrumental enrichment.* Baltimore, MD: University Park Press.

Fowler, R.L., and Barker, A.S. (1974). Effectiveness of highlighting for retention of text material. *Journal of Applied Psychology, 59,* 358–364.

Fridlund, A.J. (1994). *Human facial expression: An evolutionary view.* San Diego, CA: Academic Press.

Fulcher, G.S. (1965). *Common sense decision-making.* Evanston, IL: Northwestern University Press.

Gall, M.D., and Gall, J.P., Jacobsen, D.R., and Bullock, T.L. (1990). *Tools for learning: A guide to teaching study skills.* Alexandria,

VA: Association for Supervision and Curriculum Development.

Gardner, H. (1993). *Multiple intelligences: The theory in practice.* New York: Basic Books.

Gates, G. (1923). An experimental study of the growth of social perception. *Journal of Educational Psychology, 14,* 449–461.

Gelatt, H.B., Varenhorst, B., Carey, R., and Miller, G. (1973). *Decisions and outcomes.* New York: College Entrance Examination Board.

Glasser, W. (1965). *Reality therapy.* New York: Harper and Row.

Glasser, W. (1969). *Schools without failure.* New York: Harper and Row.

Glasser, W. (1993). *The quality school teacher.* New York: Harper-Collins.

Goffman, E. (1976). Replies and responses. *Language in Society, 5,* 257–313.

Goodlad, J. (1983). *A place called school: Prospects for the future.* New York: McGraw-Hill.

Greatsinger, C. (1976a). *Label talk.* Syracuse, NY: New Reader's Press.

Greatsinger, C. (1976b). *Signs around town.* Syracuse, NY: New Reader's Press.

Grice, H. (1975). Logic and conversation. In P. Cole and J. Morgan (Eds), *Syntax and semantics: Vol. 3. Speech acts* (pp. 41–58). New York: Academic Press.

Hall, E. (1969). *The hidden dimension.* New York: Doubleday.

Hamersky, J. (1993). *Vocabulary maps: Strategies for developing word meanings.* Eau Claire, WI: Thinking Publications.

Harper, L., and Sanders, K. (1975). Preschool children's use of space: Sex differences in outdoor play. *Developmental Psychology, 11,* 119.

Hayes, J.R. (1981). *The complete problem solver.* Philadelphia, PA: Franklin Institute Press.

Hayes, J.R. (1989). *The complete problem solver* (2nd ed.). Hillsdale, NJ: Erlbaum.

Holley, C.D., and Danserau, D.F. (1984). *Spatial learning strategies: Techniques, applications, and related issues.* New York: Academic Press.

Hunt, P., and Smith, J. (1980). Initiation of group counseling with minority female adolescents. *The School Counselor, 27,* 192–197.

Izard, C. (1971). *The face of emotion.* New York: Appleton-Century-Crofts.

Jalongo, M. (1991). *Strategies for developing children's listening skills* (Fastback No. 314). Bloomington, IN: Phi Delta Kappa Educational Foundation.

Jenkins, J. (1975). Remember that old theory of memory? Well, forget it! *American Psychologist, 29,* 785–795.

Johnson, H., Ekman, P., and Friesen, W. (1975). Communicative body movements: American emblems. *Semiotica, 15,* 335–353.

Jones, B.F., Palincsar, A.S., Ogle, D.S., and Carr, E.G. (1987). *Strategic teaching and learning: Cognitive instruction in the content areas.* Alexandria, VA: Association for Supervision and Curriculum Development.

Jones, S., and Aiello, J. (1973). Proxemic behavior of black and white first, third, and fifth-grade children. *Journal of Personality and Social Psychology, 25,* 21–27.

Kaniel, S. (1995). Strategies for improving the function of working memory. *Journal of Cognitive Education, 4*(1), 57–68.

Kelly, G. (1955). *The psychology of personal constructs.* New York: Norton.

Kendon, A. (1967). Some functions of gaze—direction in social interaction. *Acta Psychologica, 26,* 22–63.

Knapp, M. (1978). *Nonverbal communication in human interaction*. New York: Holt, Rinehart and Winston.

Knapp, M., and Hall, J. (1992). *Nonverbal communication in human interaction* (3rd ed.). Orlando, FL: Harcourt Brace College Publishers.

Kurfiss, J. (1988). *Critical thinking: Theory and research, practice, and possibilities.* (ASHE-ERIC Higher Education Report No. 2). Washington, DC: Association for the Study of Higher Education.

LaFrance, M., and Mayo, C. (1976). Racial differences in gaze behavior during conversations: Two systematic observational studies. *Journal of Personality and Social Psychology, 33*, 547–552.

Larson, M., and Dittman, F. (1975). *Compensatory education and early adolescence: Reviewing our national strategy* (Research report). Menlo Park, CA: Stanford Research Institution.

Larson, V. Lord, and McKinley, N. (1987). *Communication assessment and intervention strategies for adolescents*. Eau Claire, WI: Thinking Publications.

Larson, V. Lord, and McKinley, N. (1995). *Language disorders in older students: Preadolescents and adolescents*. Eau Claire, WI: Thinking Publications.

Lazarus, A. (1969). The inner circle strategy: Identifying crucial problems. In V. Krumboltz and C. Thoresen (Eds.), *Behavioral counseling: Cases and techniques* (pp. 19–24). New York: Holt, Rinehart and Winston.

Leathers, D. (1976). *Nonverbal communication systems*. Boston: Allyn and Bacon.

Levine, M., and Sutton-Smith, B. (1973). Effects of age, sex, and task on visual behavior during dyadic interaction. *Developmental Psychology, 9*, 400–405.

Lyman, S., and Scott, M. (1967). Territoriality: A neglected sociological dimension. *Social Problems, 15*, 235–249.

MacLennan, B., and Felsenfeld, N. (1968). *Group counseling and psychotherapy with adolescents*. New York: Columbia University Press.

Markgraf, B. (1966). Demands on listening skills of secondary school pupils. In S. Duker (Ed.), *Listening readings* (pp. 90–101). New York: Scarecrow Press.

Marzano, R.J., Brandt, R.S., Hughes, C.S., Jones, B.F., Presseisen, B.Z., Rankin, S.C., and Suhor, C. (1988). *Dimensions of thinking: A framework for curriculum and instruction.* Alexandria, VA: Association for Supervision and Curriculum Development.

Mehrabian, A. (1968). Communication without words. *Psychology Today*, 2, 51–52.

Michael, G., and Willis, F. (1968). The development of gestures as a function of social class, education, and sex. *Psychological Record, 18*, 515–519.

Michael, G., and Willis, F. (1969). The development of gestures in three subcultural groups. *Journal of Social Psychology, 79*, 35–41.

Miller, G. (1956). The magical number seven, plus or minus two: Some limits on our capacity for processing information. *Psychological Review, 63*, 81–97.

Morris, D., Collett, P., Marsh, P., and O'Shaughnessy, M. (1979). *Gestures: Their origins and distribution.* Briarcliff Manor, NY: Stein and Day.

Nelson, N. Wolf. (1993). *Childhood language disorders in context: Infancy through adolescence.* New York: Macmillan.

Nichols, M. (1995). *The lost art of listening.* New York: Guilford Press.

Nichols, R. (1957). *Are you listening?* New York: McGraw-Hill.

Nichols, R. (1991). Foreword. In D. Borisoff and M. Purdy (Eds.), *Listening in everyday life: A personal and professional approach* (pp. v–vii). Lanham, MD: University Press of America.

Nielsen, G. (1962). *Studies in self confrontation.* Copenhagen, Denmark: Monksgaard.

Parente, R. (1992, May). *Retraining memory and cognition.* Paper presented at the annual convention of the New Jersey Speech-Language-Hearing Association, Parsippiny.

Parker, C. (1968). (Ed.). *Counseling theories and counselor education.* Boston: Houghton Mifflin.

Paul, R. (1995). *Language disorders from infancy through adolescence: Assessment and intervention.* St. Louis, MO: Mosby.

Peterson, C.W. (1981). *Conversation starters for speech-language pathology.* Danville, IL: Interstate Printers and Publishers.

Project STILE. (1979). *Learning how to learn.* Lawrence, KS: Lawrence High School.

Rafoth, M., Leal, L., and DeFabo, L. (1993). *Strategies for learning and remembering: Study skills across the curriculum.* Washington, D.C.: National Education Association.

Ratner, V., and Harris, L. (1994). *Understanding language disorders: The impact on learning.* Eau Claire, WI: Thinking Publications.

Rees, N., and Wollner, S. (1982, February). *A taxonomy of pragmatic abilities.* Educational Telephone Network Conference, State of Wisconsin.

Renzulli, J., and Smith, L. (1978). *Learning styles inventory.* Storrs, CT: Creative Learning Press.

Richey, J. (1978). *Restaurant language.* Hayward, CA: Janus.

Richey, J. (1980). *Credit language.* Hayward, CA: Janus.

Ridge, A. (1993). A perspective on listening skills. In A. Wolvin and C. Coakley (Eds.), *Perspectives on listening* (pp. 1–14). Norwood, NJ: Ablex.

Rowher, W.D., Jr. (1971). Prime time for education: Early childhood or adolescence. *Harvard Educational Review, 41,* 316–341.

Sanderson, D.W. (1993). *Smileys.* Sebastopol, CA: O'Reilly.

Schnell, T.R., and Rocchio, D. (1975). A comparison of underlining strategies for improving reading comprehension and retention. In G.H. McNinch and W.D. Miller (Eds.), *Reading: Convention and inquiry* (24th yearbook of the National Reading Conference, pp. 279–284). Clemson, SC: National Reading Conference.

Schumaker, J.B., and Deshler, D.D. (1994/95). Secondary classes can be inclusive, too. *Educational Leadership, 52*(4), 50–51.

Seidenberg, P. (1988). Cognitive and academic instructional intervention for learning-disabled adolescents. *Topics in Language Disorders, 8*(3), 56–71.

Selekman, M. (1993). *Pathways to change: Brief therapy solutions with difficult adolescents.* New York: Guilford Press.

Simon, C. (1981, November). *After is-verbing: Then what?* Paper presented at the annual convention of the American Speech-Language-Hearing Association, Los Angeles, CA.

Smith, D. (1969, April). The healing art of paying attention. *Guideposts, 23,* 22–25.

Stauffer, R.G. (1942). A study of prefixes in the Thorndike list to establish a list of prefixes that should be taught in the elementary school. *Journal of Educational Research, 35,* 453–458.

Steil, L. (1991). Listening training: The key to success in today's organizations. In D. Borisoff and M. Purdy (Eds.), *Listening in everyday life: A personal and professional approach* (pp. 201-227). Lanham, MD: University Press of America.

Sternberg, R.J. (1994). Allowing for thinking styles. *Educational Leadership 52*(3), 36–40.

Sylwester, R. (1995). *A celebration of neurons: An educator's guide to the human brain.* Alexandria, VA: Association for Supervision and Curriculum Development.

Thompson, C., and Poppen, W. (1972). *For those who care: Ways of relating to youth.* Columbus, OH: Merrill.

Valletutti, P., and Bender, M. (1982). *Teaching functional academics.* Baltimore: University Park Press.

Weinberg, G. (1969). *The action approach.* Cleveland, OH: World Publishing.

Wells, G. (1974). Learning to code experience through language. *Journal of Child Language, 1,* 243–269.

Wiig, E. (1982a, May) *Identifying language disorders in adolescents.* Oral presentation at Gundersen Clinic, LaCrosse, Wisconsin.

Wiig, E. (1982b). *Let's talk: Developing prosocial communication skills.* Columbus, OH: Merrill.

Wiig, E. (1982c). *Let's talk inventory for adolescents.* Columbus, OH: Merrill.

Wolff, F., Marsnik, N., Tacey, W., and Nichols, R. (1983). *Perceptive listening.* New York: Holt, Rinehart and Winston.

Wolff, F., and Marsnik, N. (1992). *Perceptive listening* (2nd ed.). New York: Harcourt, Brace, Jovanovich.

Wolvin, A., and Coakley, C. (1982). *Listening.* Dubuque, IA: Brown Publishers.

Wolvin, A., and Coakley, C. (1993). Introduction. In A. Wolvin and C. Coakley (Eds.), *Perspectives on listening* (pp. xi–xv). Norwood, NJ: Ablex.

Wong, B. (1980). Motivation for learning in mildly handicapped adolescents and young adults: A review of related theories [Special issue]. *Exceptional Education Quarterly, 1*(2), 37–45.

World Book Encyclopedia. (1981). *The world book complete word power library* (Vol. 2). Chicago: Author.

Wyatt, N. (1989). Structuring speaking and listening in the classroom. In P. Phelan (Ed.), *Talking to learn: Classroom practices in teaching English, Volume 24.* Urbana, Il: National Council of Teachers of English.

Zimmerman, B., and Pons, M. (1986). Development of a structured interview for assessing student use of self-regulated learning strategies. *American Educational Research Journal, 23,* 614–628.

USE OUR COMMUNICATION POSTERS AS VISUAL REMINDERS OF INTERVENTION GOALS

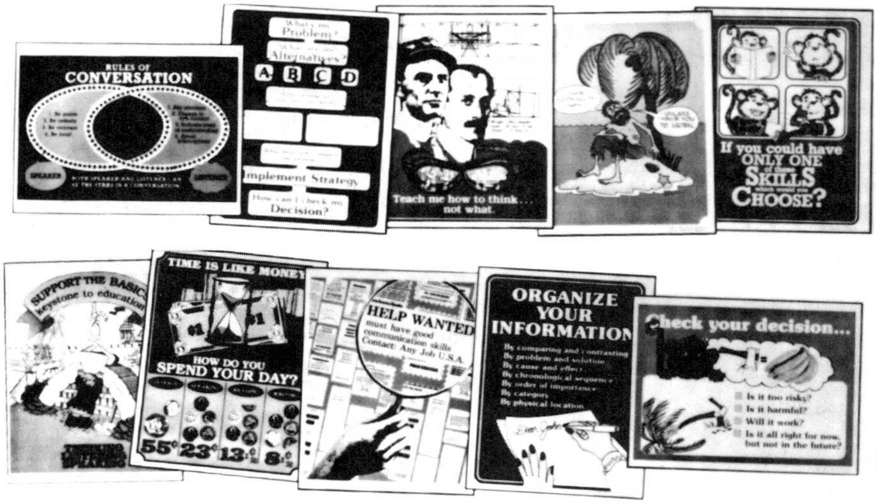

POSTERS PROMOTE THE IMPORTANCE OF THINKING, LISTENING, AND SPEAKING

PLUS THEY EXEMPLIFY LESSONS TAUGHT IN *DAILY COMMUNICATION!*

Posters are printed on heavy stock paper and are available as 17½" X 22" wall-size (sold individually or in a set) or 8½" X 11" (in a set only)

Rules of Conversation ....Item #401-BP
Problem Solving................................Item #402-BP
Not What to Think.............................Item #403-BP
Nothing to Say ....Item #404-BP
Skills—Which to Choose....................Item #405-BP
Support the Basics.............................Item #406-BP
Time is Like Money ....Item #407-BP
Help Wanted.....................................Item #408-BP
Check Your Decision ....Item #409-BP
Organize Your Information .... Item #410-BP

Set of 17½" X 22½" posters ....Item #411-BP
Set of 8½" X 11" posters ....Item #412-BP

MORE LISTENING AND SPEAKING ACTIVITIES FOR ADOLESCENTS AND YOUNG ADULTS!

Referential Communication: Barrier Activities for Speakers and Listeners (Part Two) teaches students (grades 6–12) and adults to listen and speak with more precision. Step-by-step instructions are provided for simplifying and increasing the complexity of the listening/speaking task. Activities give participants the opportunity to analyze why and how their communication is breaking down.

Includes 50 pattern cards, hundreds of die-cut forms, a teaching manual, and a sturdy file box. Item #1102-BP

Save money! Order ***Make-It Yourself Barrier Activities*** and do the work of coloring and cutting the patterns and pieces. Grades K–12 and adults Item #2401-BP

For more information about these products or to receive a catalog of other Thinking Publications products, call **1-800-225-4769**

THINKING PUBLICATIONS®
A Division of McKinley Companies, Inc.

P.O. Box 163 • 424 Galloway Street • Eau Claire, WI 54702-0163
(715) 832-2488 • FAX (715) 832-9082 • E-Mail: 74353,2124@compuserve.com • AliveAlive@aol.com